THE Pregnancy
ENCYCLOPEDIA

THE
Pregnancy
ENCYCLOPEDIA

All your questions answered

Editor-in-chief

Dr Chandrima Biswas,
Consultant Obstetrician

Editor-in-chief Dr Chandrima Biswas
Consultants Dr Anastasia Alcock, Dr Jenny Hall,
Dr Su Laurent, Professor Lesley Page
Writers Judy Barratt, Claire Cross, Susannah Steel
Senior Editors Carrie Love, Victoria Heyworth-Dunne
Senior Art Editors Nicola Rodway, Alison Gardner, Collette Sadler
Project Editors Shashwati Tia Sarkar, Victoria Marshallsay,
Dawn Bates, Hilary Mandleberg, Ruth O'Rourke
Project Designers Emma Forge, Tom Forge
Jacket Designer Nicola Powling
Jacket Editor Francesca Young
Pre-production Producer Andy Hilliard
Senior Print Producer Stephanie McConnell
Creative Technical Support Sonia Charbonnier
New illustrations Peter Bull
New photography Ruth Jenkinson
Picture Researchers Lucy Claxton, Martin Copeland
Managing Editor Lisa Dyer
Managing Art Editor Marianne Markham
Art Director Maxine Pedliham
Publishing Director Mary-Clare Jerram

First published in Great Britain in 2016
By Dorling Kindersley Limited
80 Strand, London WC2R 0RL

Copyright © 2016 Dorling Kindersley

A Penguin Random House Company

2 4 6 8 10 9 7 5 3 1
001 – 280240 – Feb/2016

ISBN 978-0-2412-1655-2

Printed and bound in China

A WORLD OF IDEAS:
SEE ALL THERE IS TO KNOW

www.dk.com

Contents

Foreword

Your pregnancy journey, the first time and each time you embark on it, is incredible and unique to you. From my professional working life in obstetrics, and seeing patients from all sorts of backgrounds, I have found there are as many different pregnancies and birth experiences as there are individual women.

Finding out you are pregnant for the first time, or indeed the second, third or fourth times, can bring on a myriad of emotions – joy, excitement, reticence, fear, awe, curiosity, and, of course, anxiety. These feelings are entirely natural, as is the need for advice. In the past, societies with large families and different social structures created a network of sisterly support to help and inform women about all matters pregnancy-related. By contrast, today we may talk about our pregnancy to only a handful of family members and girlfriends; and to our midwife or obstetrician every couple of weeks.

Often, our first step is to perform an Internet search. Here there is an abundance of information (and misinformation), and anecdotes of the pregnancy and childbirth experiences of other parents – including those that are unusually good or unusually disappointing. Sometimes search results are informative but too often they can be confusing and lead to further anxiety about our own experience.

Your questions answered

On the following pages, we have aimed to provide the balanced advice and support you need at one of the most important times of your life. We have covered every stage: pre-conception, the pregnancy, labour, birth, and even the first three months of your baby's life. We have arranged the chapters by theme, and question, helping you to find the answers you are seeking, as well as other related subjects you might want to know about. A timetable of antenatal care is outlined and expert advice is given on

Q Who are the consultants?

Editor-in-chief
Dr Chandrima Biswas
MRCOG MBBS

Dr Chandrima Biswas is Clinical Director at the Whittington Hospital in London, and is also the obstetric lead for the North Central London Maternity Network. She is a Fellow of the Royal College of Obstetrics and Gynaecology, and a former President of the Maternity and Newborn Forum of the Royal Society of Medicine. She specializes in high-risk obstetrics, in particular the problems associated with maternal obesity.

Consultant
Dr Anastasia Alcock
MRCPCH MBBS DTM&H
DPID DRCOG

Dr Anastasia Alcock is a paediatrician with specialist interests in emergency medicine and infectious diseases. She is currently working at the John Radcliffe Hospital in Oxford, having graduated from Imperial College School of Medicine, London. Anastasia is the founder of The Prenatal Classroom, which provides prenatal and postnatal advice. She is the author of *Your Baby's First Year*, which guides parents through the ups and downs of the first year.

Consultant
Dr Jenny Hall
EdD RM ADM MSc PGDip(HE)

Dr Jenny Hall has been involved with the NHS for more than 35 years, as a nurse and midwife and then as an educator. She is currently senior lecturer at Bournemouth University and researches particularly spirituality and dignity in care. She was the editor for *The Practising Midwife Journal* for ten years and is currently associate editor for *Women & Birth* journal. She is the author and co-author of a variety of midwifery articles and books.

what is likely to occur during your pregnancy, from procedures and scans to birth plans and labour techniques. You will learn about nutrition and exercise, and how to keep healthy, as well as the biological changes taking place in your body and your baby's. There are also sections on clothes to buy to accommodate your increasingly large bump, and also what to buy to prepare for your new arrival. You'll find guidance on all concerns from common complaints during the first trimester to caring for your newborn. Where you should be taking advice from a midwife or obstetrician, we have asked you to do so.

Your journey to birth and beyond

The story of the beginnings of your baby's life is told in a visually beautiful, easy-to-read, and factually accurate account. Throughout, in-depth medical information and authoritative advice will enable you to feel confident about what to expect before, during, and after the birth, while information on lifestyle, working, and wellbeing will help you have a balanced and joyful pregnancy, and look forward to meeting the newest member of your family.

To all those contemplating pregnancy, or who are already pregnant, I hope you will find that this fascinating book helps you understand and enjoy the very start of your baby's life.

Dr Chandrima Biswas

Consultant
Dr Su Laurent
MRCP, FRCPCH

Dr Su Laurent has been a Consultant Paediatrician at Barnet Hospital, London since 1993. Her special interests include asthma, and the interaction between the mind and body and how this affects physical health. She has written several books on parenting and child health. She is the medical advisor to the charity Child Bereavement UK and was the expert paediatrician for *Mother and Baby* magazine for many years.

Consultant
Professor Lesley Page CBE
PhD MSc BA RM RN
Honorary DSc HFRCM

Professor Lesley Page is president of the Royal College of Midwives. She was the first professor of midwifery in the UK at Thames Valley University and Queen Charlotte's Hospital. She is a renowned international academic, advocate, and activist for midwives, mothers, and babies. She has contributed to the development of woman centred maternity care. She has practised midwifery in the community, hospital, and home birth settings for more than 32 years.

US Consultant Editor
Dr Paula Amato
MD

Dr Paula Amato is a reproductive endocrinologist and is an associate professor at the Oregon Health and Science University (OHSU) in Oregon. She received her degree from the University of Toronto, where she also completed her residency in obstetrics and gynaecology. She was subsequently a fellow in reproductive endocrinology and infertility at the University of California. She is board-certified in obstetrics, gynaecology, reproductive endocrinology, and infertility.

How do I use this book?

The Pregnancy Encyclopedia is a one-stop reference that will guide and inform you throughout these special nine months. Presented in an easy-to-navigate question-and-answer format, the book covers all aspects of pregnancy and labour, and looks ahead to life with your brand new baby and the first few weeks of family life.

HOW EACH CHAPTER IS ARRANGED

Chapters are arranged thematically, allowing you to find the answers to all your questions on a topic in one place. Whether you want to clue up on all the pregnancy tests and scans, find out exactly what you should and shouldn't eat, explore your baby's development, or check what equipment you will need when your newborn arrives, dedicated chapters provide a complete reference on each topic.

Within each chapter, sections explore particular elements of a topic, beginning with a summary and then an accessible question-and-answer format. Special feature pages examine key questions in depth, and gorgeous visual highlight pages take a closer look at areas of interest.

Navigation A mini contents list tells you where to find the section you're looking for

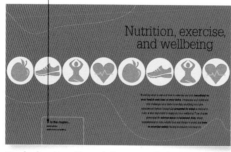

Book chapters Themed chapters make it easy to find what you need to know about a particular area of pregnancy.

Introduction An overview gives some background to questions you might have

Chapter sections Sections take aspects of the chapter's topic and explore them in detail.

Questions Informative answers from trusted professionals are given

Visual explanations Tricky concepts are made easy to understand

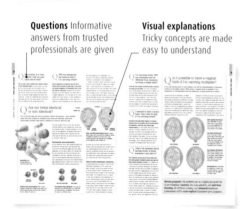

Q&A pages Find answers to your most-asked questions with this easy-to-follow format. Full of clear illustrations to help explain the information.

Single question Key topics are given a thorough treatment

Side headings At-a-glance guide to the contents of each page

Special features Feature pages look at the big questions in depth. Detailed answers and visuals give you the full picture on a variety of topics.

Steps Processes are explained through clearly marked steps

Fun facts Lists of amazing facts will fill you with awe

Highlight pages Beautiful visuals and fascinating facts celebrate the wonder of pregnancy and having a newborn baby.

THE CHAPTERS IN THIS BOOK

WELCOME TO YOUR PREGNANCY

Illustrations See how your baby grows at each week throughout your pregnancy

》 pages 10–25

Week-by-week guidance for your pregnancy

is offered in the initial chapter of this book. There are weekly digests on the progress of your baby's development in "Baby watch" and you can follow your own pregnancy journey in "Mum matters". Read about the incredible changes that take place within each week of the three trimesters. Helpful hints and reminders are given for each week, such as when to book your antenatal classes.

Timeline Follow the weeks on the timeline bar

Welcome chapter Your baby's size and weight are listed for each week, along with possible symptoms you might be experiencing

CONCEPTION

» pages 26–45

The first step in your pregnancy journey, this chapter looks at the incredible chain of events that lead to conception, with detailed explanations of how your monthly cycle prepares your body for pregnancy, and on how pregnancy is established with the implantation of the tiny embryo. From optimizing fertility to the early signs of pregnancy, this chapter helps you prepare for and navigate these first important weeks.

NUTRITION, EXERCISE, AND WELLBEING

» pages 46–75

Pregnancy comes with a bewildering array of advice on what you should and shouldn't do to keep you and your baby healthy. This chapter provides clear-cut guidelines on which foods to avoid, and explains how healthy eating can optimize your baby's early development. Sensible exercise advice and relaxation techniques help you cope with common pregnancy niggles, and develop stamina and focus for labour.

ANTENATAL CARE

» pages 76–103

The type of care you receive is a primary concern in pregnancy. This chapter details the options for antenatal care and who you can expect to look after you. It also prompts you to think about where you want to give birth, who you would like to be with you, and what type of birth you would prefer. A section on all the tests and scans you will be offered in pregnancy helps you to understand why these are done and how they can benefit you and your baby.

ALL ABOUT YOU

» pages 104–147

The changes to your body in pregnancy impact on many aspects of life, from your relationship with your partner to your ability to stay comfortable and sleep, to making travel arrangements. As well as these practical matters, this chapter also explores the many physical and emotional changes pregnancy brings, and looks at some of the common complaints and complications of pregnancy and how to manage them.

YOUR GROWING BABY

» pages 148–171

Nothing is more fascinating in pregnancy than the incredible development of your baby in the uterus. This chapter documents each step of your baby's progress, showing how, within a matter of weeks, your baby develops from a tiny bundle of cells to a recognizably human fetus. As well as her external growth and features, we look at how your baby's vital organs develop and at the unique genetic inheritance your baby holds.

PRACTICAL PREPARATIONS

» pages 172–195

From maternity and nursing bras, support belts, and pregnancy jeans, through to feeding cushions, buggies, cots, and sleepsuits, there's a whole host of items you will need for your pregnancy and your baby when he arrives. This chapter helps you to make practical choices, gives tips on what to buy when, and ensures that you have all you need to get you through pregnancy and the early weeks and months with your new baby.

LABOUR AND BIRTH

» pages 196–239

A dedicated chapter on labour and birth guides you through each stage of labour, showing you how to recognize when labour is really underway and how to chart its progress. Guidance on pain-relief options will help you to consider which techniques and medications you might prefer to use in labour. And you can find out what happens straight after the birth: how your baby is cared for, how you might feel, and how to kick-start the bonding process.

THE POSTNATAL PERIOD

» pages 240–301

During pregnancy, you will want to think ahead to life with your new baby. This chapter allows you to do just that, providing a glimpse into what you can expect, and preparing you for the everyday care of your baby. You can read up on essential areas such as feeding, washing, dressing, comforting, transporting your baby, and dealing with first illnesses. You'll also find advice and tips on how to give yourself time to heal and recover gently after the birth.

SPECIAL SITUATIONS

» pages 302–333

Sometimes pregnancy throws up painful and unexpected situations, whether the actual loss of the pregnancy, a baby that arrives too early and needs special care, or a newborn who has a particular medical concern or long-term condition. This chapter looks at some of the difficult and challenging scenarios families can face and offers advice, information, and guidance to help families understand, come to terms with, and cope with these situations.

» In this chapter...

Welcome to your pregnancy

Congratulations – **you're pregnant**, or at least you think
you might be! In this chapter you'll find a summary of **what
to expect during each week** of pregnancy. You can then
turn to the chapters later in the book for more detailed
information on each subject.

YOUR PREGNANCY
Timeline

From the moment of conception, you and your growing baby go through a multitude of extraordinary changes. Your pregnancy is dated from the first day of your last period. The average length of pregnancy is 40 weeks and it is divided into three parts, or trimesters, which last approximately three months each. Throughout this book when a "week" is referred to it means a completed week of pregnancy. This timeline of key events gives you an at-a-glance view of your pregnancy journey.

Menstruation Pregnancy is dated from the first day of your last period, so for the first two weeks you are not actually pregnant.

Supplements Take folic acid before you become pregnant, or as soon as you know you are, and continue until 12 weeks pregnant. Take vitamin D throughout your pregnancy, and beyond if you plan to breastfeed.

YOUR DEVELOPING BABY
Although no bigger than a large grape, your baby is developing rapidly. A tiny heart is beating, a little face is taking shape, and limbs are starting to form.

8-WEEK-OLD EMBRYO

THE ANOMALY SCAN
This scan checks your baby's organs, body systems, and limbs. The sonographer may also be able to tell you whether it's a boy or a girl.

First trimester													Second trimester							
0	1	2	3	4	5	6	7	8	9	10	11	12	13	14	15	16	17	18	19	20

CONCEPTION
Once a sperm fertilizes an egg, your baby begins life. After several days, it burrows into the lining of the uterus. The place where it implants will develop into the placenta.

Early pregnancy symptoms You may be experiencing symptoms such as food cravings, pregnancy sickness, extreme tiredness, and mood swings. These often fade.

Antenatal appointments Your first appointment takes place at around 8 to 12 weeks. It will be really thorough and you'll be given your medical notes to keep with you and bring to all follow-up appointments.

Telling others After the first trimester, or when you've had your first ultrasound scan, is a good time to tell the wider world about your pregnancy.

Exercise Keep active and healthy. Your regular exercise may be too strenuous now so adapt your routine and consider exercise classes especially tailored for pregnant women.

Flu vaccine Potentially harmful to you and your unborn baby, flu can be prevented through vaccination at any point during pregnancy. Ask your doctor for a flu jab.

THE DATING SCAN
When you are 8 to 14 weeks pregnant, your baby will be measured from crown to rump and you'll be given an estimated delivery date. Bear in mind, though, that there's a five-week range when birth could happen. You may be offered a nuchal translucency scan at the same time if you are 11 to 14 weeks pregnant.

You're pregnant! A pregnancy test will detect the presence of a certain hormone that will confirm you are expecting a baby.

GOOD NEWS!

YOUR BABY'S POSITION

At this late stage, your baby's growth continues to be assessed as well as the efficiency of the placenta. By this point, your baby is nearly at full-term and space is tight inside your uterus. Her head may begin to move into the pelvic cavity. Engagement occurs when the widest part of the baby's head has entered the pelvic inlet. This is one of the ways your body prepares itself for labour.

HEAD ENGAGED

Baby equipment Start thinking about the equipment you will need for your baby. You'll want to try out buggies, car seats, and slings. Think about whether your baby will sleep in a cot, crib, or Moses basket.

Your birth plan Now is a good time to confirm where you would like to give birth, who you would like to be there, and the labour techniques you might consider.

Telling your employer You are legally obliged to give notice of maternity leave at least 15 weeks before you give birth. You must also hand in your MATB1 form at this point; make sure to keep a copy.

Whooping cough vaccine This is offered to you between 28 and 38 weeks. It protects your baby from birth to her first vaccinations.

Antenatal classes Classes may start around now. They are popular, so book at least 12 weeks in advance. Your midwife will explain what is available.

Due date It's normal for babies to be born between 37 and 42 weeks so don't worry if yours hasn't arrived.

Third trimester

21	22	23	24	25	26	27	28	29	30	31	32	33	34	35	36	37	38	39	40+

COMMON SIDE EFFECTS OF PREGNANCY

Many women feel full of energy and positive in the second trimester. You may begin to experience common side effects including swollen hands and feet, bleeding gums, haemorrhoids, cramps, and skin changes. Some women get a dark line called a linea nigra on their abdomen that fades after birth.

YOUR MOVING BABY

For the last couple of weeks your baby's movements will have become more obvious; you may be able to feel her hiccups and she will be growing used to the sound of your voice. Be aware of your baby's pattern of behaviour and report unusual changes to your midwife.

The nesting instinct Try to rest as much as you can. If you feel the urge to clean and scrub, be careful not to overdo it.

Prepare your hospital bag and notes Always carry your antenatal notes with you and pack your hospital bag or organize home birth equipment. Make sure your birth partner knows where everything is.

Preparing for labour Practise exercises that might ease labour. Spend time on all fours or sitting on a birthing ball; start relaxation and breathing techniques; try massaging your perineum to make the area more supple.

KICKING INSIDE THE UTERUS

ARE YOU READY?

Watch out for early labour signs such as a "show", waters breaking, and contractions beginning. If you go over 41 to 42 weeks you'll be overdue. This is very common and you can speak to your midwife about the next course of action.

First trimester

DAYS 1–14 The countdown of your pregnancy begins with your period – the start of the fertility cycle.

Babywatch

There is no baby yet, but the ovarian follicles are working to ripen the next egg.

Mum matters

Since it is often hard to be sure of the exact date when fertilization takes place, the first day of your last menstrual period (LMP) is used as a marker. In the first two weeks the body is resetting the fertility cycle: in the first week, the previous month's uterine lining sheds; in the second week, the uterine lining has begun to thicken in preparation for the next opportunity to conceive a baby.

 ### This week...

» Start taking 400mcg folic acid daily, before conception.

» Both you and your partner should adopt a healthy lifestyle to increase your chances of becoming pregnant and having a trouble-free pregnancy - stop smoking, reduce alcohol and caffeine intake, eat healthily, and take regular exercise.

» It's worth getting your health checked by a doctor, making sure your immunizations are up to date, and seeking advice on how to get existing conditions under control.

» Obesity can result in high-risk pregnancies, and should be tackled before you conceive. It can also interfere with your hormones and lower your chances of conceiving.

2 WEEKS A mature egg is released from the ovaries and if a sperm fertilizes it, a baby is conceived.

Babywatch

Length: approximately 0.1mm (¹⁄₂₅in)
Once released, an egg can survive up to 24 hours as it waits to be fertilized. Around 200–500 million sperm are ejaculated during orgasm, but only a few hundred will make it all the way to the egg, where one winning sperm will penetrate and fertilize it. Shortly after fertilization, the outer layer of the egg thickens so that no other sperm can enter. The sperm and egg fuse their genetic material to start making your baby, which begins life as a single cell called a zygote.

Mum matters

The zygote will signal its existence to the pituitary gland in your brain. A new hormone is released called human chorionic gonadotrophin (hCG) that over-rides your usual monthly cycle.

 ### This week...

» Enjoy sex frequently to give yourselves the best chance of conceiving. Have sex at least every two to three days throughout the month.

» Make sure you find time to relax and unwind - stress may affect your ability to become pregnant. It's no wonder that many couples seem to conceive while on holiday.

3 WEEKS Amazing things are happening inside your body, and some women may experience early signs.

Babywatch

Length: >1mm (¹⁄₃₂in)
Your baby-to-be is now a ball of around 100 cells called a blastocyst. It burrows into the lining of the uterus, which has become sticky to help it attach securely. The place where it implants will eventually develop into a placenta; for now a yolk sac is forming to nourish your baby in the earliest stages.

Mum matters

Hormones, including oestrogen and progesterone, surge through your body to help the blastocyst settle safely. It's possible to experience very early symptoms such as sore breasts and tiredness. When the egg implants, it can cause some slight bleeding or "spotting", but this bleeding should be light, brief, and not painful.

 ### This week...

» While you are waiting to find out whether you are pregnant, avoid alcohol, smoking, and caffeine and eat a balanced diet. This will give your baby a great start.

» You may be able to find out whether you are pregnant this week using an extra sensitive pregnancy test.

» Consult your doctor about whether or not it is safe to carry on taking any existing medication.

The first trimester is a crucial time, during which all the major organs are formed. The pregnancy is supported by hormones from the ovary until the placenta takes over at around 10 weeks.

KEY

 Average height:
Up to 20 weeks crown to rump
From 20 weeks crown to heel

 Average weight

4 WEEKS
If you miss a period this week, it could be the first time you wonder, "Am I pregnant?".

Babywatch

Length: 2mm (¹⁄₁₆in)

Your tiny baby has begun life as an embryo and is currently a disc of layered cells that is developing fast. It is floating in a fluid-filled amniotic sac. A basic blood circulation system has been established, and the brain and nervous system have begun to develop.

Mum matters

You might experience a variety of pregnancy symptoms, including pregnancy nausea and sickness. The levels of human chorionic gonadotrophin (hCG) hormone the fertilized egg is producing are high enough now that a pregnancy test will register positive.

This week...

» Take a pregnancy test.

» Start taking 400mcg folic acid and 10mcg vitamin D daily, if you aren't already.

» Find out about stopping your contraception, if your pregnancy wasn't planned.

» Call your doctor to make an appointment for antenatal care.

» Stop drinking alcohol, smoking, and limit caffeine to no more than 200mg per day.

5 WEEKS
You won't be looking pregnant but as your body adapts to the pregnancy, you might well be feeling it.

Babywatch

 4mm (⅛in)

The embryo now resembles a tiny tadpole. The body has lengthened, and a row of dark cells has formed along the back, which is the beginning of the spinal cord. Dark spots on the face are the earliest hints of eyes, and bud like growths will become limbs. The heart is growing fast and by the end of this week it will start beating.

Mum matters

Common first trimester symptoms could be in full swing now. Most of the time they fade after 12 weeks. If you are suffering from pregnancy sickness try eating plain foods and taking ginger. If you can't keep anything down, speak to your doctor.

This week...

» Learn about what to eat for a healthy pregnancy and avoid foods that can cause food poisoning, such as undercooked egg and meats, pâté and liver, and unpasteurized dairy products and soft cheeses.

» If you have a hazardous or physically strenuous job, tell your employer about your pregnancy so he or she can make provisions for you.

» Be safe when using cleaning products – wear protective gloves and open windows so that you don't inhale fumes.

6 WEEKS
Although there is no visible bump, it doesn't mean your body isn't changing in other ways.

Babywatch

 8mm (⅜in)

Your baby has doubled in length and resembles a small prawn. The head and brain are growing at an incredible rate, and dark spots that will develop into eyes have appeared on the sides of the head. Primitive retinas are already forming.

Mum matters

Your metabolism speeds up, your lungs are working harder, and your blood volume is already increasing. Don't be surprised to find a little weight gain already, even though there's no sign of a bump. Your blood pressure drops as your blood vessels relax; this can cause dizziness so try to avoid standing up for long periods. Your nipples and the circles of skin around them (the areolae) may be darker and a mucus plug in the cervix seals off the uterus to protect the baby from infection.

This week...

» You may be offered an early scan to check your pregnancy if you have had any bleeding or a previous miscarriage.

» Be aware of toxoplasmosis, which can be found in cat faeces, undercooked meat, and contaminated soil.

» Keep up with or take up some gentle exercise – the fitter you keep yourself, the easier labour and delivery will be.

During this time your baby is evolving into a recognizably human baby. Development is rapid, and by the end of the first trimester, all the major organs and body systems are in place.

7 WEEKS Though you still cannot feel the baby inside you, the heart can be seen beating on a scan now.

Babywatch

 1.6cm (⅝in) 1g (¹⁄₃₂oz)

Major organs are now being formed; the digestive system and bowel are taking shape and your baby's lungs have begun to develop. The head is proportionally larger than the rest of the body. The embryo is covered in a thin layer of skin and the fingers and toes are primitive. The placenta is growing stronger and will be ready to take over in a few weeks.

Mum matters

Your uterus is gradually expanding, and you may find that your waistline is thicker. Your breasts will be heavier and may feel tender as they start to adapt for breastfeeding. Hormonal surges can also bring skin changes, and you may find you suddenly become spotty, or that your skin dries.

 ## This week...

» Start practising pelvic floor exercises.

» Be attentive to kitchen hygiene as you are more vulnerable to food poisoning in pregnancy.

» Think about what type of antenatal care you would like, and compile questions to ask at your booking appointment.

» Start to budget for when the baby arrives.

8 WEEKS As your body adapts to the hormonal swings of pregnancy, you may find your moods change abruptly.

Babywatch

2.3cm (⅞in) 2g (¹⁄₁₆oz)

Your baby is about the size of a large grape, and a tiny nose is now visible. The limbs resemble paddles, though the fingers and toes have not formed yet. The eyes are now larger and darkening with pigment. The yolk sac starts to shrink as the embryo increasingly gets oxygen and nutrients from you.

Mum matters

These first weeks are commonly marked by nausea, complete exhaustion, and mood swings. These are caused by hormonal and physiological changes that support your growing baby. Frequent trips to the loo are due to the increased production of urine by certain hormones and the growing uterus putting pressure on your bladder. Many women also have strange food cravings, or develop strong aversions to some foods.

 ## This week...

» Make an appointment with the dentist (dental treatment is free in the UK during pregnancy) to check your gum health as gums soften and bleed in pregnancy.

» If your breasts feel fuller, get your bust measured by an experienced fitter and buy a supportive maternity bra.

» Get a flu jab at any time to protect your baby and yourself.

9 WEEKS Your tiny baby is starting to move around, though you won't yet be able to feel this exciting action.

Babywatch

3cm (1¼in) 4g (⅛oz)

Now the size of a prune, your baby continues to develop. The webbed fingers start to separate and tiny toes are emerging. Early facial features are in place. Soft cartilage makes up the skeleton, which will later harden into bone. The sex organs and external genitalia begin to form, though it's not possible to tell your baby's sex yet. Buds from the bladder connect with tissue cells that will eventually form the kidneys.

Mum matters

Your respiratory system adapts rapidly to help your body meet the demands of pregnancy. The ribs expand and the diaphragm moves up, enabling the lungs to take in more air, increasing oxygen absorption. You may feel the heat as the blood supply to the skin increases; to counter this, blood vessels dilate, dispersing heat and controlling your blood pressure.

 ## This week...

» Your first antenatal visit, the booking appointment, can take place between eight and 12 weeks of pregnancy. At this appointment your medical notes will be compiled, you will be weighed, and your blood pressure will be checked. You will also be offered blood tests and urine checks.

10 WEEKS Though not obvious to others, you may start to notice that your body is beginning to look pregnant.

Babywatch

4.1cm (1⅝in) **7g (¼oz)**

Your baby is now classed as a fetus. The limbs are growing and the neck has lengthened, enabling your baby to make kicking and squirming movements, though it will be a few weeks before you feel them. The heart now has a basic structure, with four chambers, and it beats rapidly, up to 160 beats a minute, as it circulates blood around the body.

Mum matters

Your uterus starts to move up and out of the pelvis as it grows. This shift in its position means less pressure on your bladder. Your breasts continue to grow, and you may go up two or three bra sizes by the end of this trimester. It is normal to feel increasingly breathless – your body needs to take in more air, which is directed towards the baby, uterus, and placenta – but do mention it to your doctor or midwife if you are alarmed.

 This week...

» Check out your maternity rights and benefits with regards to your employment status.

» If your breasts are tender, wear a softer bra at night.

» Start looking into antenatal classes to sign up for.

11 WEEKS You may see your baby for the first time on your dating scan. It's the start of your love affair!

Babywatch

5.4cm (2⅛in) **14g (½oz)**

Your baby is roughly the size of a lime. The brain is forming left and right hemispheres, and at the same time, primitive reflexes are developing. You baby may move in response to pressure on the abdomen. Facial features are developing. The eyelids are fused together and will remain tightly shut until about 26 weeks, but the eyes and ears are not quite in their final position.

Mum matters

You may need to adjust your waistband or opt for looser-fitting garments. Pregnancy hormones can mean your nipples and areolae darken and become bigger. By now, up to a quarter of the blood pumped around your body is being sent to the uterus to support the rapid growth of your baby and the placenta.

 This week...

» A dating scan is carried out between 8 and 14 weeks. Various measurements are taken and you are given an estimated delivery date (EDD). The scan also checks whether you are having one baby or more.

» You may have first screening tests to assess your baby's risk of chromosomal and genetic conditions. Your healthcare professional will talk to you about what is available.

12 WEEKS With nausea and tiredness fading away, you are likely to feel more invigorated.

Babywatch

7.4cm (2⅞in) **23g (¾oz)**

By the end of this first trimester, the head is still large in proportion to the body, taking up about half the crown-rump length. The heart is fully functional, but the heart rate slows down. As the chest wall forms, your baby starts to practise breathing movements, and may also hiccup and swallow. The mouth, stomach and intestines are now linked. The placenta is ready to take over the job of nourishing your baby.

Mum matters

Some of the more unpleasant symptoms of early pregnancy may start to recede, and you may feel great relief as your appetite returns, and your energy levels increase. The hormone hCG falls significantly now, which may be behind the nausea subsiding. For some women, nausea can continue to around week 20. If this is the case, rest assured that your baby will still be taking all the nutrients she needs, even if you are suffering!

 This week...

» If you've been waiting until your first scan to tell family and friends, have fun breaking the good news.

» You may be offered the nuchal translucency scan around now (often at the same time as your dating scan). This is used to help assess your baby's risk of Down's syndrome.

Second trimester

13 WEEKS
Changes inside your body mean that you are glowing now. Sit back and enjoy this settled period.

Babywatch
 8.7cm (3⅜in) 🐾 43g (1½oz)

Your baby will begin to look more in proportion as the trunk starts to lengthen. The hands and feet are no longer webbed, toenails continue to develop, and the numerous bones of the hands and feet start to form.

Mum matters

The hormone relaxin is softening your joints and ligaments in preparation for birth. The downside is the added strain on your ligaments; you may start to feel some discomfort. As your blood volume continues to increase, your skin may start to take on the characteristic pregnancy "glow"; this, together with your more noticeable bump can start to signal to others that you're pregnant.

✎ This week...

» Now is a great time to take a holiday if you wish, while you feel more energetic and are not uncomfortably big. Most airlines don't let women fly in advanced pregnancy, so check their latest dates for flying before you book.

» Keep a diary or photo journal of your pregnancy. You can record your growing bump, feelings, and changing symptoms.

» Keep up your regular exercise if it is gentle enough. Walking and swimming are ideal, and moderate jogging is fine if you're used to this.

14 WEEKS
Your pregnancy may be becoming obvious, and you may feel an incredible sense of wellbeing.

Babywatch
 10.1cm (4in) 🐾 70g (2½oz)

The umbilical cord, your baby's lifeline, is growing thicker and longer as it transports an increasing volume of oxygen-rich blood and nutrients to your baby. In baby girls, the ovaries are forming thousands of eggs, and the ovaries themselves are moving down into the pelvis. The external genitalia are increasingly visible now, and could possibly be seen on an ultrasound scan.

Mum matters

It's not uncommon to have a permanently stuffy nose, nosebleeds, and sinus headaches. These are caused by the extra blood flow to the mucous membranes. New symptoms may emerge such as constipation and indigestion. These are thought to be side effects of the hormones that make your digestive system sluggish.

✎ This week...

» You may need to shop for a few pregnancy clothes as waistbands may be growing too tight.

» If you have been referred for diagnostic tests such as CVS or amniocentesis, they could be carried out around this time.

» You are not obliged to tell your employer about your pregnancy yet, but discussing it sooner means you can talk through plans. You will be protected by employment laws.

15 WEEKS
It is normal to have mixed feelings about your changing body shape and curves.

Babywatch
 11.6cm (4⅝in) 🐾 100g (3½oz)

Your baby's kidneys are functioning and can filter blood and eliminate waste from the body. The messages from the baby's brain and the rest of the body travel with more speed, allowing for more coordinated actions, including slow eye movements.

Mum matters

As well as glowing skin, you may also find that your hair is fuller and more glossy as hormonal conditions prolong the growth phase of hair and less hair falls out on a daily basis than usual. Nails become healthier and stronger too.

✎ This week...

» If you don't already exercise, put into place a gentle, regular exercise regime. Now is a good time to start an antenatal yoga class.

» It's not too early to start thinking about your birth plan – where you would like to give birth, who you would like to be with you, and birthing techniques you might consider.

» Enrol in antenatal classes this week if you haven't done so already, if you wish to attend a course. These don't start until later in pregnancy but can get booked up quickly. Your midwife can give you details of hospital and private classes.

» Try to set aside time for you and your partner.

Your pregnancy is well-established as the risk of miscarriage drops significantly, and you may enjoy a resurgence of energy now. The fetus grows dramatically, and your abdomen will soon develop a rounded bump.

16 WEEKS You will definitely start to look pregnant now, even if you don't feel that different.

Babywatch
 13cm (5⅛in) 140g (5oz)

The fetus is now larger than the placenta. The trunk and limbs are growing quickly, and head growth slows, so the fetus looks more in proportion. You may hear your baby's heartbeat for the first time now as your midwife listens in with a special device called a Doppler sonicaid that is placed on your abdomen to measure sound waves.

Mum matters

A rise in the production of melanin, the pigment that gives your skin and hair its colour, can create temporary skin changes. Dark patches, called "chloasma", may appear on your cheeks, forehead, upper lip, and neck. You may develop a dark vertical line down your abdomen, called a linea nigra. These lighten or disappear after birth.

This week...

» Your midwife will talk to you about the mid-pregnancy anomaly scan due soon. If blood tests revealed you were anaemic, you may be offered iron supplements.

» If you wear contact lenses, you may find your eyes are drier than usual. Your optician can give you special drops.

» Dieting isn't recommended in pregnancy; try to stick to fresh, healthy foods.

17 WEEKS The bloom of pregnancy may be showing in your skin, and even in your mood.

Babywatch
14.2cm (5⅝in) 190g (6¾oz)

The baby's sexual organs are well developed now and will be clearly visible. By the end of this week, all your baby's milk teethbuds have formed and are nestled in place under the gums.

Mum matters

Your heart is now working at twice its normal rate to pump the increased blood volume around your body. To cope with this extra volume of blood and stop your blood pressure rising, your blood vessels become more flexible and dilate. As more blood is diverted to the skin, you may look positively glowing and healthy. You may have a renewed interest in sex, helped by the increased blood flow to the pelvic area.

This week...

» Due to hormonal changes you may feel hotter than usual; dress in breathable fabrics or layers you can adjust.

» Support your baby's developing nervous system by eating foods containing omega-3 fatty acids, such as flaxseed, olive oil, and oily fish. However, limit your consumption of oily fish, especially those high in mercury, such as tuna and mackerel, to no more than two portions per week (see p.52).

» While your energy levels may have picked up, be careful not to overdo things. Plan plenty of relaxation time.

18 WEEKS You may experience your baby's early, fluttering movements. These are known as "quickening".

Babywatch
15.3cm (6in) 240g (8½oz)

Your baby increasingly resembles the little person you will meet. Facial features are well formed and unique fingerprints have begun to develop. Though the eyelids are still shut, the eyeballs can move from side to side.

Mum matters

You may feel your baby move for the very first time from this point. These early movements are known as "quickening" and can feel like a fluttery sensation. Each week your uterus grows around 1cm (⅜in), and the top of the uterus (the fundus) is almost level with your belly button. The ligaments that support the pelvic area stretch and thin, which can cause hip and back pain.

This week...

» Your mid-pregnancy scan takes place around this time, so think ahead as to whether or not you want to discover your baby's sex.

» As your bump becomes ever more prominent, you may attract comments on your appearance and people may want to touch your bump. It is fine to ask people not to.

» Your changing shape and size means your centre of gravity shifts, and you may feel a little wobbly. It may be time to put your high heels to one side.

By the end of this second trimester, your baby has doubled her weight, and the major organs continue to develop apace. You will look obviously pregnant now, and are likely to feel a calm sense of wellbeing.

19 WEEKS You are almost halfway through your journey. Congratulations!

Babywatch

 16.4cm (6½in) 300g (10½oz)

The legs are longer than the arms, and areas of hard bone continue to form. Your baby's senses of sight, sound, taste, touch, and smell are developing in the brain.

Mum matters

Your weight gain accelerates in this trimester. On average, women gain 0.5–1kg (1–2lb) per week from now up until delivery. Your baby accounts for only some of this extra weight; the rest is increased blood volume, breast size, amniotic fluid, and fat stores. As your uterus continues to move upwards, pressing into the stomach, and progesterone relaxes the abdominal muscles, digestion can become sluggish. You may suffer with heartburn, indigestion, and constipation, or existing symptoms may worsen .

This week...

» Include plenty of fibre in your diet and drink plenty of fluids to help keep your stools soft and avoid uncomfortable constipation.

» Start thinking about baby names, and compile a list of your favourites.

20 WEEKS Your scan gives you a glimpse of your well-formed baby.

Babywatch

 26.7cm (10½in) 360g (12¼ oz)

The skin is covered in fine, downy lanugo hair and fat is beginning to be deposited under the skin. The skin forms two distinct layers, the epidermis and the dermis. Your baby is regularly swallowing more amniotic fluid and the kidneys are processing this, and she is urinating. Your baby's skin begins to release a white, waxy substance called "vernix caseosa", which forms a protective coating on the skin.

Mum matters

Your tummy is increasingly rounded – your bump sits just below your belly button. Your extra blood volume helps supply the organs, which are working harder now to support you and your baby.

This week...

» You will be offered an "anomaly" scan between 18 and 22 weeks. This takes various key measurements of your baby and checks her organs and body systems, and if you wish you can ask the sonographer to reveal your baby's gender. The position of your placenta will also be checked.

21 WEEKS You are becoming more aware of your lively baby.

Babywatch

 27.8cm (10⅞in) 430g (15oz)

The nerves and tiny bones in your baby's inner ear are developed enough for her to detect sounds. As the nervous system develops, your baby's movements become more deliberate: she kicks and may suck her thumb.

Mum matters

A large proportion of your increased blood volume is sent to your uterus, and this change in the distribution of your blood can make you feel dizzy at times. Your baby's movements become more obvious. Once you become aware of your baby's pattern of movement (rather than the actual number of movements), this becomes a good indicator of fetal wellbeing. If you don't feel any movement for 24 hours, contact your midwife.

This week...

» Pick up a MATB1 form from your midwife soon. You will need to give it to your employer to claim maternity pay.

» Continue to eat a healthy diet, and avoid fatty, rich foods to counter indigestion.

22 WEEKS You may see some unwanted, though usually temporary, side effects.

Babywatch

 28.9cm (11⅜in) 501g (1.1lb)

Bathed in amniotic fluid and with just a little subcutaneous fat, your baby looks a little wrinkly. The skin cells start to produce a protective layer of keratin. Tiny nails start to emerge at the base of the nail beds, hair might be appearing on the scalp, and your baby now has eyelashes and eyebrows.

Mum matters

As the uterus expands, thinning the skin's collagen and elastin fibres, stretch marks may appear. These fade from red or dark purple to a shiny, paler colour after pregnancy. Your skin may feel very dry and itchy. Keeping hydrated and using an umperfumed moisturizer can help. Painful leg muscle cramps are a common symptom during this time, with spasms often occurring at night. Flexing the foot and massage can relieve cramps.

This week...

» Anecdotally, foods containing potassium (such as bananas) or calcium may help to reduce the incidence of cramps. Staying well hydrated also helps prevent them.

23 WEEKS
Keeping active means you will be well prepared for the birth, and primed for a rapid recovery.

Babywatch

30cm (12in)   600g (1lb 5oz)

Your baby's lungs start to produce a substance called surfactant now, which supports the tiny air sacs (alveoli) in the lungs, strengthening them in preparation for breathing outside of the uterus. In the inner ear, the cochlea is fully developed and allows hearing. Your baby may startle at loud noises and turn her head in response to sounds. She is also becoming familiar with your voice, which she'll recognize at birth.

Mum matters

Regular gentle exercise will help to keep your muscles and ligaments strong and supple. This will also help to relieve pregnancy complaints such as backache. There's also some evidence that women who exercise have a shorter labour, and that the fetal heartbeat is stronger. Pelvic floor exercises are very important too, helping to strengthen the hammock of muscles that support the pelvic area and organs, including the uterus.

This week...

» If you haven't already done so, think about how to tell an older child about the baby's arrival. A young child may have little concept of timings, though, so keep explanations simple. There are also books you can use to introduce the idea.

» Good sources of protein such as lean meat, pulses, eggs, and cheese are essential for the healthy growth of your baby.

24 WEEKS
Your baby might be active when you want to sleep – kicking, yawning, and even hiccupping.

Babywatch

34.6cm (13⅝in)   660g (1lb 8oz)

Your baby is starting to develop a primitive memory as the brain becomes more complex, and brain waves now are similar to those of a newborn's. You may notice your baby's hiccups now, and your baby may yawn as she develops a cycle of sleeping and waking. The nostrils are open, and the adult teeth buds are developing in the gums. By the end of this trimester, the fetal heartbeat has slowed to 140–150 beats a minute.

Mum matters

You will notice your abdomen expanding quickly as it stretches to accommodate your rapidly growing baby. As your bump protrudes outwards and rises up, it presses on your diaphragm, and you may feel breathless. It also nudges against your stomach, which can lead to heartburn and acid reflux.

This week...

» As your bump gets bigger, you may feel off-balance. Be aware of compensating for this with bad posture that puts an additional strain on your back.

» You are legally obliged to tell your employer this week (at least 15 weeks before your due date) of the date you want to start your maternity leave.

» Your MATB1 form (which claims maternity pay) must be handed in to your employer by this point of your pregnancy. Make sure you take a copy before you hand over the original.

25 WEEKS
At the close of the second trimester, your thoughts might turn to the birth.

Babywatch

35.6cm (14in)   760g (1lb 10¼oz)

With fully formed hands, your baby can grasp anything she comes into contact with. She may have discovered the pleasure of thumb sucking. There's still room in the uterus for quite a bit of movement; some babies make a pedalling motion akin to walking. In boys, the testes start to move down from the lower abdomen into the scrotum.

Mum matters

Your uterus continues to move upwards. Your organs are compressed by the expanding uterus, and you could feel a bit cramped inside. Blood volume has increased to around 5 litres (8¾ pints), and your heart is working hard to pump it around. The blood vessels have relaxed as far as possible, so blood pressure may rise a little now. It is normal for your hands, feet, and ankles to swell as a result of fluid retention (oedema). Severe swelling will need to be monitored.

This week...

» You may have an antenatal appointment this week. The midwife will measure the height of your uterus (the fundus) to check that your baby is growing as expected.

» If you have had a previous late miscarriage, you may be offered a scan now to check the length of your cervix.

» As your digestive system is squashed, it may be easier to eat smaller, more frequent meals instead of the usual three large meals.

Third trimester

26 WEEKS It's the home stretch.
Your bump is a source of pride, and you will marvel as it grows.

Babywatch

36.6cm (14⅜ in)   875g (1lb 14½ oz)

Your baby's eyelids open for the very first time around now. He is sensitive to light passing through the abdominal wall, though at the moment he can see only in black, white, and greys. As the kidneys mature, more urine is produced and excreted into the amniotic sac. The waxy vernix that is coating your baby helps prevent his skin from being irritated by the urine.

Mum matters

Don't be surprised if your breasts start leaking a little fluid now. This pre-milk, called colostrum, is produced in pregnancy, ready for your baby straight after birth. You may feel a sense of relief as your reach the third trimester.

 This week...

» Talking to your unborn baby now can kickstart the bonding process as your voice becomes familiar to him.

» If you are suffering with haemorrhoids, keep up your fibre intake to keep stools soft.

» If varicose veins are a problem, wear support tights and put your feet up as much as possible.

» Make a checklist of everything you will need for your baby. Start doing research on which big items to borrow or buy and begin purchasing things if you feel comfortable doing so.

27 WEEKS Reassuringly, babies
who are born at this stage in pregnancy have a 90 per cent survival rate.

Babywatch

37.6cm (14⅞ in)   1kg (2lb 4oz)

Your steadily growing baby fits ever more snugly in the uterus, but he can still manage to turn and flex his limbs. Your baby's muscle and organ development is supported by amino acids (the building blocks of protein) passed on from your blood. Baby boys start to outgrow girls now. Creases form on the palms of the hands and in the toothbuds, enamel and dentine develop.

Mum matters

With the production of amniotic fluid slowing and your baby becoming increasingly active, you're likely to feel plenty of kicks. Note your baby's pattern of activities; if there are changes in his normal behaviour (such as slowing down or stopping completely), you should report them to your healthcare professional. Some women develop a pregnancy "waddle" as they grow, caused by their changing shape and the loosening of ligaments and tissues. This might become more exaggerated over the coming weeks. Many women find they become clumsier at this stage. Take care on slippery surfaces such as the shower or bath.

 This week...

» Take care with your movements to avoid putting a strain on your back.

» Monitor swollen hands and feet.

28 WEEKS At this point,
you may not remember how you felt without a bump.

Babywatch

38.6cm (15⅛ in)   1.2g (2lb 8oz)

Vital development is continuing in the lungs, preparing your baby to breathe at birth. The folds of the brain have increased to house millions of new brain cells, and the cerebral cortex can send electrical impulses.

Mum matters

Your breasts are gearing up for feeding your baby. Pregnancy hormones increase the blood flow to the breasts and cause changes to the tissue, the veins become more prominent, and they may increase in size. The nipple area, or areola, also continues to grow and darken. You may notice small bumps known as Montgomery's tubercules forming around your nipples.

This week...

» You may have an antenatal appointment this week. Your midwife may offer you bloods tests to check for anaemia and pregnancy-induced gestational diabetes.

» If your blood group is Rhesus negative, you will be offered an anti-D treatment to avoid complications in this and future pregnancies.

» If you're suffering with restless leg syndrome, avoid caffeine late in the day, and eat foods containing the amino acid tryptophan, such as pumpkin seeds and yogurt, that triggers the release of the calming brain chemical serotonin, promoting good sleep.

Though your baby could survive in the outside world with assistance if born now, the uterus is still the best place for him as his lungs and digestive system mature and the brain continues to develop.

29 WEEKS You may start to feel sharp kicks from your baby.

Babywatch

39.9cm (15⅝ in) 1.3kg (3lb)

Your baby makes practise breathing movements as he swallows amniotic fluid. His nervous system is becoming more complex, refining his movements and developing his sucking reflex. He starts to fill out more as muscle and fat are laid down. Between now and the end of pregnancy, his weight will double.

Mum matters

Your lung capacity has increased and your ribs have spread out sideways to help your lungs to work harder. There is pressure on your other organs, and you may find symptoms such as heartburn, constipation, and palpitations worsen, and you experience twinges, aches, and pains.

 This week...

» You will be offered the whooping cough vaccine between 28 and 38 weeks to protect your unborn baby from this virus.

» If it's hard to stay comfortable at night, position pillows to support your bump. V-shaped pillows are helpful.

30 WEEKS It's worth reviewing your birth plan. It's not too late to make changes.

Babywatch

41.1cm (16⅛ in) 1.5kg (3lb 3oz)

The skin is developing a pinker hue as fat builds up underneath and your baby will now be able to regulate his own body temperature. Although he is increasingly cramped for space, your baby is very flexible and can easily bring his feet up to his head, and even suck on his toes!

Mum matters

Although labour is a couple of months off, your uterus is preparing for the event by making practise "Braxton Hicks" contractions – you may start to notice tightening sensations around your abdomen around now or in later weeks. These range from being mild to a stronger cramp like feeling, but their irregularity and the fact they aren't very painful means this isn't the real thing.

 This week...

» Antenatal classes start around this time. Encourage your partner to attend so he knows what to expect. It's the perfect chance to start building a support network.

31 WEEKS Your baby may be lying in any number of positions.

Babywatch

42.4cm (16⅝ in) 1.7kg (3lb 10oz)

As your baby exercises his limbs, his muscle mass increases and muscle tone improves, so his movements become stronger and more purposeful. His practice breathing movements are regular and rhythmic, moving his diaphragm and chest wall.

Mum matters

Your blood volume peaks around this time. This extra volume is largely down to an increase in the plasma and fluid content of the blood, while the number of red blood cells remains the same. This means the red blood cells become less concentrated, a common cause of anaemia in late pregnancy. There's no need to worry about the baby, though, as he will still receive all the nutrients and oxygen he needs to thrive.

 This week...

» You may have a routine antenatal appointment where your blood pressure and urine are checked, and your uterus will be measured. Signs of pre-eclampsia will also be checked for.

32 WEEKS Now is a good time to start thinking about practical preparations.

Babywatch

43.7cm (17⅛in) 1.9kg (4lb 3½oz)

Fine tuning is taking place in your baby's nervous system as brain cells are gradually coded into distinct areas that will control specific functions. Your baby will now be looking more substantial and plump as the wrinkles start filling out.

Mum matters

The size of your bump puts pressure on your veins; this can lead to varicose veins. Gentle exercise, rest, and support tights can bring relief, and symptoms should settle after the birth. Your tummy button may pop out around now. If this bothers you, rest assured that it should go back after the birth.

 This week...

» Spend time on all fours, sitting on a birth ball, or leaning over a bean bag or ball to move your baby into the best position.

» Check out the route to the hospital now. Find out how long the journey is at different times of day.

» Talk to your midwife and partner about any anxieties you have about the approaching labour.

In these final weeks, your baby continues to lay down insulating fat deposits for life outside of the uterus, and the lungs are ready to take their first breath. Your baby will settle into his final position, ready for the birth.

33 WEEKS Each day, your baby is preparing for survival in the outside world.

Babywatch

45cm (17⅝ in) 2.1kg (4lb 11½oz)

Your baby is increasingly awake and active, and is becoming more aware of her surroundings, as she touches her face and pulls on the umbilical cord. Her sucking reflex is strong enough now that if born this early, she should be able to feed independently. Her fingernails are reaching the tips of her nail beds, and may need a trim at birth.

Mum matters

Your heart works extra hard now as you approach the home run – your heart rate increases by 10 to 15 beats a minute and the heart works up to 50 per cent harder. It's not uncommon to experience fluttery palpitations; these are usually harmless, though mention them to your midwife if accompanied by breathlessness or chest pain.

 This week...

» Regularly massaging your perineum can help make this area more supple and reduces your risk of tearing during the delivery.

» Start to think about who will support you once the baby is here, and also in the future.

34 WEEKS Practising relaxation techniques will help you prepare for labour.

Babywatch

46.2cm (18⅛ in) 2.4kg (5lb 5oz)

Your baby looks far more in proportion, and is nicely plump. In the limbs, the bones continue to harden. Waste from the amniotic fluid is building up in the gut, forming a sticky substance called meconium, which will be your baby's first greeny-black poo after the birth.

Mum matters

Your baby is most likely to be lying vertically by this stage of pregnancy, though occasionally, babies are in a diagonal or horizontal position. As your baby gets bigger, her movements are likely to feel stronger, more frequent, and have a recognizable pattern now rather than seeming like isolated kicks.

 This week...

» If you are Rhesus negative, you may have a second anti-D treatment if the first was a small dose.

» Pack your hospital bag and keep your antenatal notes to hand. Make sure your partner knows where everything is, too.

35 WEEKS Your body is well and truly gearing up for the big day.

Babywatch

47.4cm (18⅝ in) 2.6kg (5lb 10oz)

Your baby may have stationed herself in a head-down position, ready for her exit later this month. She is still busy laying down fat to insulate her after birth. At the same time, she will shed her lanugo hair, and may have just a few patches left over the back and shoulders.

Mum matters

With labour approaching, your baby's head may begin to "engage" (descend into your pelvis), and your bump may sit lower. The release of pressure on your diaphragm makes it easier to breathe. This is known as "lightening". The baby's head now presses on your bladder, which means frequent loo stops and broken sleep. Aches and pains in the pelvic area may well increase.

 This week...

» Have a fitting for a nursing bra now and get equipped for breastfeeding.

» Have your handover notes ready at work if you're starting maternity leave.

» Keep practising your pelvic floor exercises regularly to avoid stress incontinence later.

36 WEEKS Make sure you have a plan ready for when you go into labour.

Babywatch

48.6cm (19⅛ in) 2.9kg (6lb 5oz)

Your baby is almost full term, and the lungs are fully developed now, which means she could breathe without help if born from this point. She is losing the waxy vernix, though some may linger at birth.

Mum matters

Braxton Hicks contractions may be occurring with increasing regularity, and production of the hormone relaxin increases, helping to relax the pelvic ligaments and to soften the cervix. A combination of hormonal surges, anxiety about labour, lack of sleep, and aches and pains may leave you feeling a little vulnerable. Mood swings are quite common in these final weeks.

 This week...

» You will have an antenatal appointment this week. Your blood pressure and the baby's growth and position will be checked. Your midwife will talk to you about your options if you pass your due date, and will discuss the hospital's policy on inducing labour.

» Finalize your birth plan.

37 WEEKS At this point you are probably as big as you are going to get.

Babywatch

49.8cm (19⅝in)   3.1kg (6lb 10oz)

Space is at a premium for your baby, and she may draw her legs and arms into her body in the classic fetal pose. The skull bones aren't fused, which allows the bony plates to overlap and elongate to help your baby squeeze through the birth canal.

Mum matters

Your movement may be slowing as your size makes it difficult to move quickly and maintain balance. Your breasts are ready to feed your baby at birth. The milk ducts have branched off, creating a transport system to deliver milk to your baby.

 This week...

» Keep an eye on the strength and pattern of your baby's movements and report any changes to your midwife.

» Learn about the of signs of labour so that you know what to expect, and feel confident about when to call your midwife.

» Make a few home-cooked dishes to pop in the freezer for after the birth.

» Make sure everything is ready if you are having a home birth.

38 WEEKS Double check your birth plan; it's not too late to make changes.

Babywatch

50.7cm (20in)   3.3kg (7lb 3oz)

The grey matter of the brain, the cortex, develops in layers of cells. As each layer is complete, more connections are made between cells, which help to fine-tune your baby's movements. Thanks to antibodies from your blood, your baby has some protection from infection, and after birth she can continue to receive antibodies from your breast milk.

Mum matters

You may feel very fatigued in these final stages as you carry all the extra weight of the fetus, uterus, and extra fluid. Your heart is working at full capacity. Having a lie down increases the blood flow to your baby, and helps you rest and recuperate.

 This week...

» You may have a late burst of energy now and an urge to clean and scrub. If the "nesting" urge hits you, by all means go with it, but be careful not to overdo it.

» Practise breathing and relaxation techniques to help reduce anxiety.

39 WEEKS Make sure you are clear on how to recognize the signs of labour.

Babywatch

51.2cm (20⅛in)   3.5kg (7lb 11oz)

With her arrival imminent, your baby is well prepared for life on the outside. Eyebrows, eyelashes, and nails are all in place, and her organs and body systems are sufficiently developed, though many of these will continue to develop after the birth.

Mum matters

It's best to take it easy now and conserve your energy for labour. Combine rests with periods of gentle activity. You are likely to feel a mounting pressure in your pubic region and your baby may be partially or fully engaged in your pelvis, although in second and subsequent pregnancies, this often happens later on.

 This week...

» You will have an antenatal appointment this week where your midwife can check if the head is engaged and assess your baby's wellbeing.

» Relieve backache with warm baths and a soothing massage.

40 WEEKS Very soon you will be holding your new baby in your arms.

Babywatch

51.2cm (20⅛in)   3.5kg (7lb 11oz)

At 40 weeks your baby has little space to move around. You're likely to feel her limbs protruding or her hiccupping. If she is born after 40 weeks she will have some vernix on her skin and may have less amniotic fluid surrounding her.

Mum matters

Approximately 45 per cent of women haven't given birth at 40 weeks. However, the majority deliver during the next week and only 15 per cent go above 41 weeks. You might be offered a "sweep" to induce labour. This encourages the release of hormones that help to start contractions.

 This week...

» Keep your maternity notes and birth plan with you at all times. Your packed hospital bag should also be close to hand.

» Make sure you have fuel in your car, coins for parking, and a fully charged phone and camera in your bag.

Conception

The moment you conceive a baby is **incredibly special**. You may not even realize conception has taken place, but **life is stirring deep inside you**. If you have only just decided to try for a baby then there are steps you can take to improve your fertility and chances of getting pregnant. This chapter includes detailed explanations on how the male and female **reproductive systems** actually work. It also answers questions and concerns surrounding fertility, assisted conception, and unexpected pregnancy.

If you have decided to **try for a baby,** you may be excited but unsure about what to do next. There are ways to **maximize your fertility** and prepare for pregnancy, but once you've done those things, relax and **let nature take its course.** If you don't conceive quickly, try not to get disheartened. It is normal for it to take some time.

Trying for a baby

Preparing for pregnancy

Once you've decided to get pregnant, there are some practical steps you need to take – from stopping any birth control and making lifestyle changes to checking your immunity to certain infections. Taking these actions before you conceive will put you in the best possible health for pregnancy.

During pregnancy, the focus is understandably on the woman. However, at this preconception stage it really is about both of you. Men, as well as women, can do much to improve their fertility by making dietary and lifestyle changes, with the added advantage that when the baby arrives he will have two fit and healthy parents.

You can maximize your chances of becoming pregnant by tracking your menstrual cycle and knowing the optimal time to conceive. As well as using an ovulation prediction kit, you can learn to spot the natural signs that you are ovulating. Be aware, though, of the importance of relaxing and enjoying the process of getting pregnant. Becoming too focused on conceiving and feeling stressed can spoil your enjoyment of this special and exciting time, and actually adversely affect your fertility. It can also negatively affect your relationship if your lovemaking is all about getting pregnant.

Couples who have been trying to get pregnant for some time may want to investigate why they have had no success so far. This is especially true of older couples, who may want to seek advice sooner rather than later. There is a great deal of help available, starting with basic fertility tests, such as blood tests and ultrasound scans, to rule out any physical problems. Sometimes knowing that your reproductive organs are in good health can help you to relax and actually improve your chances of conceiving.

For couples who are considering having fertility treatment, this chapter outlines the options available, such as in vitro fertilization (IVF). There is a wide range of fertility treatments available and success rates are improving gradually all the time.

Getting pregnant again

If you are trying for another baby, the preparation is the same. Although it is harder to prioritize yourself once you are a mother, being in good shape will benefit your conception chances and provide the energy to care for more children. If you had any problems conceiving or during previous pregnancies, discuss these with your GP so you can go into this pregnancy feeling happy and confident.

Q I want to have a baby. Should I just stop using birth control?

It depends on which type of birth control you use. Condoms and spermicides can be stopped immediately. If you are on the pill or mini-pill, finish the course so you have a bleed. Although it may take a few months for ovulation to return to normal, you can conceive immediately after stopping without any risks to your baby.

If you have an IUD or IUS fitted, or an implant, book an appointment for it to be removed. If you are on injections, simply stop renewing them and the hormones will gradually decrease. It can, however, take a year for your cycle to return to normal.

Whichever contraception you use, you may want to make diet and lifestyle changes and have medical checks before you get pregnant. It may be worth doing this preconception preparation before you stop your birth control in case you fall pregnant quickly.

Q Why should I have my immunity checked before conceiving?

Some infections are dangerous to catch in pregnancy, so it is wise to get your immunity checked before you conceive. Your GP can arrange blood tests for this purpose. If you are not immune to certain infectious diseases, you can be vaccinated before you get pregnant, but not afterwards. Rubella (German measles) is most dangerous to the fetus in the first 16 weeks, capable of causing miscarriage, stillbirth, or abnormalities such as hearing loss and brain damage. Chickenpox can cause miscarriage and birth defects. Vaccination prevents rubella and lessens the chance of chickenpox developing, and makes it milder if you do contract it.

Hepatitis causes liver disease and can be passed to your baby; if you are at high risk of infection you should be immunized. Checks can also be done for group B streptococcus and chlamydia.

Toxoplasmosis is a parasitic infection that can be present in cat faeces and undercooked meat. Wash your hands thoroughly after gardening, changing cat litter, or handling raw meat. Wash all vegetables and fruit before you eat them. If you think you may be at risk of toxoplasmosis (see p.108), ask your doctor to test you.

Q Can we do anything to improve our chances of getting pregnant?

Improving your diet and lifestyle will put you in the best possible position to conceive – and that works for both of you. Sperm and egg cells both take three months to mature fully, so taking action early will produce the healthiest cells.

To be in the best shape for fertility and parenthood, remove unhealthy indulgences such as fast food, refined carbohydrates, alcohol, caffeine, and tobacco from your life. Eat foods that nourish you (see pp.48–55), and limit toxins by eating fresh, local, and organic produce if possible. Exercise to help maintain a healthy weight and to manage your stress levels.

TIPS FOR MALE FERTILITY

Improve the health of your sperm and be in the best shape for parenthood:

 » Take a multivitamin: choose one that includes selenium, zinc, and folate for optimal sperm production and health.

 » Clean up your diet: eat plenty of fruit and vegetables as their antioxidants promote sperm health.

 » Maintain a healthy weight: too much or too little body weight can inhibit the production of reproductive hormones and affect sperm quality.

 » Quit smoking tobacco or marijuana: both substances can affect fertility. Seek help to quit if necessary.

 » Limit alcohol: too much can affect sperm quality.

 » Enjoy a caffeine boost: there's nothing wrong with an occasional coffee.

 » Exercise moderately: cycling a lot could compress the testes, but cycling in moderation is fine.

 » Reduce stress: being stressed may affect certain hormones required for sperm production.

TIPS FOR FEMALE FERTILITY

Prevent hormone imbalances and help to regulate your menstrual cycle:

 » Take folic acid: take 400mcg a day, either as a single supplement or as part of a preconception multivitamin.

 » Eat well: ensure your diet is well balanced to maximize essential nutrients.

 » Maintain a healthy weight: being overweight or underweight can affect fertility. Stay at a healthy weight by eating a balanced diet and exercising moderately.

 » Watch what you drink: alcohol and caffeine can affect fertility. If you don't want to give these up, drink them moderately. Drink alcohol only occasionally and limit your caffeine intake to 200mg a day (that's two cups of instant coffee – coffee-shop varieties are stronger). Remember, soft drinks, energy drinks, and tea also contain caffeine. Choose decaffeinated and herbal alternatives.

 » Quit smoking: the toxins in cigarettes age your ovaries, damage your eggs, and adversely affect fertilization and implantation. Seek help to quit if necessary.

 » Manage stress: find ways to relax. Try your best not to make getting pregnant your main focus.

Being relaxed can double your chances of becoming pregnant within a year – so have fun and enjoy trying for a baby!

Q At which point in my menstrual cycle should we have sex in order to get pregnant?

The best way to maximize your chances is to have sex regularly – every two to three days throughout the month – but if you wish you can also try tracking your ovulation.

You are most likely to conceive in the five to six days leading up to and including ovulation (when your body releases an egg). This is called the "fertile window". Aside from charting your monthly cycle, there are a few ways to work out when you might be ovulating.

Monitor your cervical mucus

Just before the fertile window, a sticky, thick, cloudy white mucus appears. It turns thinner, clearer, and stretchy at ovulation. After ovulation, the mucus decreases and disappears. To check the mucus, wash your hands and insert your fingers into your vagina or wipe yourself with toilet paper. Stretch the mucus between your fingers. Note the colour and consistency.

Use an ovulatory predictor kit

An ovulation kit helps predict your fertile window by measuring levels of luteinizing hormone (LH), the hormone that releases your egg. You simply test your urine to detect LH surges up to two days before ovulation, which is useful if you have an irregular cycle.

Measure your basal temperature

Your basal body temperature (BBT) changes throughout the month. Before ovulation, your BBT is usually about 35–37°C (96–98°F). Just after ovulation, the progesterone released into the body raises your body temperature slightly (approximately 0.2°C/0.4°F) until your next period. So you can determine when ovulation has happened, but not predict it, using BBT.

If you chart your temperature changes over a few months, you may see a pattern forming of when ovulation is likely. Buy a special basal body thermometer from a pharmacy. Note down your temperature at the same time every morning before you eat or drink.

There are lots of apps available for monitoring your monthly cycle.

CHANGES DURING THE MENSTRUAL CYCLE

This graph shows a 28-day menstrual cycle and the changes that help predict the fertile window, which is in the middle of the cycle and lasts five to six days. If your menstrual cycle is not 28 days long (most are between 21 and 35 days), the fertile window will still fall roughly in the middle.

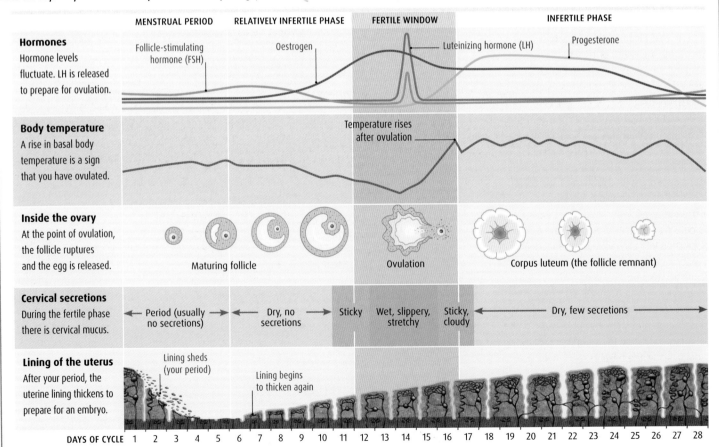

MENSTRUAL PERIOD   **RELATIVELY INFERTILE PHASE**   **FERTILE WINDOW**   **INFERTILE PHASE**

Hormones
Hormone levels fluctuate. LH is released to prepare for ovulation.

Follicle-stimulating hormone (FSH)   Oestrogen   Luteinizing hormone (LH)   Progesterone

Body temperature
A rise in basal body temperature is a sign that you have ovulated.

Temperature rises after ovulation

Inside the ovary
At the point of ovulation, the follicle ruptures and the egg is released.

Maturing follicle   Ovulation   Corpus luteum (the follicle remnant)

Cervical secretions
During the fertile phase there is cervical mucus.

← Period (usually no secretions) →   ← Dry, no secretions →   Sticky   Wet, slippery, stretchy   Sticky, cloudy   ← Dry, few secretions →

Lining of the uterus
After your period, the uterine lining thickens to prepare for an embryo.

Lining sheds (your period)   Lining begins to thicken again

DAYS OF CYCLE 1 2 3 4 5 6 7 8 9 10 11 12 13 14 15 16 17 18 19 20 21 22 23 24 25 26 27 28

Q Are there any sexual positions that might help us conceive?

No, there is no scientific evidence that having sex in a particular position increases your chances of conception. There are unsupported claims that it helps to have sex in the missionary position so that the man is on top, or in positions that allow deep penetration, and that a female orgasm can help to pull sperm further into the cervix. You don't need to lie on your back with your legs raised after sex to give the sperm the best chance of success either! However, it certainly doesn't hurt to give any of these methods a try – simply having sex, in whichever position you like, will improve your chances of getting pregnant.

Q I've got two daughters. How can I improve my chances of conceiving a boy?

It would be nice to think that you can influence the gender of your baby, but unfortunately there is no evidence that you can. Whether your baby is a boy or a girl is dependent on whether the sperm that fertilizes the egg carries an X chromosome (for a girl) or a Y chromosome (for a boy), and this is purely a matter of chance.

Nevertheless, you are not the first to ask this question and there are lots of old wives' tales about it! In the 1960s, a theory called the Shettles Method claimed that X-bearing sperm survive longer in the cervix but move more slowly than faster, smaller, though less healthy, Y-bearing sperm. With this in mind, the theory suggested that you should have sex as close to ovulation as possible for a boy, but two to three days before ovulation for a girl. There are some sex-selection kits available online that utilize this theory, but this method has not been scientifically proven.

Another theory for natural sex selection, also not scientifically proven, is the Whelan Method. This advises having sex two to three days before ovulation for a girl and four to five days before the basal body temperature rises to conceive a boy – which is the opposite advice to the Shettles Method. The Whelan Method also advocates eating a diet that is high in calcium and magnesium for a boy, and eating lots of salty and potassium-rich foods for a girl.

Q How long will it take for us to get pregnant?

The time it takes will depend on many different factors, but be aware that it is normal for even a fertile couple to take a year, or even two, to conceive.

Figures reveal that on average more than 80 per cent of couples under the age of 40 get pregnant within a year if they have regular unprotected sex; more than 90 per cent achieve pregnancy in two years. Naturally, it is frustrating if conception is taking a long time for you, but the figures show that it is worth keeping going.

Whatever your age, you can both make dietary and lifestyle changes to improve your chances of conceiving (see pp.50–51). You can also monitor when you ovulate to increase your chances of success (see opposite).

However, some experts argue that staying relaxed and not focusing too much on tracking ovulation will help you to conceive.

If you have been having unprotected sex for a year without success, consider seeing your GP about your fertility.

If you are a woman aged over 35 and you haven't conceived after six months of regular unprotected sex, seek medical advice at this point (statistically, fertility rates drop at age 35). You should also seek advice if you have irregular periods or are worried about your Fallopian tubes due to your medical history.

Make sure you are having sex on a **regular basis**. Some couples simply don't have sex often enough to get pregnant!

AVERAGE CONCEPTION RATES IN FERTILE COUPLES

After a year of trying, 93 out of 100 couples in a US study achieved a pregnancy, at the rates set out below.

MONTH	1	2	3	4	5	6	7	8	9	10	11	12
PERCENTAGE OF COUPLES PREGNANT	20	36	49	59	67	74	79	83	86	89	91	93

Q We have one child and know we want another. How long should we wait before trying to get pregnant?

This may depend on your experience first time round. If you had a normal pregnancy with no complications, there is no reason not to conceive again once you feel ready. However, consider factors such as whether you have the energy to care for a young baby while pregnant and whether you want some time to enjoy the child that you have.

If it took a while for you to conceive, you may want to start trying for a baby as soon as you feel ready, though be prepared that you could conceive more quickly this time round. Conversely, if you conceived quite quickly last time, it is not unusual for it to take longer to get pregnant again.

If you had a Caesarean section with your first baby, wait for at least a year before getting pregnant again. This is to give your body enough time to recover – becoming pregnant sooner can double the risk of complications in the next pregnancy. Waiting a year also gives your scar a chance to heal. If you would like a vaginal birth next time and the scar isn't properly healed, there is more chance of it rupturing during a VBAC (vaginal birth after Caesarean section).

Any medical complications experienced in your first pregnancy, such as severe sickness (hyperemesis gravidarum), pre-eclampsia, gestational diabetes, or a premature birth, could reoccur. You may want to discuss the likelihood of this with a medical professional before you begin trying for another baby.

Becoming pregnant is a complex biological process. Firstly, it requires the release of an egg from the ovary. This egg must then be fertilized by a sperm in the Fallopian tube. Once fertilized, the egg becomes a ball of cells that must travel down the Fallopian tube and implant in the lining of the uterus. When this occurs, you have conceived and are pregnant.

Creating new life

You will have the best chance of conceiving if your reproductive organs are healthy and functioning well. Sperm are produced in a man's testes. Once matured in the epididymis, the sperm travel into a tube, the vas deferens, which leads to a sac-like structure. When a man ejaculates, semen – a fluid containing the sperm – discharges into the urethra inside the penis. In a woman, the ovaries are positioned either side of the uterus. They contain the eggs, or ova, that are released each month (ovulation).

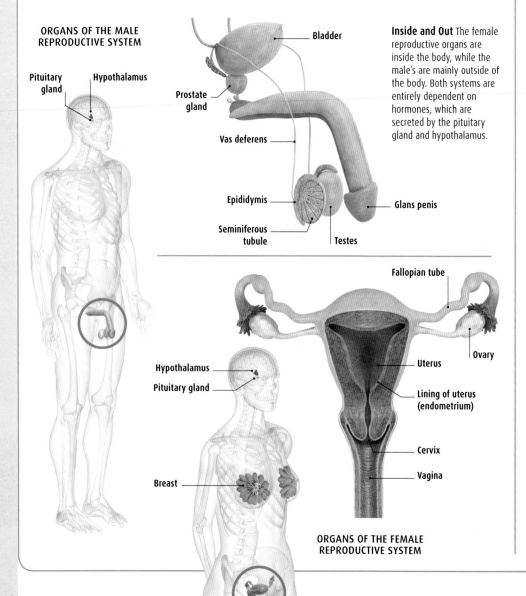

ORGANS OF THE MALE REPRODUCTIVE SYSTEM

Pituitary gland
Hypothalamus

Bladder

Prostate gland

Vas deferens

Epididymis

Seminiferous tubule

Testes

Glans penis

Inside and Out The female reproductive organs are inside the body, while the male's are mainly outside of the body. Both systems are entirely dependent on hormones, which are secreted by the pituitary gland and hypothalamus.

Hypothalamus

Pituitary gland

Breast

Fallopian tube

Uterus

Lining of uterus (endometrium)

Cervix

Vagina

Ovary

ORGANS OF THE FEMALE REPRODUCTIVE SYSTEM

The egg's journey

All the eggs in an ovary are exposed to follicle-stimulating hormone (FSH) each month in order to mature, but only about 20 develop. Eggs mature within follicles, fluid-filled structures that enlarge in response to FSH. Usually only one follicle matures fully and releases an egg, while the other follicles shrivel and their eggs are lost.

If a woman has a non-identical twin pregnancy, it means two of her follicles have matured and each one released an egg that month.

Ovulation triggers

The mature egg is surrounded by cells that produce the hormone oestrogen. This stimulates the growth of tissue in the breasts, thickens the uterine lining, and nourishes the egg. As the levels of oestrogen rise, the hypothalamus in the brain triggers a burst of luteinizing hormone (LH) that works to release the egg from its follicle: ovulation occurs.

The Fallopian tube

At the point of ovulation, the newly released egg is wafted into the nearby Fallopian tube by delicate frond-like strands called fimbriae. It is encouraged down the tube towards the uterus by tiny hair-like projections, known as cilia, in the lining. This can take five days or more. If a woman has sexual intercourse around this time, the egg may be fertilized by a sperm while it is in the Fallopian tube.

2 FERTILIZATION

A single sperm penetrates the outer layers of the egg to fertilize it, while it is in the Fallopian tube. The 23 chromosomes (which contain DNA, the genetic information needed for the development of a cell) in the sperm join with the 23 in the egg. Together these 46 chromosomes create a blueprint that makes your baby unique.

The fertilized egg, now called a zygote, divides into two identical cells. Within hours, the zygote divides multiple times into a microscopic ball of cells (morula) as it heads towards the uterus.

Uterus At this stage the uterus is the size of a plum, but will expand as your developing baby grows

Fallopian tube

Path of egg

Zygote Once fertilized, the egg is known as a zygote

Morula Around three to four days after fertilization, a ball of around 16 cells heads towards the uterus

Fimbriae Finger-like projections sweep the egg into the Fallopian tube

Ovary A mature egg is released from the ovary

Blastocyst By the time it implants in the uterus, about a week after fertilization, what was a single cell is now a ball of up to 100 cells

3 IMPLANTATION

About a week after fertilization, the ball of cells, now known as a blastocyst, implants itself in the lining of the uterus. The blastocyst has an outer layer of cells, which will develop into the placenta, and an inner mass of cells that will become the embryo.

Once implanted, the blastocyst begins to secrete the pregnancy hormone hCG, which helps to maintain the thick lining of the uterus and prevents it shedding (your monthly period). This is the hormone that can be detected in your urine when you take a pregnancy test.

1 OVULATION

The ovaries typically alternate in releasing an egg during each monthly cycle, so ovulation takes place from just one ovary. One – or occasionally more than one – fully mature egg is released from an ovary and is wafted into a nearby Fallopian tube.

Once the egg begins its journey, the ovaries produce the hormone progesterone, which causes the uterine lining to thicken and ripen in anticipation of a possible pregnancy. It also produces the nutrients necessary to support a developing embryo, and causes the breast lobules (milk glands) to swell.

FROM OVULATION TO IMPLANTATION

Q I had an abortion when I was younger. Can I still get pregnant?

If your abortion was conducted before 14 weeks of pregnancy, and as long as your Fallopian tubes were not damaged for any reason, you should still be able to get pregnant. If your abortion was between 14 and 24 weeks, there may be a slight risk of premature delivery if you fall pregnant again. If you have been trying to conceive for a year or more, or for six months if you are over 35, you may want to see your GP to have some basic fertility tests.

Q I'm on long-term medication. Will this affect my fertility?

Some medication prescribed for long-term medical conditions may affect your ability to conceive. If you have an existing medical condition, it's important to talk to your GP before you try to get pregnant.

Such conditions include asthma, diabetes, heart disease, inflammatory bowel disease (IBD) lupus, epilepsy, migraine, mental health problems, acne, high blood pressure, anaemia, obesity, and being underweight. The type or dose of prescription drugs, vitamins, herbal medicine, or other supplements you take may need to be adjusted before and during pregnancy. Don't stop taking any medication you've been prescribed until advised to do so by your doctor. Don't forget to mention any allergies and over-the-counter medications too.

You may need to take a higher dose of folic acid if you are at risk of having a pregnancy affected by a neural tube defect (see p.49). This may be the case if you take anti-epileptic medication, you are diabetic, if you had a neural tube defect in a previous pregnancy, or there is a history of neural tube defects in your family.

Q I think my partner and I have fertility issues. What should we do?

The first thing to do is make an appointment with your GP, especially if the female partner has irregular or painful periods, feels pain during intercourse, has previously had a pelvic infection or operation, or if there's any reason the male partner might have abnormal semen.

Q What is genetic screening and should we have it before we conceive?

Genetic screening may be carried out to find out if couples who are planning to conceive are carrying a particular altered gene that could lead to their baby inheriting a specific medical condition. It helps couples to prepare for the likelihood of their child having the condition.

Some genetic disorders are more common in particular ethnic groups. Sickle cell disease is most common in those of African descent, while most cases of Tay-Sachs disease and cystic fibrosis affect Ashkenazi Jews and northern white Europeans respectively. Contact your GP to be referred for screening.

The test usually involves giving a blood or sample tissue so that your DNA can be analyzed. It may take weeks, or sometimes months, to get the results. It is vital to remember that screening is not foolproof or conclusive. Genetic counselling is often provided to inform and support parents.

Sickle-cell anaemia
In this example both parents are carriers – they each have one sickle-cell gene. If the baby inherits a sickle-cell gene from each parent, he will have sickle-cell anaemia. If he inherits only one, he will be a carrier. He may inherit neither of the sickle-cell genes.

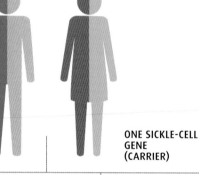

Both genes
A child who inherits both sickle-cell genes will have the condition

ONE SICKLE-CELL GENE (CARRIER)   ONE SICKLE-CELL GENE (CARRIER)

NO SICKLE-CELL GENES   ONE SICKLE-CELL GENE (CARRIER)   ONE SICKLE-CELL GENE (CARRIER)   PAIR OF SICKLE-CELL GENES (SICKLE-CELL ANAEMIA)

Your doctor will ask you how long you have been trying to conceive, the current state of your health, and about any past health issues. If appropriate, he or she will suggest a range of tests that may establish the cause.

For women, the possible causes include damaged or blocked Fallopian tubes, failure to ovulate, endometriosis, fibroids, cysts on the ovaries, and pelvic inflammatory disease. The most common tests are blood tests to check levels of hormones linked to ovulation, ultrasound scans to look at the reproductive organs, and X-rays of the uterus and Fallopian tubes. For men, the causes include poor sperm count, blockage of the tubes, and infections.

Tests will assess sperm quality, hormones, the reproductive organs, and chromosomes.

Depending on the situation, there are various treatment options such as medicines and drugs to assist fertility, surgical procedures, and assisted conception. Although the tests may discover the root of the problem there are occasions where fertility can be unexplained.

Going through these investigations can be extremely stressful and frustrating. During this time, it is vital to learn everything you can about your medical situation, so ask your doctor or specialist if you have any questions or concerns, and communicate with your partner about your feelings.

Q Is it still possible to have a baby in our forties, or have we left it too late?

Women are increasingly having babies in their forties, particularly if they have assisted conception. Statistically, the odds aren't in your favour, but it depends on your individual circumstances and health.

Talk to your GP if you haven't conceived after having unprotected sex for six months. He or she will begin initial investigations (see opposite) to check whether you have any problems that could be affecting your fertility.

Do all that you can to maximize your fertility by making diet and lifestyle changes (see p.29). As well as improving your chances of conceiving naturally, these changes will also ensure you are in the best possible health for pregnancy and parenthood.

You may be advised that your best option of conceiving is to have fertility treatment. Using donated eggs is often an effective treatment for women who are in their forties. After the age of 40, you may be offered one cycle of in vitro fertilization (IVF) on the NHS, but only if you meet strict criteria. It may also depend on where you live. If you go to a private clinic for IVF, be aware of the costs, and budget for the fact that you may need to have more than one cycle of treatment.

> The number of babies born to women who are aged 40 and over has **more than quadrupled** over the last three decades.

AVERAGE RATES OF INFERTILITY IN WOMEN

Women are most fertile in their 20s, with only a 3 per cent likelihood of being infertile. By age 35 this has risen to 15 per cent and by age 40, a woman has a 32 per cent chance of infertility. Women in their late forties have a 69 per cent likelihood of infertility.

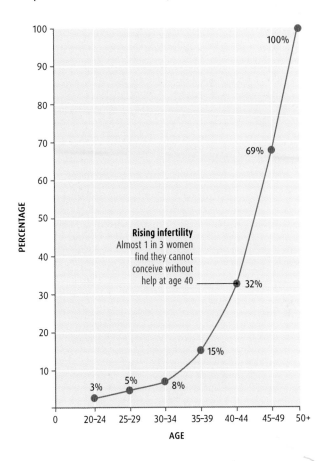

Rising infertility
Almost 1 in 3 women find they cannot conceive without help at age 40

Biological clock As this graph shows, a woman is nearly twice as likely to have fertility issues at age 35 as she did at age 30. That likelihood doubles again by 40.

KEY
● Likelihood of infertility

Q Is it true that it's more common to have twins when you are older?

Since women over the age of 35 are more likely to release more than one egg per cycle, yes, they do have a higher chance of conceiving a multiple pregnancy. Another reason is the number of older women who are taking advantage of assisted conception, which carries with it the possibility of a multiple pregnancy because the treatments sometimes use more than one embryo at a time. Multiple pregnancy is the biggest risk factor to an unborn baby, due to the high chance of premature birth.

Q My partner is a few years older than I am. Will this affect how long it takes us to conceive?

Male fertility begins to decline after the age of 40, when the quality of the sperm deteriorates. This can affect the health of the children born to the man as well as having an impact on his rate of fertility. Statistically, the average time for a man to conceive with his partner if he is aged under 25 is just four-and-a-half months; if the female partner is aged under 25 and the man is 40, it is likely to take nearly two years – five times as long – to conceive.

Q We've been trying to get pregnant for six months. Do we need to see a doctor?

If you are under 35, the recommended time to wait before consulting your GP is one year. In the meantime, try not to worry, maintain a healthy lifestyle, and keep having sex regularly.

If you are over 35, or have a history of gynaecological issues, you are more likely to have problems conceiving. See your doctor if you've been unsuccessful after six months of trying for a baby so that the necessary tests and investigations can be carried out.

Q We are considering IVF. How successful is it and what does it involve?

The live birth rate from IVF is increasing gradually. In 2012, UK success rates were 32.8 per cent for women aged under 35; 27.3 per cent for 35–37 years; 20.7 per cent for 38–39 years; 13.1 per cent for 40–42 years; and 4.4 per cent for 43 years plus.

1 in 50

babies **in the UK** are **born as a result of IVF treatment** (2014).

IVF is the process by which an egg and sperm are mixed together in a Petri dish outside the body. Following fertilization, an embryo (possibly more than one) is transferred to the uterus. The process is extremely time-consuming and involves many appointments. You are also required to take medication by injection and undergo a minor surgical procedure. Before beginning IVF, it is crucial to prepare yourself for the fact that it can be an extremely fraught and draining experience. It can put an enormous amount of pressure on a couple and it is vital, therefore, that both partners are in complete agreement about the course of action.

Before embarking on the treatment, speak to your GP and consider doing your own research into hospitals, clinics, and the procedure. IVF is appropriate in some medical situations, but not in others. There are also some couples for whom IVF is likely to be of little help, so a full understanding of what it involves is essential.

WHAT HAPPENS WHEN?

A number of eggs are usually required to increase the likelihood of conceiving a viable embryo. IVF treatment involves injections to encourage the ovaries to ripen more than one egg. Your progress is monitored with scans and a specialist will choose an optimum point to collect the eggs for fertilization.

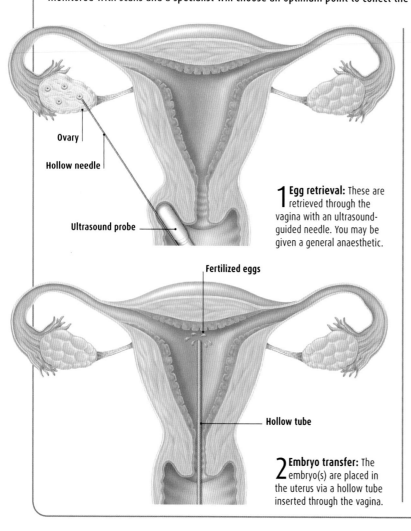

Ovary

Hollow needle

Ultrasound probe

1 Egg retrieval: These are retrieved through the vagina with an ultrasound-guided needle. You may be given a general anaesthetic.

Fertilized eggs

Hollow tube

2 Embryo transfer: The embryo(s) are placed in the uterus via a hollow tube inserted through the vagina.

THE STAGES OF IVF

Stage 1 – Suppression

In some treatments, the ovaries are suppressed before stimulating them to produce multiple eggs. This stage can begin one week before your period is due or the day after it begins. You take a nasal spray or inject a drug for one to two weeks to suppress your natural cycle. This prevents the pituitary gland from producing follicle-stimulating hormones (FSH). Other treatments go straight to stimulation (see below) and suppress the release of mature eggs afterwards.

Stage 2 – Stimulation

An ultrasound scan is done to confirm that the ovaries are not active. Following this, you take FSH as a daily injection for 10 to 12 days. This increases the number of eggs your ovaries produce. During this time regular hormone tests are done to indicate how well the follicles are responding to the FSH. A last injection given approximately 36 hours before egg collection helps the eggs to mature.

Stage 3 – Egg retrieval

This is usually done using a vaginal ultrasound that gives an image of each ovary. The eggs are sucked into a test tube and given to an embryologist who places them in special fluid to be examined.

Stage 4 – Embryo selection

The male partner produces semen and his sperm are mixed with the eggs and placed in an incubator. The embryos are assessed 48 hours later and checked to ensure they look normal. The ideal time to transfer the embryo is after about five days when it has developed into a blastocyst. This gives a higher chance of pregnancy.

Stage 5 – Embryo transfer

An embryo is put into a fine plastic tube and this is inserted through the cervix into the uterus.

Q My doctor said we might want to consider having ICSI rather than normal IVF treatment. What is it?

This is only different from IVF at the point of fertilization. Instead of the egg and sperm being left to fertilize naturally in a Petri dish, one healthy sperm is selected and injected directly into a mature egg.

ICSI (intra-cytoplasmic sperm injection) is recommended to couples if the man has a very low sperm count, for example, or other sperm problems that mean the egg is unlikely to be fertilized naturally. This treatment may be recommended if you have had low – or even zero – fertilization rates in a previous IVF cycle – the eggs that have been collected have failed to turn into embryos in the first 24 hours.

The process of stimulating the ovaries to produce more eggs and egg collection is the same as for IVF. Following the ICSI fertilization procedure, the IVF treatment continues as normal in that the embryo is placed into the uterus (see opposite). Be aware that if you are paying for your IVF treatment, there is an additional fee for ICSI.

ICSI

In the ICSI procedure, the sperm and egg are brought together instead of being left to fertilize naturally.

Pipette This holds the egg still

Fine needle A single sperm is injected directly

Egg

Q I know someone who got pregnant by having IUI. What exactly is it?

IUI stands for intrauterine insemination and is a procedure where sperm is placed directly into the uterus. Before being considered for IUI, your Fallopian tubes are tested to ensure that they are open. You are given a blood or urine test to detect ovulation. As soon as the egg is mature, a hormone injection is given to release it. Then 36–40 hours after this your partner provides a sperm sample. The fastest-moving, least-sluggish sperm are selected and inserted into your uterus using a catheter. It is a quick and painless procedure.

The rest is left to nature in the hope that one sperm fertilizes the egg. You may be advised to have up to six cycles of IUI. You may be recommended to opt for IUI if you have ovulation problems, your partner is impotent, or you are trying for a baby using donated sperm. IUI is not normally offered by the NHS but is available privately.

Q We're using donor eggs. Will my body naturally accept them?

If you are not ovulating (an inability to produce eggs is not rare) and require a donated egg, the lining of your uterus probably won't be thick enough for an embryo to implant in it. You will need a cycle of hormone replacement prior to the egg being implanted to ensure the uterine lining can nourish the embryo. This is the main key to a successful pregnancy from a donated egg. The principle risk for you is a multiple birth if you have more than one fertilized egg transferred.

Q I've heard that some women freeze their eggs. Is this something I should consider doing?

Freezing and storing your eggs may enable you to use them for treatment in the future. As many women are leaving child-bearing to later in life, egg-freezing is becoming more common. Apart from preserving fertility, it is something that is recommended for women under 40 who need cancer treatment that may make them infertile or for those who cannot wait for another IVF attempt (due to age or illness) if the first one fails. The procedure for collecting eggs is the same as the first stages of a cycle of IVF treatment where drugs are used to stimulate the ovaries to produce follicles (which contain the eggs). When the follicles are large enough, the eggs are retrieved and placed in storage in liquid nitrogen. Until relatively recently, using eggs that had been frozen carried certain risks and the success rate had been poor. Due to improved freezing methods (vitrification), this is now changing.

Women undergoing IVF or ICSI often have a number of unused embryos. Some people choose to have these frozen for use in another treatment cycle if the first fails, to attempt another pregnancy with a sibling embryo, or to donate to others. The chances of a successful pregnancy using a thawed frozen embryo are not affected by the amount of time the embryo is stored and frozen. However, not all embryos survive the thawing process. The clinic will advise you on the best procedure for using your frozen embryos. There are options depending on your personal and medical circumstances.

For both egg and embryo freezing, you will need to give your consent. Similarly, you, your partner, or the donor can withdraw consent at any time before the treatment begins or before the embryos are used. If one person withdraws their consent, then there is a period of a year in which you can decide what happens to the embryos.

Q Did you know...

Eating oysters is good for male fertility. They are high in zinc, which helps sperm count, sperm motility (the way sperm moves), and increases testosterone levels. If you can't stomach oysters, other good sources of zinc are legumes, nuts, spinach, and lean beef and lamb, or you could take a daily zinc supplement.

Discovering that you are pregnant will be one of the most **transformative and memorable** experiences of your life. Even if the pregnancy is planned, you are likely to feel a range of **emotions** from joy to trepidation. Take time to adjust and then start to learn about the many miraculous changes taking place **inside your body**.

Pregnant!

Finding out that you are pregnant

Congratulations! You are now on an amazing, life-changing journey. Perhaps you have missed your period, or noticed symptoms such as sore breasts, nausea, and extreme tiredness. Maybe you know just how far along you must be, or it has taken weeks to realize you could be pregnant. Whether you have been actively trying for a baby, have been undergoing fertility treatment, or your pregnancy was unplanned, enjoy the moment of discovery – there is no more exciting and momentous news.

Most women find out they are pregnant by doing a home pregnancy test as these are so accurate and reliable. In some circumstances, a blood test or ultrasound scan may be needed to confirm a pregnancy.

One or both of you may feel overwhelmed that you are going to be parents. It is quite normal to have a number of questions and concerns – about your stage of pregnancy and when your baby is due, and whether your baby is in good health. You may look to the future and wonder about how much life will change, but try not to get too anxious – you have plenty of time until your baby is born.

If you are a single parent, whether you have an unexpected or a planned pregnancy, you may be experiencing some anxiety, as well as shock or delight.

There is no right or wrong time to tell people that you are having a baby. You may want to confide only in immediate family members until you are into your second trimester and the likelihood of miscarriage is minimal. Otherwise, trust your instincts and tell those close friends and family members whom you know will actively support you through the first weeks of pregnancy.

If you work, you may want to wait until you have had your first ultrasound scan before you tell your boss. However, if you are experiencing symptoms such as nausea and sickness it can be more difficult to hide your pregnancy. Also, if your job involves chemicals or heavy lifting then you will definitely need to tell your manager.

What to expect

It is worth familiarizing yourself with the common symptoms of early pregnancy, such as tiredness and nausea, and finding ways to cope with them. Equally, be reassured that you may not have any symptoms and this is normal for some women.

Many of the more difficult symptoms, such as vomiting and fatigue lessen by early in the second trimester and you may find at that time you begin to relax and enjoy your pregnancy a bit more.

Q I think I may be pregnant. How do I find out for sure?

A urine test is the quickest and simplest way to measure whether you have high levels of the pregnancy hormone human chorionic gonadotrophin (hCG) in your body, which starts rising several days after conception.

You can buy a pregnancy testing kit from a pharmacy or a supermarket to use at home, or you can ask your GP or family planning clinic to perform a free test for you.

Most home testing kits can be used on the first day of your missed period; any earlier, and the test is less reliable (see graph, below). However, some brands claim to provide an accurate result up to four days before your period is due.

If you have irregular periods and you aren't sure when the first day of your missed period will be, do a test three weeks after you last had unprotected sex.

How to test

It is advisable, but not essential, to do the test soon after you wake in the morning as your urine has the highest concentration of hormones at that time. You simply pee on the test stick for a few seconds and wait for the positive or negative symbol or the words "Pregnant" or "Not Pregnant" to appear on the screen. The result should show on the screen within a couple of minutes. If you follow the instructions correctly, a positive result means you are almost certainly pregnant. If you have a negative result and your period still hasn't arrived, you may have tested too early. Although any delay can feel incredibly frustrating, it's worth waiting a few days before testing again.

GPs accept pregnancy home testing kits as accurate. If there is any doubt, a blood test may be done to detect the exact levels of hCG in your body, even if those levels are still low. This may be recommended if you are undergoing fertility treatment.

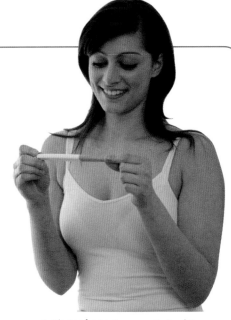
Testing at home Pregnancy testing kits are usually easy-to-use sticks that test the hormone levels in your urine.

HCG LEVELS IN PREGNANCY

The hormone that signals you are pregnant is called hCG. As the graph shows, hCG levels start rising a week after conception – a little at first and then steadily until your baby is well-established in the uterus. The other main pregnancy hormones, oestrogen and progesterone, surge later on.

KEY
— Human chorionic gonadotrophin (hCG)
— Oestrogen
— Progesterone
● Conception

Increased hormones Note the huge surge in hCG (the purple line) following conception.

Q My home pregnancy test result is positive. Can I be sure it's right? What happens next?

A positive pregnancy test result means you have raised levels of the pregnancy hormone hCG in your body. Even if the positive symbol or words on the test screen are quite faint, you are still likely to be pregnant. Many women often do another test just to make sure (many home pregnancy tests come as a double pack), though this isn't necessary.

Make an appointment with your GP as soon as you can to let him or her know that you are pregnant. At the appointment you will find out about your antenatal healthcare and have the opportunity to ask questions. If you don't want to wait to see your doctor you can fill out a self-referral form for your local midwifery unit.

Your doctor will want to discuss nutrition and lifestyle with you and ensure you know about taking folic acid (see p.49). He or she will also discuss your medical history in case you need additional antenatal screenings or need to adapt any current medication.

Your doctor will give you an estimated delivery date (EDD). You can use a due-date calendar to work out your EDD yourself (see p.42). They are most useful if you have a regular menstrual cycle: simply look up the first date of your last menstrual period to find your EDD. However, it's an estimate and only 4 per cent of women give birth on their EDD. Ultrasound scans aren't usually done until you're 8–14 weeks pregnant but in some cases – if you've had a miscarriage, have a suspected ectopic pregnancy (see p.308), or you're experiencing bleeding – an earlier scan may be recommended.

The accuracy of **home pregnancy tests is more than 99 per cent.** So if it says "pregnant" on that little screen, you can be fairly certain that you are!

A CLOSER LOOK
When sperm meets egg

This is the moment of the miracle: when a single sperm from the 200–500 million contenders in a single ejaculate penetrates a mature egg that only survives for 24 hours. The journey has taken the tiny sperm around 5–20 minutes, and most of its brothers have fallen by the wayside in the vital race.

A long, whip-like tail propels the sperm on its swim towards the egg.

The midpiece houses a spiral mitochondrion – it's the powerhouse that provides the sperm with energy.

1 **This sperm has beaten millions** of others to reach the egg in the Fallopian tube. Only around 200-300 sperm made it this far. The others bind to the surface of the egg, but this winning sperm pushes through the egg's layers to penetrate it.

The sperm head contains the male DNA – including the X or Y chromosome that will determine whether your baby is a girl or boy.

2 **The sperm is able to enter** the egg's corona radiata and zona pellucida layers with the help of enzymes in its acrosome – a cap-like structure on its head. The acrosome will shed when the job is done, allowing the sperm to fuse with and fertilize the egg.

The egg is encased by a thick transparent double membrane called a zona pellucida.

Layers of corona radiata cells surround the egg to form the outermost protective coat.

3 **As soon as the head of this sperm** pushes through the zona pellucida, it triggers a reaction that causes this outer layer of the egg to block all other sperm from entering.

4 **Fertilization takes place** when the sperm reaches the innermost part of the egg (the oocyte) and fuses with its nucleus. Since the sperm and egg contain 23 chromosomes each, this fusion creates a single nucleus with the full 46 chromosomes that make up the DNA for a new baby.

FASCINATING FACTS

About the size of a grain of sand, the egg is one of the largest cells in the human body. The sperm is one of the tiniest.

500 million

In one ejaculation there can be 200–500 million sperm, but only 200–300 will survive the journey to the egg.

7 million

This is the number of immature egg cells a female baby grows while in utero. She will have these by 20 weeks.

400,000

A girl's ovaries contain about 400,000 eggs by the time she reaches puberty. Each menstrual cycle, 1,000 eggs are lost.

100 days

The man's testicles generate a new complement of sperm cells every 100 days.

36 hours

The average life span of sperm is between one and two days.

Q When will my baby arrive? Can I find out before I see my GP?

It is easy to calculate the estimated birth date of your baby as long as you know the first day of your last menstrual period.

Before your first ultrasound scan, your GP or midwife will use the first day of your last menstrual period (known as LMP) as a marker for the start of your pregnancy. This means you can calculate the estimated date of delivery (EDD) yourself using a due date calendar, such as the one below. It is wonderful to have an actual day to work towards, but try not to get too tied to it since the due date is only an estimate after all. Almost 50 per cent of babies are born before the EDD and about the same again are born after the EDD. You will reach full term at 37 weeks and if you haven't given birth by 41 weeks you will be offered an induction to reduce the risk of having an overdue baby.

4%
of babies are born on their **due date.**

WHEN WILL YOUR BABY BE BORN?

To work out your estimated date of delivery (EDD) - also known as the due date - find the date you started your last menstrual period (LMP) on the upper lines of the chart, then see the dates in bold below to discover when your baby is expected. For example, if your last LMP was August 16, then your baby will be due on 23 May.

JANUARY	1	2	3	4	5	6	7	8	9	10	11	12	13	14	15	16	17	18	19	20	21	22	23	24	25	26	27	28	29	30	31
OCT/NOV	8	9	10	11	12	13	14	15	16	17	18	19	20	21	22	23	24	25	26	27	28	29	30	31	1	2	3	4	5	6	7
FEBRUARY	1	2	3	4	5	6	7	8	9	10	11	12	13	14	15	16	17	18	19	20	21	22	23	24	25	26	27	28			
NOV/DEC	8	9	10	11	12	13	14	15	16	17	18	19	20	21	22	23	24	25	26	27	28	29	30	1	2	3	4	5			
MARCH	1	2	3	4	5	6	7	8	9	10	11	12	13	14	15	16	17	18	19	20	21	22	23	24	25	26	27	28	29	30	31
DEC/JAN	6	7	8	9	10	11	12	13	14	15	16	17	18	19	20	21	22	23	24	25	26	27	28	29	30	31	1	2	3	4	5
APRIL	1	2	3	4	5	6	7	8	9	10	11	12	13	14	15	16	17	18	19	20	21	22	23	24	25	26	27	28	29	30	
JAN/FEB	6	7	8	9	10	11	12	13	14	15	16	17	18	19	20	21	22	23	24	25	26	27	28	29	30	31	1	2	3	4	
MAY	1	2	3	4	5	6	7	8	9	10	11	12	13	14	15	16	17	18	19	20	21	22	23	24	25	26	27	28	29	30	31
FEB/MAR	5	6	7	8	9	10	11	12	13	14	15	16	17	18	19	20	21	22	23	24	25	26	27	28	1	2	3	4	5	6	7
JUNE	1	2	3	4	5	6	7	8	9	10	11	12	13	14	15	16	17	18	19	20	21	22	23	24	25	26	27	28	29	30	
MAR/APR	8	9	10	11	12	13	14	15	16	17	18	19	20	21	22	23	24	25	26	27	28	29	30	31	1	2	3	4	5	6	
JULY	1	2	3	4	5	6	7	8	9	10	11	12	13	14	15	16	17	18	19	20	21	22	23	24	25	26	27	28	29	30	31
APR/MAY	7	8	9	10	11	12	13	14	15	16	17	18	19	20	21	22	23	24	25	26	27	28	29	30	1	2	3	4	5	6	7
AUGUST	1	2	3	4	5	6	7	8	9	10	11	12	13	14	15	16	17	18	19	20	21	22	23	24	25	26	27	28	29	30	31
MAY/JUNE	8	9	10	11	12	13	14	15	16	17	18	19	20	21	22	**23**	24	25	26	27	28	29	30	31	1	2	3	4	5	6	7
SEPTEMBER	1	2	3	4	5	6	7	8	9	10	11	12	13	14	15	16	17	18	19	20	21	22	23	24	25	26	27	28	29	30	
JUNE/JULY	8	9	10	11	12	13	14	15	16	17	18	19	20	21	22	23	24	25	26	27	28	29	30	1	2	3	4	5	6	7	
OCTOBER	1	2	3	4	5	6	7	8	9	10	11	12	13	14	15	16	17	18	19	20	21	22	23	24	25	26	27	28	29	30	31
JULY/AUG	8	9	10	11	12	13	14	15	16	17	18	19	20	21	22	23	24	25	26	27	28	29	30	31	1	2	3	4	5	6	7
NOVEMBER	1	2	3	4	5	6	7	8	9	10	11	12	13	14	15	16	17	18	19	20	21	22	23	24	25	26	27	28	29	30	
AUG/SEPT	8	9	10	11	12	13	14	15	16	17	18	19	20	21	22	23	24	25	26	27	28	29	30	31	1	2	3	4	5	6	
DECEMBER	1	2	3	4	5	6	7	8	9	10	11	12	13	14	15	16	17	18	19	20	21	22	23	24	25	26	27	28	29	30	31
SEPT/OCT	7	8	9	10	11	12	13	14	15	16	17	18	19	20	21	22	23	24	25	26	27	28	29	30	1	2	3	4	5	6	7

Q How can I find out my stage of pregnancy?

You will have your first ultrasound scan, known as a dating scan, at around 8-14 weeks. The due date is based on your last menstrual period, but does not tell you when you conceived. Dating scans are a more accurate indicator of your stage of pregnancy and due date. You may find you are further along than you thought.

Q Is it important to know which trimester I'm in?

It helps to understand the trimesters, so you know what to expect at each stage. The first trimester lasts from the first day of your last period to 12 weeks pregnant (you conceive at two weeks). During this trimester you may experience lots of symptoms (see opposite). It can also be an anxious time because the risk of miscarriage is highest in the first trimester. In the second trimester - from 13 weeks to 25 weeks pregnant - you may have fewer symptoms, but will probably feel more pregnant because your bump will be showing. The final trimester, up to 42 weeks, can be very tiring, due to the weight of the baby, broken sleep, and symptoms such as backache. While this can be a tough stage, it is exciting too as you begin all the preparation for your baby's arrival.

Did you know...

Twin pregnancies can bring additional nausea and sickness. While it doesn't happen for every expectant mum of twins, there is an increased risk of nausea and sickness due to the higher hCG levels (see p.39) in a twin, or other multiple, pregnancy. There are also higher levels of the hormone progesterone with twins, which can cause shortness of breath. In later pregnancy, carrying multiple babies can lead to more fatigue, constipation, heartburn, and back pain for mum-to-be.

Q I'm pregnant but I have no symptoms. Should I be worried?

It's normal for some women to experience few or no symptoms in early pregnancy, even though hormones are flooding the body and changes are underway. This is nothing to worry about – you are just as pregnant as a woman who has nausea and sickness, for example, but just not as sensitive to the hormonal changes that are taking place.

Even though you may not feel the tiredness associated with early pregnancy, be sure to rest and take good care of yourself.

Q Are there any pregnancy symptoms I should be concerned about?

Although concerning symptoms are not common in early pregnancy, seek medical advice if you have any of the following symptoms.

» Vaginal bleeding: light spotting is common but you must report it to your GP or midwife. Heavy bleeding, especially if you also have stomach cramps, can be a sign of a threatening miscarriage. Bleeding and lower abdominal pain can also signal an ectopic pregnancy (see p.308).

» Severe vomiting: seek advice if you are vomiting to the point of dehydration and can't keep any fluids down for more than 12 hours.

» A fever: you may have an infection.

» Vaginal discharge and itching: this may mean you have an infection such as thrush. It can be treated to offer relief from the symptoms.

Q I'm five weeks pregnant. I feel OK, but what symptoms might I get?

Most women experience some symptoms in early pregnancy due to the hormonal changes taking place. Thankfully many of these pass, especially morning sickness, by the end of the first trimester or early in the second trimester.

EARLY PREGNANCY SYMPTOMS

All women are different, but here are some of the symptoms you may experience in early pregnancy.

» Feeling dizzy and faint: in early pregnancy, this may be caused by low blood pressure.

» Headaches: these can be caused by increased blood circulation in early pregnancy.

» Sore breasts and tingly nipples: there may also be visible breast changes (see p.125).

» Fatigue: as your body adapts to support the pregnancy, it is normal to feel totally exhausted.

» Craving/disliking foods: a heightened sense of taste makes you love, or completely avoid, some foods.

» Mood swings: even if you are happy, you are likely to feel emotional and be easily upset.

» Sense of smell: you may become much more aware of and averse to everyday smells.

» Nausea and sickness: vomiting and/or nausea can happen at any time of day.

» Loss of appetite: this is likely if you have had a lot of nausea and vomiting.

» Peeing more often: this may also cause sleep disruption if you need to pee during the night.

The most reliable sign of pregnancy is a **missed period**. If your period is late, do a pregnancy test.

» A burning sensation when you pee: this can be the sign of urinary infection, which will need to be treated with antibiotics.

» Leg or calf pain, swelling on one side, and/or a severe headache: these are signs of a blood clot, which is more likely to occur in pregnancy, though it is rare.

» A flare-up of a current medical condition: let your GP or specialist know of any symptoms that you have experienced since being pregnant.

7 in 10
women **experience nausea or vomiting** or both during pregnancy.

Q I've been taking the pill – but I'm pregnant. Will my baby be OK?

The risks to your baby are low. If you are on the pill or mini-pill, stop taking it if your pregnancy test is positive – you don't need to finish the cycle.

It's understandable that you may not have been aware you are pregnant for a while. Some of the side effects of this form of contraception, such as feeling nauseous and having tender breasts, can also be early pregnancy symptoms. The results of a pregnancy test won't be affected by the pill itself as the test only reacts to hCG readings.

Try not to worry, but take action immediately to stop whichever type of contraception you are using, as outlined in the chart, right. The hormones in the pill don't last long in your system and trials indicate that there isn't an increase in the risk of birth defects. There is, however, a slightly greater chance of an ectopic pregnancy (see p.308); the mini-pill can alter the motility of the Fallopian tube – affecting the ability of an egg to move through it.

Make an appointment to see your GP as soon as you can to let him or her know that you are pregnant and that you conceived while you were still taking a contraceptive pill. Your doctor can refer you for an ultrasound to rule out an ectopic pregnancy.

 Did you know...

Some couples rely on the withdrawal method as a form of contraception. This is when the man pulls his penis out of the woman before he ejaculates. While this can be effective for some couples who are adept in the method, it shouldn't be relied upon to prevent pregnancy. Some experts claim that pre-ejaculate can pick up sperm that's in the man's urethra from a previous ejaculation, which can lead to pregnancy.

CONTRACEPTION FAILURES AND EFFECTS

While some contraception is more effective than others, no contraception is a 100 per cent barrier to pregnancy. This table explains what to do if your contraception has failed.

TYPE OF CONTRACEPTION	WHAT DOES IT DO?	HOW SHOULD I STOP?
Combined pill	Contains oestrogen and progestogen. Oestrogen inhibits ovulation and progestogen thickens cervical mucus to make it difficult for a sperm to reach an egg and an egg to implant in the uterus.	Stop taking the pills straight away. There is no need to finish the cycle.
Mini-pill	Contains just progestogen, not oestrogen. The progestogen thickens cervical mucus to make it difficult for a sperm to reach an egg and an egg to implant in the uterus.	Stop taking the pills straight away. There is no need to finish the cycle.
Emergency contraceptive pill (also called the morning after pill)	Works by preventing or delaying ovulation.	Do not take any more emergency contraception.
Injections	Contains progestogen, which thickens cervical mucus to make it difficult for a sperm to reach an egg and an egg to implant in the uterus.	Simply stop renewing your injections.
Implants	Inserted under the skin of your upper arm, the flexible tube slowly releases progestogen to stop sperm from reaching an egg and the uterus from supporting a fertilized egg.	A specially trained doctor will need to remove the implant, and an ultrasound scan may be necessary to locate it.
IUD coil	Positioned in the uterus, the coil prevents a sperm and egg, or a fertilized egg, from implanting in the uterus or Fallopian tubes.	There is a risk of miscarriage and ectopic pregnancy because of the presence of a foreign body in the uterus, possible inflammation, and an increased risk of infection. If the coil is visible, it's best for a specialist to remove it; if not, it is best left where it is for the pregnancy.
Spermicide	Available in different forms (including gels and foams), spermicide contains chemicals that stop sperm from moving.	Do not use once you are pregnant.
Sterilization	The Fallopian tubes are tied to prevent an egg reaching the uterus.	N/A

WHAT ELSE SHOULD I KNOW?

There is no scientific evidence that the hormones oestrogen and progestogen contained in this product affect a developing embryo and fetus.

There is no scientific evidence that the progestogen in this product affects a developing embryo and fetus.

This contains the same components as the combined and mini-pills, so there is no risk to the developing embryo and fetus. Neither does it cause an abortion.

There is no scientific evidence that the progestogen in this product affects a developing embryo and fetus.

There is no scientific evidence that the progestogen in this product affects a developing embryo and fetus. If the implant can't be located and removed, there is no need to worry.

You need to request a scan to rule out an ectopic pregnancy. If the coil stays in position while you are pregnant, it is usually delivered with the placenta after the birth.

There is no scientific evidence that this product affects a developing embryo and fetus.

You should make an appointment with your GP promptly: your Fallopian tubes are likely to have been damaged by the sterilization procedure and you may be at risk of an ectopic pregnancy (see p.308).

Q Is there anything I should do now I know I am pregnant?

These practical steps are some of the first things to do on your pregnancy journey.
≫ Make an appointment with your GP
≫ Start taking 400mcg folic acid a day (available from a pharmacy) if you're not already taking it
≫ Limit caffeine and avoid drinking alcohol, smoking, and taking drugs (see p.53)
≫ Eat healthily
≫ Exercise moderately
≫ Find ways to relax
≫ Become informed by reading about the stages of pregnancy, how your baby is developing, and understanding the tests and scans you will be offered in the coming months.

Q I didn't plan to get pregnant, but I am. What should I do?

You are probably deep in shock at the news, but it's worth remembering that many women have mixed emotions when they find out they are pregnant, even when it is planned. Firstly, take the pressure off yourself and your partner, if you have one, and take time to adjust to the situation. You will probably want to talk to trusted family members and friends for support, but if you feel overly anxious or fearful, tell your GP. You may also want to seek professional advice about making changes to your housing arrangements or your finances when you feel ready. The magnitude of change may seem huge, but take a deep breath and start taking steps to ensure you have a healthy pregnancy.

Q I drank and smoked before realizing that I was pregnant. Will that have harmed my baby?

You probably won't have harmed your baby if you had a couple of drinks and the odd cigarette, but you must stop straight away to reduce risk of damage to you and your baby. Alcohol and drugs have their greatest effect during organ development, which doesn't begin until week five. As soon as you know you are pregnant, however, you should abstain from all alcohol and stop smoking during pregnancy. If you drink or smoke heavily and you continue throughout your pregnancy, you are at risk of damaging both your health and that of your baby. Smoking can directly affect the placenta's growth, and in later pregnancy it can reduce the supply of oxygen and nutrients to the baby, resulting in a lower birthweight and more chance of a premature baby. Smoking doubles the risk of stillbirth. Regular or heavy drinking can lead to fetal alcohol syndrome (see p.325), which damages the baby's nervous system and inhibits his ability to thrive after birth.

Q I'm not as happy as I thought I'd be about being pregnant.

Whether planned or not, a pregnancy can raise deep emotional issues that you have never been aware of before. You may be facing a whole range of emotions, including disbelief, feeling overwhelmed, and you may be at a loss about what to do next. Give yourself permission to go along with whatever you are feeling for the next few weeks until you have begun to adjust to this new role in life, and don't feel guilty. If you continue to feel negative about the pregnancy, seek support and reassurance from loved ones or speak to your GP or midwife.

Q What if my partner isn't pleased about the pregnancy?

If you are in this situation, accept your partner's feelings and give him plenty of time to adjust to what is, after all, life-changing news. On hearing the news, he may feel upset and angry, and panic, especially if the pregnancy is unplanned. Try not to take his reaction personally. Hopefully it will become a constructive part of processing the news and coming to terms with the future. In the meantime, try to plan some short-term goals that you can enjoy together, or book out some proper time together in the diary, to build on your relationship as a couple.

Taken properly, the combined contraceptive pill is **more than 99 per cent effective.**

Nutrition, exercise, and wellbeing

Knowing what to eat and how to exercise are both **beneficial to your health and that of your baby**. Pregnancy and childbirth will challenge your body more than anything you have experienced before. Being fully **prepared in mind** as well as in body is also important to maintain your wellbeing. This chapter gives specific **advice about a balanced diet**, which supplements to take, which food and drinks to avoid, and **how to exercise safely** during pregnancy and beyond.

From pre-conception to birth, what you eat and drink can **affect your pregnancy**: how quickly you **conceive**, **your health** during pregnancy, your experiences of **pregnancy** and **labour**, and the **health of your baby** – not only while he is growing inside you, but also long into his future.

Nutrition

Eating to stay healthy

There are few experiences in your life that will demand as much of your body as pregnancy and childbirth. Preparing yourself by eating as well as you can is hugely beneficial – a healthy body helps to make your experience of conception, pregnancy, and labour a positive one.

Our diets have changed dramatically over the course of the last 50 years; it seems normal now to regularly eat ready-made, processed, and refined foods rather than always making meals and snacks from scratch ourselves. However, eating enough of the right nutrients is one of the most positive things you can do in pre-pregnancy and pregnancy, and is something you can easily take control of. Good nutrition need not be any more complicated than the general principles of eating a healthy, balanced diet – just be aware that what you stock in your cupboards and fridge and put on your plate is even more important than usual, both for your fertility and energy levels and for the health of your developing baby. You don't have to follow a rigid diet or eat unpleasant foods: it's all about eating twice as well (and not twice as much) to ensure you receive the best nutrients from every mouthful.

Eating well at every stage

As soon as you conceive, you become the lifeline to your baby – everything you eat, drink, and breathe is broken down into molecules containing valuable nutrients and oxygen and transported through your bloodstream and placenta to the fetus. So it's important to have good habits in place from the start. This section gives advice on how you can prepare for and aid conception, including what supplements to take. Once you have conceived, you can read about eating for energy and health, what your baby needs, the best approach if you have an intolerance or you follow a special diet for personal or medical reasons, which foods to avoid, and advice on smoking and drugs. After the birth, you can learn about how to boost your recovery through good nutrition.

Q What is folic acid and why do I need to take it?

Folic acid is a B-group vitamin that is key to the formation of your baby's spine, brain, and nervous system. These organs are some of the very first to develop, which is why you are encouraged to take folic acid even before you conceive.

The neural tube is the part of the embryo that develops into your baby's brain and spinal chord. Ensuring you have good levels of folic acid in your system throughout pre-conception, conception, and the first three months of pregnancy will help to minimize the risk that your baby will develop neural tube defects by 72 per cent. In dads-to-be, good folate levels can reduce the instance of sperm abnormalities.

Essential supplement

Folic acid is the synthesized version of vitamin B9. When it occurs naturally in food, it is known as folate and is present in leafy green vegetables such as cabbage. Studies show that our bodies are better at using the synthesized version so look for supplements that contain 5-methyltetrahydrofolic acid, which is already "biologically active". When you are hoping to conceive, ideally both of you should start taking a daily supplement of 400mcg folic acid before you stop contraception. When pregnant, keep taking it until you are at least 12 weeks pregnant. If you are considered high risk (if either of you has a medical or family history of a neural tube defect; if a previous pregnancy was affected; if you are over 35; or if you are diabetic or epileptic), you may be advised to take a higher dosage of 5mg daily.

Whether you're already pregnant or trying for a baby, start taking **folic acid** as soon as you can.

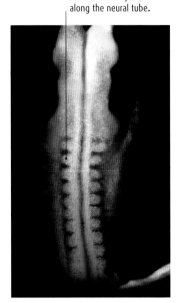

Somites run in pairs along the neural tube.

Neural tube By week five of pregnancy, there is a neural tube running down the middle of the embryo, complete with somites that will become vertebrae.

NEURAL TUBE FORMATION

In the earliest stages, your baby forms from three primary layers of cells. These layers fold to create the basic structures of the body, including the important neural tube.

Neural groove in ectoderm layer

Notochord in mesoderm layer

1 **A neural groove begins to form** when the top layer (ectoderm) sinks towards a column of cells called the notochord in the middle layer (mesoderm).

Neural folds meet

Site of future spinal cord

2 **As the groove deepens**, its edges come together to make a tube shape. This tube extends along the embryo's back, eventually forming the spine and brain.

Neural folds fuse and neural tube is complete

3 **Folic acid helps the folds of the tube to fuse.** If the tube doesn't close fully, it can result in birth defects such as spina bifida.

Q We are trying for a baby. Do we need to change what we eat or drink?

If you lead a healthy lifestyle and eat a good, balanced diet, you've already established the right pattern. If not, make positive changes to your nutrition now to help the health of your sperm and eggs (which each take three months to develop) and establish the necessary stores of nutrients for a healthy pregnancy. Also eliminate, or reduce to within guideline levels, alcohol and caffeine, which have a detrimental effect on conception. Eat more phytoestrogens – found in linseed, wholewheat, and lentils – to balance hormones in both partners, and eat a colourful range of antioxidant-rich foods to boost the quality and motility of sperm.

Q Is it true that what you eat can affect how long it takes to conceive? We have fertility issues.

Anything – including diet – that can affect hormones and the health of the woman's eggs, the man's sperm, the Fallopian tubes, and the uterus can have an impact on how long it takes to get pregnant. So yes, your diet can adversely affect your internal chemistry.

Your weight – whether overweight or underweight – is also an important factor if there are fertility issues, as it can determine whether or not you have too little or too much oestrogen to ovulate. For a man, being underweight can affect the quality of his sperm. Eat the right balance of healthy, nutritious,

unrefined foods from the main food groups, avoid the "empty calories" of junk food, and have three regular meals a day to help you regulate your hormones and boost your chances of conception in the months ahead.

Some women may be advised to take a **prenatal multivitamin** in addition to folic acid, but in general you should be able to get all the **nutrients** you need from your diet.

Q What is a healthy, balanced diet and how can I eat enough nutrients?

A healthy diet is comprised of the right balance of nutritious foods from several main food groups: protein, fruit, vegetables, unrefined carbohydrates, and healthy fats. You should eat foods from these groups in their most natural, unprocessed state to receive the maximum number of nutrients.

Whether you are still at the stage of planning conception or are already pregnant, you need to ensure your diet includes the correct balance of the main food groups. A balanced diet allows your body to store enough of the right nutrients for a healthy pregnancy and feel in peak condition. Eating in a consistent and measured way also helps you to keep your weight within healthy limits, which is a factor for successful conception. Once you become pregnant, the benefit of eating a balanced diet is that you will be supplying your body with the best possible diet for fetal growth and development and providing yourself with enough energy to cope with the pregnancy.

HEALTHY EATING

Eat a variety of foods from each of these groups in the right proportions for optimum nutritional benefits at every meal. The breakdown of these healthy foods equates to approximately five to six portions of fresh vegetables, two portions of fresh fruit, and three portions each of protein and unrefined carbohydrates per day.

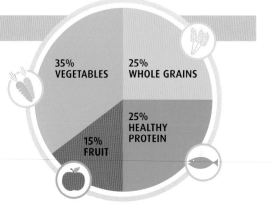

35% VEGETABLES

25% WHOLE GRAINS

25% HEALTHY PROTEIN

15% FRUIT

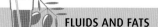

FLUIDS AND FATS

» **Stay hydrated:** often feelings of hunger are in fact symptoms of thirst. Water is best.

» **Enjoy healthy fats:** dairy produce (also a source of calcium) and oils (such as olive oil) are good for you in moderate amounts.

 VEGETABLES

The more vegetables – and the greater the variety – the better. Steaming is the best way to prepare vegetables if you don't eat them raw.

 FRUIT

Eat fresh fruit of all colours. Fruit contains fructose, a type of sugar, so a couple of portions a day will give you fibre and vitamins without overloading on sugar.

 HEALTHY PROTEINS

Choose fish, poultry, beans, and nuts; limit red meat and avoid bacon and processed meats. Steam, grill, or bake fish and meat.

 WHOLE GRAINS

Eat a variety of whole grains (such as wholewheat bread, wholegrain pasta, and brown rice). Limit or avoid refined grains (such as white rice and white bread).

Fresh fruit and vegetables
When it comes to fruit and vegetables, the more colourful the better. Strong colour is a sign that they are rich in vitamins and minerals, and high in protective antioxidants, which help to fight free radicals in the body. Eat a wide colour range of vegetables and fruit for the maximum benefits.

Q Should I take an iron supplement in case I become anaemic?

It is usually better to get your iron needs from your diet. This is because iron tablets can have the side effect of causing constipation, which pregnant women are already susceptible to. Eating iron-rich, high-fibre foods is good for tackling both constipation and low iron levels. Include more green leafy vegetables, lean red meat, nuts such as peanuts, and dried fruit in your diet. It's usual during pregnancy to feel more tired than normal, particularly in the first and last trimesters. However, if you are extremely lethargic, pale in colour, and suffering from heart palpitations and/or shortness of breath, you could be anaemic. If you are, a healthcare professional will discuss iron supplementation. In addition, consider cutting out caffeine altogether as this can hamper iron absorption.

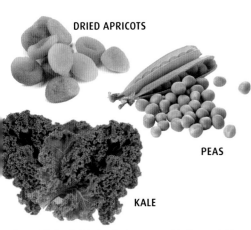

DRIED APRICOTS

PEAS

KALE

Iron-rich foods Dried apricots, peas, and leafy vegetables such as kale are great sources of iron. Vitamin C helps with iron absorption, so drink orange juice with your meal.

Q Do I need to take a multivitamin supplement now that I am pregnant?

The most important supplement you need to take is folic acid. Healthcare professionals advise a vitamin D supplement (10 mcg daily) to help your body metabolize calcium for the benefit of maintaining your own bones and teeth as well as your baby's developing bones. The other elements in a multivitamin supplement aren't strictly essential if you are eating a balanced diet. If you do choose to take a supplement formula, make sure it is right for pregnancy. Never take a supplement containing vitamin A, as too much can harm your baby.

Q Could my weight affect my chances of having a healthy pregnancy?

Unfortunately, being either obese or underweight can have a negative impact on both your ability to conceive and your health in pregnancy. If you can, take action to ensure your weight is within healthy limits before getting pregnant.

It is best to achieve a healthy weight before you think about conception. For both partners, you need a certain level of body fat to produce the right levels of hormones for healthy sperm production and ovulation to occur. In obese people, excess oestrogen can decrease sperm levels and hamper or even prevent ovulation, while underweight people can have too few fat stores in their bodies to conceive. If you are underweight, there is a greater risk of your baby having a low birthweight or being premature. Gain and maintain weight healthily by eating an extra 200-300 calories a day until your weight improves. During pregnancy, obesity can affect the health of your baby, and it is known to increase the risk of conditions such as gestational diabetes and pre-eclampsia (see pp.144-45) – factors that can cause complications during pregnancy and the birth.

BODY MASS INDEX (BMI) CHART

This chart is appropriate for women over the age of 18. Body mass index (BMI) gauges whether you are a healthy weight in relation to your height. A BMI of 30 or more is considered obese, while a BMI of less than 18.5 is deemed underweight.

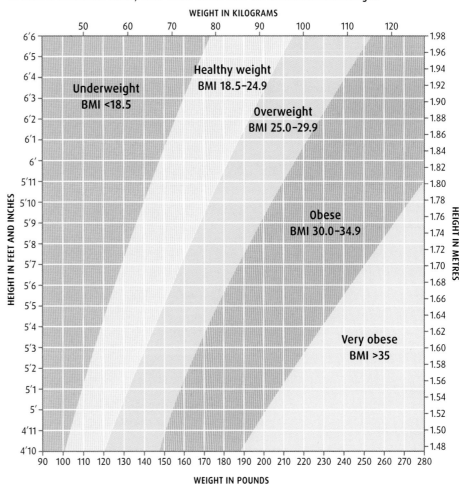

WEIGHT IN KILOGRAMS

Underweight BMI <18.5

Healthy weight BMI 18.5–24.9

Overweight BMI 25.0–29.9

Obese BMI 30.0–34.9

Very obese BMI >35

HEIGHT IN FEET AND INCHES

HEIGHT IN METRES

WEIGHT IN POUNDS

Knowing what foods and drinks to avoid helps your health and the safe development of your baby. Some foods contain, or may contain, bacteria or substances that may make you ill or be harmful to your baby. While this may seem very alarming, it's worth remembering that the risks are very low.

Health and hygiene

You are more vulnerable to infections while pregnant, so being aware of what you eat and drink and following good food hygiene principles are necessary precautions.

Food hygiene is straightforward if you are vigilant. Always check the use-by dates on food product labels and reject any food that smells off or looks suspect. Wash your hands before and after handling food, and rinse fruit, salads, and vegetables to remove traces of soil and pesticides. Take extra care with raw poultry and meat: use separate chopping boards and knives, and wash them afterwards with detergent in very hot water. Defrost frozen foods carefully according to the instructions on the packaging, and if you reheat cooked food in the microwave, ensure that the whole dish is piping hot.

Avoid foods (listed below) that may carry harmful bacteria, parasites, or cause food poisoning; some herbal teas and sugar substitutes; smoking; recreational drugs; alcohol; and limit caffeine. If you drank alcohol or smoked before you discovered you were pregnant, don't be anxious but do stop now. The fetus will start being supported by the placenta from 12 weeks, although it can't protect an unborn baby against all infections and bacteria.

FOODS TO LIMIT OR AVOID

Although there is usually only a small risk that foods such as these may prove harmful to your baby, they are best avoided or limited while you are pregnant.

Banned foods Cured meats and unpasteurized cheeses should be avoided.

FOOD	YOU SHOULD AVOID	RELATED PROBLEMS	YOU CAN EAT
Cheese	≫ Any unpasteurized cheese. ≫ Soft mould-ripened cheeses (with a "white rind"), such as Camembert and brie. ≫ Uncooked soft blue cheeses, such as Roquefort and gorgonzola.	In rare cases, cheese may carry the listeria bacteria. Listeriosis (listeria infection) may cause only mild, flu-like symptoms in you, but it can be harmful to your baby and in severe cases can lead to brain damage.	≫ Hard cheeses and hard blue cheeses (such as Parmesan, gouda, Cheddar, and Stilton). ≫ Soft cheeses made with pasteurized milk – for example cottage cheese, cream cheese, mozzarella, feta, and ricotta.
Meat	≫ Raw or undercooked red meat. ≫ Cured meats (salami, chorizo, Parma ham). ≫ Liver or other organ meats, and liver pâté – they contain high levels of vitamin A.	Undercooked meat may be infected with the toxoplasmosis parasite and cured meats may contain listeria. Both may harm your baby. Too much vitamin A can cause birth defects and harm your baby's liver.	≫ Meats that have been pre-packed (such as ham) are fine, as are any meats (including cured meats) that have been frozen and fully defrosted, or that have been cooked.
Seafood	≫ Uncooked shellfish. ≫ Avoid shark, marlin, and swordfish, which contain high levels of mercury.	Food poisoning from seafood is unpleasant for you, but it doesn't pose any health risks to your developing baby. High levels of mercury, found in certain fish, can be harmful to your baby's nervous system.	≫ Oily fish, but only once or twice a week, as it may contain toxins such as PCBs and dioxins (as well as lots of good nutrients). ≫ Cooked shellfish.
Eggs	≫ Raw eggs and raw egg products such as mayonnaise and mousse. ≫ Undercooked eggs – eat only if the yolk and white are solid.	There is a tiny risk that raw eggs may contain the salmonella bacteria. A salmonella infection is not thought to be harmful to an unborn baby, but can cause vomiting and diarrhoea for you.	≫ Choose eggs stamped to show that they have been laid in conditions following the strictest hygiene.

The placenta protects the fetus from most (but not all) infections and bacteria, and it can't prevent substances such as alcohol from passing across it.

Umbilical cord

Your baby receives all its oxygen and nutrients from the placenta via the umbilical cord.

SUGAR SUBSTITUTES

Most artificial sweeteners are considered safe in moderation during pregnancy, including sucralose and aspartame. However, avoid saccharin, which can cross the placenta and has been linked to certain types of cancer. (Though there is no firm evidence to suggest it is unsafe in pregnancy, why take the risk?) Some countries have banned cyclamates, as they may cause cancer. Avoid them during pregnancy – and beyond.

HERBAL TEAS

Although herbal teas contain no caffeine, they have other properties that are not always safe for pregnancy. Experts agree that the safest option is to choose a specialist "pregnancy herbal tea", which comes pre-blended. Two individual herbs deemed safe for drinking during pregnancy are mint and lemon balm, both of which can help with feelings of nausea and help relax you if you're feeling anxious.

ALCOHOL

We know that alcohol crosses the placenta, meaning any alcohol you drink can make its way into your baby's system. Because the liver is one of the last organs to develop in the fetus, your baby can't detoxify the effects. This raises the concentration of alcohol in the baby's blood and starves the baby of oxygen.

⚠️ **Alcohol-related problems** in babies exposed during development include:

» **low birthweight**
» **premature birth**
» **In extreme cases fetal alcohol syndrome**, which can cause malformed facial features, learning difficulties, kidneys, and heart defects.

✓ **Abstention from alcohol** is the only clear way to be sure you are minimizing the risks to your baby.

CAFFEINE

This is present in much more than just coffee and tea – chocolate, carbonated drinks, and energy drinks, to name a few. Guidelines are that, during pregnancy, women shouldn't drink more than two cups of instant coffee a day.

⚠️ **Caffeine-related problems** in babies exposed during development include:

» **low birthweight**
» **raised heart rate**
» **raised blood pressure**
» **miscarriage in rare cases**

✓ **Switch to decaffeinated alternatives** for tea and coffee (at least 97 per cent caffeine-free) and consider herbal or fruit teas – but proceed with caution, as not all herbal teas are safe (see left).

SMOKING, DRUGS, AND MEDICATIONS

⚠️ Cigarettes and recreational drugs (such as cocaine and marijuana) are known to pose significant health risks to an unborn child, resulting in:

» **low birthweight**
» **brain or lung damage**
» **miscarriage**
» **babies born with "addiction"**

✓ **The advice is clear** – do not smoke or use drugs. Seek advice before using e-cigarettes, patches, or gum. Consult your doctor if you take prescription drugs, and don't take over-the-counter medicines without advice.

Q I am gluten intolerant. What does this mean for my baby?

A gluten-free diet can be low in calcium, iron, fibre, zinc, B-vitamins, vitamin D, and magnesium. If you're coeliac, it's important that you continue with your gluten-free diet, as studies show that pregnant coeliac women who reintroduce gluten to their diet can be at increased risk of miscarriage and low birthweight. There are no specific dietary guidelines to follow other than eating a healthy balanced diet, but the fact that you are gluten-free means you could be lacking nutrients – specifically iron, vitamin B12, and calcium. You may require some supplementation in addition to what you eat in order to meet the recommended daily amounts of these missing nutrients. Talk to your healthcare professional, who will be able to assess your diet and give you individual advice. In the meantime, increase quantities of potatoes, rice, corn, nuts, beans and lentils, red meat, chicken, fish, eggs and dairy produce in your daily diet, which will all help to boost your intake of those nutrients that are otherwise present in gluten foods.

Q Should I start shopping for organic foods now that I'm pregnant?

We are exposed to chemical pesticides and fertilizers in all manner of ways – in the air, in cleaning products, and in the food we eat. Pesticides work by attacking the nervous systems of insects. Concern for unborn babies centres on the effects these chemicals may have on neural development, because studies have found tiny amounts of "expressed sequence tags" (ests) or DNA clones in amniotic fluid.

Although risks from food are smaller than those from airborne pollutants, anything you can do to minimize your exposure can only be a positive thing. If you aren't able to switch to an entirely organic diet, select wisely. For example, it's better to spend extra on organic meats as unorganic meats may have hormones and antibiotics within the flesh that are impossible to remove through cooking – than on organic fruits and vegetables, which you can wash and peel (in most hard fruits and vegetables, pesticides remain primarily on the outer skin and leaves). Do, though, choose organic soft fruits, which are less likely to have residues beneath the skin.

> **If you aren't able to switch to an entirely organic diet, select your organic purchases wisely and include meat and soft fruit.**

Q I'm vegetarian. Can I carry on eating as I usually do?

It is perfectly possible to remain vegetarian or vegan while pregnant and have a healthy baby, but be prepared to supplement any nutrients you may be lacking.

Ensure that you're aware of the nutrients your vegetarian or vegan diet does and doesn't give you, and discuss your diet with your healthcare professional. If you need extra nutrients, he or she may advise you to take supplements for the duration of your pregnancy (especially important for iron). For your own peace of mind, do check first that any supplements are not animal-derived. You may also need to plan your meals a little more carefully, but you should remain in good health throughout your pregnancy.

PREGNANCY REQUIREMENTS

Combining fresh foods with supplements is a good idea if you are vegetarian or vegan.

Milk Provides calcium

Olive oil Source of omega-6 fat

Cabbage High in fibre

Almonds Source of omega-3 fat

Balanced diet As a vegetarian or vegan, make sure you get all your major food groups: grains, protein, fruit and vegetables, dairy, and fats.

» Iodine: you may need to take supplements of iodine, which – among other things – is essential for maintaining pregnancy to term, a healthy birth, and improved brain function in your baby.

» Vitamin B12, essential fats, iron, and vitamin D: these are all essential. They can be obtained through food or in a supplement form.

» Essential amino acids: daily quantities of beans, peas, or other legumes; corn or wheat products; grains; seeds; nuts; brewer's yeast and soya; cheese, milk, eggs or other dairy produce; and a broad colour-spectrum of vegetables should provide all the amino acids you need.

» Iron: if you don't need to supplement, good sources are green leafy vegetables (spinach and kale are good), fortified breakfast cereals, dried fruits, and wholemeal bread. Drink orange juice at the same meal to aid iron absorption from these foods.

» Omega fats: flax seeds, walnut oil, and soya beans are all good sources of omega-3 fats; nuts, grains, safflower, sesame, and sunflower oils are all good sources of omega-6.

» Calcium: if you're vegan, ensure you get enough calcium. Leafy green vegetables, sesame seeds (and derivatives such as tahini), and pulses are all sources. Look for calcium-fortified vegan products such as tofu, soya, rice, oats, and bread.

Q I am lactose-intolerant. What can I do about my calcium intake?

Your ability to digest lactose may actually improve while you are pregnant, or you may need to take a calcium supplement to ensure you get enough calcium.

Calcium is crucial: it helps to build your baby's bones and teeth and prevents your bones from weakening. Interestingly, studies show that lactose intolerance eases off in around 30 to 50 per cent of pregnancies. So, in the first instance, consult your healthcare professional about how to reintroduce a tiny amount of cow's milk into your diet and measure its effects, and follow his or her guidance before you begin supplementation. If you remain intolerant, you may need to take a calcium supplement, as well as vitamin B$_{12}$ and D supplements, which are also found in dairy foods. In the meantime, increase your intake of other calcium-rich foods.

CALCIUM-RICH FOODS TO EAT IF YOU ARE LACTOSE-INTOLERANT

Include a few of these calcium-rich foods in your diet each day; the daily recommendation is 1,000 milligrams of calcium.

BROCCOLI

CRESS

FOOD	SERVING AMOUNT	CALCIUM CONTENT
Canned sardines	60g (2oz)	240mg
Cress	120g (4oz) raw	188mg
Wakame	100g (3$^1/_2$oz) raw	150mg
Haricot beans	200g (7oz) cooked	132mg
Tofu	120g (4oz) raw	126mg
Broccoli	120g (4oz) raw	112mg
Rhubarb	120g (4oz) raw	103mg
Chickpeas	200g (7oz) cooked	99mg

Q I'm Muslim and I plan to observe Ramadan. Will fasting harm my baby?

Any kind of fast is not recommended during pregnancy – your body and your baby need a constant supply of nutrition and water in order to remain healthy and develop properly. Studies show that fasting can lead to premature birth, low birthweight, and neurological problems in babies. However, many Muslim women choose to observe the Ramadan fast. First, consult your healthcare professional to discuss your individual situation and your baby's health, and then fast only if you have a healthy weight, good energy levels, no known conditions, and you feel strong. Islamic law does permit pregnant women not to fast; you can make up the days after the birth or compensate by giving to charity. So, if at any time you feel dizzy, dehydrated, or otherwise unwell, or if you think your baby has stopped moving, stop the fast immediately and consult your doctor.

Q Is there anything special I need to worry about as a pescetarian?

This semi-vegetarian diet, which excludes meat and poultry and may include dairy products and eggs in addition to fish and shellfish, shouldn't exclude any natural nutrients from your diet. Fish is an ideal form of protein; it is rich in B-complex vitamins, calcium, potassium, iron, zinc, phosphorous, and selenium, and the omega-3 fats that oily fish such as halibut, salmon, tuna, mackerel, and sardines contain are crucial for heart and brain health. However, the current medical advice is that you eat only two portions of oily fish per week (and four medium-sized cans of tuna per week) as it contains mercury, which can be harmful to your unborn baby's development in large amounts. In addition, you should avoid eating swordfish, shark, and marlin, and raw shellfish altogether. There is no need to limit the amount of white fish and cooked shellfish you eat.

Q I've been following a low-carb diet. Is it safe to continue this diet?

Without good medical reason (such as an allergy, intolerance, or other food-related auto-immune condition), there is no justification for restricting or eliminating any major nutrient during pregnancy. Carbohydrates are an important source of energy, fibre, iron, and B-vitamins, which makes them essential for your health and that of your baby. If you're worried about weight gain, remember that, gram for gram, carbohydrates have fewer calories (1g of carbohydrate gives 4 calories of energy) than fat-rich foods (9 calories per gram). Carbohydrates also keep you feeling fuller for longer, so they will actually help prevent any tendency you may have to snack.

Q I'm overweight. Would it make sense to eat fewer calories now that I'm pregnant?

Usually, dieting to lose weight while pregnant is not advised because it can deprive your baby of essential nutrients, but if your BMI was over 30 to begin with (see p.51), it can be a good idea to manage your weight. If you were already obese, there are specific risks to pregnancy – such as gestational diabetes, pre-eclampsia, having a large baby, stillbirth, and increased likelihood of Caesarean section. Work with your healthcare professional to set a programme to maintain your weight throughout your pregnancy. Too much calorie restriction is not ideal – especially if you were underweight before becoming pregnant – as this increases the risk of having a small, or low birthweight baby, which is linked to developmental issues.

Carbohydrates are essential: if your **body** doesn't get enough **fuel** from carbs, it begins to metabolize your fat stores and release toxins called PCBs that may harm your **baby's development**.

Q I feel permanently exhausted. What can I eat to give me more energy?

If this is your first or third trimester, your body is working extra hard to either form a baby or enable it to grow enough to be ready for labour and the birth. Choose foods that are rich in protein or fibre to give your body the fuel it needs.

The primary energy-giving nutrients you need are iron, complex carbohydrates, and protein. Try mapping your energy needs over a day and eat appropriately to combat the times when you typically have an energy drain. Aim to load up with protein and complex carbs at breakfast and lunchtime to give you slow-burning energy for up to three to four hours at a time, and make supper the lightest meal, but still nutritious – think healthy salads, for example. Include a healthy mid-morning and mid-afternoon snack, and don't reach for caffeine and sugary foods. Apart from the fact that these aren't good for you, the energy hit they provide will be short-lived, and you'll soon feel more tired and depleted than you did before.

NUTRIENTS YOUR BODY NEEDS FOR SUSTAINED ENERGY

Include foods containing these energy-enhancing nutrients in your meals and snacks so that you can cope with your day. Eat little and often to stave off hunger pangs and maintain energy levels.

NUTRIENT	ENERGY EFFECTS	FOOD SOURCES
Iron	Improves the health of cells so that oxygen reaches all the body systems efficiently.	Green leafy vegetables (spinach, kale etc.); shellfish; lean meat; dried fruit; nuts and seeds; pulses and legumes; whole grains.
Complex carbohydrates	These foods release energy at a steady pace into your body in the short and medium term, preventing the energy spikes that refined carbs (simple carbohydrates) and sugary foods cause.	Whole grains (including brown pasta and rice); oats; fresh fruit and vegetables (particularly starchy vegetables, such as potatoes, corn, green peas, and parsnips); legumes (including beans, peas, and lentils).
Protein	The process of breaking down protein into energy is a long one – first your body separates the protein into its constituent amino acids, which it then converts into glucose (your body's fuel). This means that protein gives you a slow energy release over several hours.	Lean meat; fish; dried legumes (such as beans, peas, and lentils); nuts and seeds; eggs; milk; and yogurt.

Q I often feel thirsty. Is this normal? Can I drink what I like?

It's very normal to find yourself drinking more while pregnant, because your body requires extra fluids to cope with the demands of your growing baby. Your body needs water to flush out toxins and waste – both your own and those generated by your developing baby – from your body. You also need water to produce the extra healthy blood cells needed during pregnancy. These blood cells carry essential nutrients to your baby through the placenta.

Staying well hydrated during pregnancy is also essential for helping to prevent water retention (oedema), dry, itchy skin, tiredness, constipation, urinary tract infections, and complications in pregnancy associated with dehydration.

Unless your body requires more, or it's a hot day or you live in a warm climate, around 2.2 litres (3½ pints) of fluid a day should be sufficient (this is the recommended amount for a healthy adult). If you feel thirsty – or even hungry – you're probably slightly dehydrated,

Stay hydrated Drink at least 8 glasses of fluid a day – water and milk both provide effective hydration.

An app is a great way to check if you are eating enough calories a day by **monitoring your calorie intake** if you want to stabilize your weight. There are lots of free food-diary apps available to help you log your food and drink intake. Aim for **2,200 calories** a day in the first trimester and **2,300 calories** a day during the second and third trimesters.

Coping with exhaustion There may be times when you feel too exhausted to move, but try to eat for energy and stay hydrated.

TOP TIPS

Having a glass of freshly pressed orange juice or eating other vitamin-C-rich foods at the same time as eating iron-rich foods will help iron absorption.

Start your day with a bowl of porridge topped with a handful of berries, such as blueberries or raspberries; or with two slices of brown toast topped with a poached egg to keep you going through the morning.

Aim to have protein at breakfast and lunch, so that you feel the energy benefits during the day when you need them the most.

so take it as a sign to drink a glass of water straightaway. Another sign of whether you are dehydrated or not is the colour of your urine: the paler it is (ideally pale or straw-coloured), the better hydrated you are. If your urine is dark, drink more water. Get into good habits to help stay hydrated: carry a water bottle with you and sip it little and often; put a glass of water beside you whenever you sit down; and drink a glass of water each time you go into the kitchen. Remember that milk, juices, and herbal teas (see p.53) count towards your daily intake, but caffeine and carbonated drinks don't.

Q I'm starving all the time – is it okay to eat more than I did before I became pregnant?

Healthy expectant mothers only need a small proportion of extra calories a day. To ensure optimal health for yourself and your baby, you should expect to increase your calorie intake by

200 calories per day in the first trimester, and by 300 calories per day after that. However, you are burning lots of energy while "building" your baby so it's not surprising that you feel hungry. Follow the advice given in the table (left) to try to stabilize your energy levels, and therefore any food cravings, so that you feel fuller for longer. You should also be able to maintain more consistent energy levels if you remember to eat little and often – three meals, with two small (healthy) snacks in between. For quick snacks, try dried fruit with a few nuts, trail mix, rice cakes, oatcakes, or raw vegetable sticks (carrots or broccoli) with hummus, for example. If you feel hungry all the time, try switching to six small meals over the course of the day (see p.58), taking care not to overeat when you do so. Try to remember to check your weight gain at your next check-up (you might need to ask to be weighed, as this doesn't necessarily happen at every appointment) and increase your calorie intake appropriately if your weight is below healthy limits.

Q What can I do to change my eating habits? I want to lose my pregnancy weight after the birth.

Pregnancy, the start of a new life, is a great time to assess poor lifestyle choices and replace them with better ones – particularly when it comes to food. Imagine your plate of food as three separate sections to be filled. Allocate the biggest section of the plate – nearly half – to vegetables, which contain fibre (and so are filling) and are packed with nutrients, but are light on calories. Divide the remainder of your plate evenly between proteins (such as lean meat, fish, and pulses) and unrefined complex carbohydrates (such as potatoes, or brown pasta, or rice). It is a good idea to get your partner on board with the new eating habits, too – now is a good time to reinforce the notion that you are in this together.

Have a clear-out of your kitchen cupboards as well. Empty them of any refined foods that are high in fat or refined sugar, give the cupboards a thorough clean, and replace their contents with healthy alternatives, especially healthy snacks (see p.60). Do the same with your fridge and freezer, so that you are not tempted to indulge in the wrong kinds of food. If you find yourself reaching for a sugary snack, stop, and have a drink instead: pour yourself a

Weight gain You will put on most of your extra weight after 20 weeks of pregnancy. This is mainly due to your growing baby, but you will also be storing fat ready to produce breast milk.

glass of fruit juice, sugar-free squash, water, or herbal or fruit tea (as long as the tea is safe for pregnancy – see p.53). You could also try making juice lollies, which last longer and can feel more satisfying than a drink.

Did you know...

Unless you are allergic to peanuts yourself, there is no evidence to suggest that eating peanuts while pregnant will contribute to your baby's chances of developing a peanut allergy (including having any impact on asthma or eczema risk). Although high in calories, peanuts are more filling than many other snacks; eat in moderation.

Q I feel so sick that I can only stomach dry crackers. Is my baby getting everything he needs?

If you are suffering from pregnancy sickness and finding it hard to keep anything down, try changing what you eat and when. Your baby won't suffer.

Your hormones slow your digestive system during pregnancy so that your body can take the maximum nutrients from whatever food you eat. Furthermore, your body prioritizes your baby, drawing reserves of major nutrients such as calcium and protein from your own body if it needs to. As long as you eat a little, your baby should be fine. If you're worried or vomiting frequently, however, talk to your healthcare professional.

EATING DURING THE DAY

If you are suffering from pregnancy sickness, try these suggestions to help you change the repertoire of what you eat or drink and when.

» Eat little and often: Try eating six small meals a day (right) rather than attempting three meals and two snacks.

» Make your food starch-rich: As well as being bland, which is all you might be able to face, potatoes, rice, pasta, and couscous contain good quantities of nutrients (B-vitamins, iron, protein, and fibre among them).

» Eat raw foods: Your queasy response to food is often to do with the smell of it rather than the taste. Raw (or cold) foods tend to have less of an aroma, which might make them more palatable for you.

» Nibble on snacks: Unroasted skinned almonds, which are nutrient-dense but plain to taste, are ideal.

» Sip water: Try adding a slice of lemon or two, or try hot water with a few mint leaves (which contain potassium, iron, and folate, among other nutrients). Drinking ginger tea can help to suppress nausea.

Sip water infused with a slice of lemon (which provides antioxidants and vitamin C).

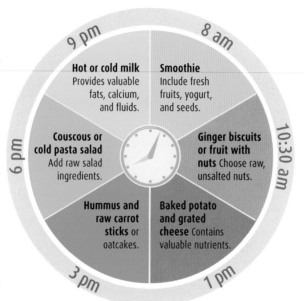

9 pm — **Hot or cold milk** Provides valuable fats, calcium, and fluids.

8 am — **Smoothie** Include fresh fruits, yogurt, and seeds.

10:30 am — **Ginger biscuits or fruit with nuts** Choose raw, unsalted nuts.

1 pm — **Baked potato and grated cheese** Contains valuable nutrients.

3 pm — **Hummus and raw carrot sticks** or oatcakes.

6 pm — **Couscous or cold pasta salad** Add raw salad ingredients.

Six small meals Break your food intake down into more palatable, manageable mini meals such as these to help you consume enough nutrients each day.

Q I love chocolate and I can't resist eating it. Does this mean my baby will have a sweet tooth?

If you like chocolate, your baby may have a preference for the smell and taste of chocolate. However, as long as your diet is healthy, with chocolate as a small and occasional indulgence (choose organic, dark varieties that are high in flavanols), your overall influence is a good one. A French study at the European Centre for Taste Science in 2012 concluded that what a mother eats, particularly during the final stages of her pregnancy, can significantly influence a newborn baby's preference for certain foods. It's thought that the flavours of foods pass through the amniotic fluid and into the baby's newly forming olfactory nerves so that when the baby is born, he will turn towards the smell of food that is familiar (and away from food that isn't). Perhaps the most important thing to remember is that any foods you consume that are high in saturated fat and sugar are low in nutritional value. Studies show that a pregnancy diet that is high in sugar and saturated fat can lead to higher birthweight babies and have a long-lasting effect on your baby's own dietary choices.

Q Does the fact that I'm skinny and petite mean that I will have a low birthweight baby?

No, not necessarily. The evidence shows that as long as you eat healthily, you will have a full-term baby who is just perfect for his genes. Low birthweight is a medical term meaning that your baby weighs less than 2.5kg (5½lb) when he is born. In a healthy pregnancy without complications, there are two main influences on a baby's birthweight. The first is what you eat while your unborn baby is growing (and, in fact, what you ate before you got pregnant because your previous weight is a factor). A study conducted in Oxford, UK, in 2014 compared the birthweights of 60,000 babies from across the world and concluded that nutrition, even more than the mother's size or her ethnicity, impacted the size of her baby at birth. The second is down to genetics. If you're petite and were yourself a small baby, it's possible (and normal) that your baby will inherit your petite size. Of course, your baby's

Q What does "eating for two" mean exactly? If I'm having twins, do I need to eat for three?

The adage "eating for two" does not mean that you need to eat twice as much as you did before you got pregnant. You just need a small increase in calories, and slightly more still if you are carrying twins or triplets.

If you are pregnant with one child, your optimal calorie intake during pregnancy should increase by only 200 daily calories during the first trimester, and by 300 daily calories during the second and third trimesters. The list of suggested snacks (right) shows what 200 calories looks like in practice. If you are carrying multiples, you should increase your calorie intake per baby. So, for twins, you need to add 400 calories at the start of your pregnancy and 600 calories during the middle and the final stages of pregnancy. The other crucial thing to remember is that you need to optimize the nutritional value of the food you "share" with your growing baby, so try to ensure these extra calories are nutrient-dense – don't forget quality in your quantity.

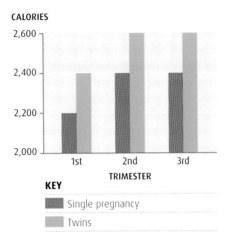

CALORIES

TRIMESTER

KEY
- Single pregnancy
- Twins

Optimum calorie intake The recommended guidelines on this chart ensure that you will give yourself and your baby enough nutrients and energy.

Ensure that the small increase in extra calories you need to eat during pregnancy are nutrient-dense so that you have quality in your quantity.

CALORIE EQUIVALENT

How can I eat an extra 200–600 calories? Choose from these options or look for other healthy alternatives.

200 calories = 1 slice of bread and 1½ tablespoons of peanut butter

APPROXIMATELY 200 CALORIES:

» 4 tablespoons of trail mix

» 4 tablespoons hummus and 4 baby carrots

» Boiled egg and toast without butter

APPROXIMATELY 400 CALORIES:

» 200g (7oz) low-fat yogurt and 1 apple

» 200g (7oz) avocado on 1 slice of toast

» Cheese sandwich

---

father's genes will come into play, too. If he is tall and broad, your baby may just as likely be long and heavy at birth – or somewhere in between the two of you. Tell your healthcare professional if you or your partner were particularly small at birth and discuss whether anything in your family histories might be reason for concern in your own baby's weight.

Q Do I have excessive cravings? I seem to want foods and drinks I've never thought of having.

If you are suddenly desperate for foods you may previously have had little interest in, you are following a typical pattern in pregnancy. During early pregnancy in particular, your senses seem to be heightened due to your high

hormone levels: you may crave new foods and find that others – including tea, coffee, or fast foods – become repellent. This may be due to your sense of smell being more sensitive or a strange, perhaps metallic, taste in your mouth. Experts suggest that your taste buds play a role in how you interpret you body's needs. Nobody really knows what causes cravings in pregnancy since scientific studies cannot easily quantify or measure them. Some studies have suggested a potential link between certain cravings – salty foods such as olives, sour fruits such as lemons, or vegetarians eating meat – and maternal diet deficiencies. Researchers are unsure if a deficiency occurs because of abnormal eating habits in pregnancy, or the cravings occur because of a deficiency in your diet. Most cravings don't represent a threat to you or your baby unless you have the condition Pica, when you crave non-food items such as clay.

If you have persistent **pregnancy sickness**, have food **cravings** such as drinking milk only, or have **lost your appetite** in late pregnancy, don't stress about whether your **baby is receiving enough** nutrients. **Stress** can prove to be more detrimental to you and your baby than **eating lightly** for a period of time.

Q What should I eat to optimize recovery after the birth?

The energy demands of new motherhood are immense, and yet at the same time you are still recovering from the birth and likely to feel sleep-deprived and time-poor. You many not have time to cook properly, but you can eat well.

Ensuring you get enough proper nutrition is immensely important. Your body is recovering from the tremendous physical exertion of the birth, and you are no doubt exhausted. You may even find you are anaemic if you lost blood during the birth, or if you've had more than one baby.

Although diet can't compensate for any sleep deprivation, eating enough nutrient-rich snacks and meals will hasten your physical recovery, help to combat any nutritional issues such as constipation, provide your body with fuel to give you the stamina to care for your baby, and help you feel better.

Healthy habits

If you established good shopping and eating habits in pregnancy, you should already be in the right mindset for continuing to eat a balanced diet. If not, this is a key time to avoid "empty calories" such as junk food and sugary snacks. They supply very little nutritional value and provide only a temporary boost of energy, leaving you feeling more tired than before. Include a wide variety of colourful fresh fruit and vegetables, whole grains, lean protein, and dairy products in your diet (see p.50). If you

are lacking iron, your healthcare professional may recommend that you restore your iron levels through both diet and supplement, so choose iron-rich sources such as lean red meat, spinach, and chick peas. If you have constipation, eat lots of fruit and vegetables, drink more water, and eat plenty of fibre: choose oats, wholegrain breads, brown rice, bran, and other high-fibre cereals. If you had a Caesarean section or surgery after the birth, increase your intake of Vitamin C, which contributes to wound healing, and protein, helping your body to repair itself.

All this may sound good in theory, but in practice you might have little time to cook and rely on snacking instead. There's nothing wrong with snacking, as long as you eat healthily (see box, right). Your nutrient intake will be fine if you can eat a good breakfast – porridge with berries or poached eggs on wholemeal toast – have nutritional snacks throughout the day, and sit down to one simple main meal – perhaps a plate of pasta (try crème fraîche with lemon juice and chopped smoked salmon) with steamed vegetables. As you find your rhythm, the time and energy to cook will return.

Include a wide variety of **colourful fresh fruit** and **vegetables,** whole grains, lean protein, and dairy products in your diet.

Snacks and superfoods

Keep your snacks healthy and include plenty of "superfoods", such as blueberries, broccoli, tomatoes, oily fish, and oats. These give you much-needed vitamins, minerals, and antioxidants. Stock up on fresh fruit – especially bananas, which contain slow-release energy, and berries. Dried fruit, raw vegetables (such as carrots, broccoli, celery), cherry tomatoes, unsalted rice cakes, breadsticks, oatcakes, hummus, and guacamole are also great. Try making a tasty dip by whizzing cooked broad beans and cannellini beans with olive oil and garlic. Store it in the fridge, and eat with vegetable sticks or spread on oatcakes.

Finger food Easy to reach for and to eat with one hand, nutrient-rich snacks are ideal in the early days of caring for your baby.

Sit down to **eat your meals;** eating on the run contributes to fatigue and can lead to overeating. If your **baby wants to be held**, put her in an infant sling so you are **hands-free** to eat.

Q I want to lose my baby weight. Is it okay to start dieting now?

Dieting too soon after the birth can delay your recovery and sap your energy levels, but if you eat sensibly and healthily, you will gradually lose your baby weight. You will find that you shed some weight quite quickly after the birth as you lose "extras" such as the amniotic fluid and any water retention. Now that you are caring for a baby, you should find yourself more active than in the last stages of pregnancy and

will be burning off more energy. However, it's recommended that you wait until you have had your six-week check before you start watching your calorie intake if you are not breastfeeding, and even then the advice is that you must not go on a crash diet. If you eat healthy, nutrient-rich foods in sensible amounts and exercise moderately every day so you lose fat and not muscle, you will gradually lose the weight and keep it off. Breastfeeding requires extra calories, so it's vital that you don't even think about restricting your calorie intake until after you have weaned your baby.

Q Do I need to change my diet now I'm breastfeeding?

You don't need to eat any special foods while you are nursing, but everything you consume passes through to your baby, so there are some things to avoid.

The wonderful thing about breastfeeding is that you don't have to do or eat anything different or special to breastfeed successfully – once your baby has learned the art of latching on, your milk will naturally deliver the best possible nutrients to her. However, as you are the primary source of nourishment for your baby while you breastfeed her, it makes sense to eat a healthy diet and drink plenty of water.

Straight to baby

Everything you eat and drink passes through your breast milk to your baby in small amounts. Because of this, experts recommend that you take precautions with some food and drink and other consumables. The advice for eating oily fish in pregnancy remains the same while you breastfeed: eat only two portions of oily fish a week to limit the amount of mercury you consume. Alcohol passes through to babies in very small amounts, as does caffeine, which may keep your baby awake. An occasional small drink may not harm your baby, but in general it's best to avoid caffeine and alcohol along with nicotine and medications (unless it is prescribed by your doctor).

Breastfeeding is demanding on your energy levels so you need plenty of fuel both to cope with looking after your baby and to produce enough milk. You need to increase your calorie intake by 500 calories a day for as long as you breastfeed. You may want to incorporate an extra snack during the day to ensure you consume enough calories, or have a slightly bigger portion at mealtimes.

Spotting sensitivity

You may notice your baby develop a strong reaction to your breast milk. This could simply be a one-off dislike of the taste due to something you've consumed that day, or it could possibly be the sign of a food intolerance. Irritability after feedings, cold symptoms and congestion, a rash, hives, itchy skin or eczema, digestive problems such as constipation or diarrhoea, abdominal discomfort, swelling of the lips or eyes, and colic (see p.285) are all possible symptoms of a food intolerance, although they are not all necessarily caused by diet. If you think your baby is sensitive to or unsettled by certain foods you eat, talk to your doctor, especially if you have a family history of allergy.

It's useful to be aware of the most common food triggers so that you can watch your diet and keep a close eye on your baby for any signs that what you've been eating doesn't agree with him or her. Garlic, chilli or spicy foods, cow's milk, orange juice, soya products, wheat, corn, eggs, peanuts, tomatoes, or shellfish are all common culprits. If you can identify a specific food that you think is causing discomfort, eliminate it from your diet for several days to see if that's the trigger, but be aware that some products, such as cow's milk, can stay in your body for up to two weeks. It's important that you continue to eat a balanced diet, so always consult your doctor before making significant changes to what you eat.

Breastfeeding Make healthy food and drink choices to benefit your baby and make sure you are eating enough to help you produce sufficient milk.

WHAT TO AVOID

It's worth avoiding some substances so that your baby isn't affected in any way. Enjoy herbal teas, decaffeinated tea and coffee, mineral water, and an occasional glass of fruit juice instead.

AVOID	EXAMPLES
Alcohol	Alcohol is not advised in more than moderate, occasional quantities (1–2 units every now and then is unlikely to harm your baby). If you want to drink one night, express milk beforehand so your baby isn't affected.
Nicotine	Smoking is not advised near or around babies: breathing in secondhand smoke is known to be bad for your baby's long-term health and increases the risk of SIDS. If you smoke and breastfeed, you may slow your baby's weight gain, as nicotine reduces the amount of milk you produce.
Medicines	All medicines, including prescription drugs, over-the-counter drugs, oral contraceptive pills, and vitamin, dietary, and herbal supplements pass through your breast milk in small amounts, and while some may not have an effect on your baby, you should talk to a healthcare professional before you take any kind of medicine, herbal or otherwise.
Caffeine	Caffeine is present in coffee, chocolate, tea, and some soft drinks and energy drinks, as well as some cold and flu remedies. Babies' bodies can't get rid of caffeine very well and may not be able to cope with you having too much caffeine in your diet.

Feeling **physically and mentally happy** goes a long way towards having a great pregnancy experience. Addressing any concerns you have about **life changes** and enjoying an **active pregnancy** safely is **beneficial** for both you and your unborn baby.

Exercise and wellbeing

A positive frame of mind

It's usual to feel apprehensive as well as excited about impending parenthood and such issues as the birth, money, and changing relationships. Accepting your worries as a first step can help you move forward and start to enjoy your pregnancy, and find solutions (see pp.69–73). Staying physically active contributes to your sense of wellbeing, helping to improve your moods, sleep patterns, and body image.

Your pregnant body

During pregnancy, your musculo-skeletal system changes, affecting the way you exercise and the amount you do. To prepare for birth, the hormones relaxin and progesterone almost immediately begin to loosen the ligaments in your pelvic cradle (and elsewhere). This makes your joints more flexible so the baby can pass through, but you may feel unstable as you walk. As your bump grows, your "core" abdominal muscles, which stabilize your back, stretch and become thinner to accommodate your baby, thus making them weaker. You may also feel off-balance as you adjust (and re-adjust) to a changing centre of gravity as your baby grows and your weight shifts forwards. In addition, a growing baby puts pressure on your bladder and pelvic floor muscles, making certain types of exercise uncomfortable to do, and on your lungs, causing breathlessness even if you are normally very fit.

How much to exercise

Exercise eases a range of pregnancy problems (nausea, aches and pains, and low energy) and lowers the risk of haemorrhoids, varicose veins, and even gestational diabetes. You are the best judge of what level of exercise suits you, but as a rule of thumb don't exert yourself more than you were used to before pregnancy. If you haven't exercised before, you can start some gentle activites in your first or second trimester. It's also normal to feel very tired during early pregnancy, so get plenty of rest as well. Consult your healthcare professional before any exercise, especially if you have high or low blood pressure, are anaemic, a heavy smoker, have a BMI greater than 40 or lower than 12, or are expecting more than one baby.

Q What are the best types of exercise during pregnancy?

Low- or no-impact exercise is ideal while you are pregnant, as it is kindest on your joints. Don't forget that any exercise that doesn't require you to try to maintain your balance over uneven or slippery ground is best.

The main aim of exercising through pregnancy is to strengthen your muscles, improve your circulation, ease any backache, and help you feel well. It's important to avoid any exercise or activities that require jumpy and jerky movements, take sharp changes of direction, or is so vigorous that it raises your core temperature or puts excessive strain on your cardiovascular system or joints. In addition, impact sports and sports that involve a risk of falling – such as squash, horse riding, downhill skiing, and contact sports – are not advisable. Some good choices are listed below.

Ligaments Relaxin loosens this connective tissue

Pubic symphysis Stretches in childbirth

Softer joints The hormone relaxin acts on the soft tissues connecting the bones of your pelvic cradle. This is great preparation for labour, but can cause aching pain beforehand. Be kind to your joints when exercising.

GREAT WAYS TO EXERCISE

Keep supple and elevate your heart rate without causing stress to your body with these options. Warm up gently, and stretch after.

» Running, power-walking, and walking: if you are already running regularly, continuing is perfectly safe. Don't try to train for an event though. Run just below your usual fitness levels, and listen to your body if it tells you you've had enough. If you haven't previously been a runner, walking and power-walking are great alternatives.

» Cycling: a low-impact form of exercise, cycling is good for your breathing and circulation. After the first trimester, when your sense of balance starts to shift, you may become unsteady, so continue into your second trimester only if you are really confident on your bike. Otherwise consider a stationary bike, which is just as good for you. A recumbent bike, on which you sit back, not upright, puts less pressure on your perineum, and may feel more comfortable as your baby grows and bears downwards.

» Swimming: as long as the pool is at a normal temperature (not higher than 32°C/90°F), swimming is fantastic, as the buoyancy of the water supports your body. Best of all, as long as you feel comfortable, you can keep swimming right up until the moment you go into labour. An aquanatal class will be specially suited to your pregnant body.

» Stretching and strengthening techniques: exercise such as Pilates and yoga, when specially adapted for pregnancy, can be gentle on your muscles and ligaments, increase strength and flexibility, and improve your breathing to help you through labour. They are also good for easing back and hip pain (normal side effects of loosened ligaments) and preparing your body for birth. Always find a qualified teacher, as there are certain yoga postures and forms of Pilates that aren't suitable during pregnancy.

Softened ligaments All the ligaments in your body become looser as a result of relaxin, which makes you more prone to injury and backache

Uterus Relaxin is thought to relax the uterine wall muscles to inhibit contractions, allowing the uterus to expand. It may help to determine the timing of your labour

Pelvis The ligaments at the front of the pelvis in particular relax in preparation for childbirth. Your hips may feel more achy as a result and your pelvic cradle is less stable

Cervix and vagina Near the end of the pregnancy, relaxin widens and softens the cervix and vagina to ease delivery

Blood pressure Relaxin influences your blood pressure by relaxing the blood vessels to increase blood flow, so helping more oxygen and nutrients reach the fetus

How your body changes Relaxin is produced by the ovaries, placenta, and other tissues to help you cope with your pregnancy and prepare for childbirth. Once released into the bloodstream, it affects your body in different ways at different times.

Q How can exercise make my pregnancy easier?

If you are one of the 70 per cent or so of women who experience backache and other physical discomfort in pregnancy, you may think that resting will help. Instead, practise safe, low-impact exercises to decrease the muscle spasms.

It's not just the extra weight of your baby as she grows that puts a strain on areas such as your back. The aches you experience increase because the hormone relaxin loosens your ligaments, especially those in your pelvic cradle. This makes way for your growing baby and prepares for birth; in fact all your ligaments soften due to the high concentrations of relaxin required to loosen the pelvic joints. Your baby's increasing size also stretches the transversus abdominis (TVA) muscles, which act like a corset to support and stabilize your lower back from the sides and front. As your centre of gravity shifts forwards with the baby's weight, it's

likely that your posture will change to compensate, increasing the strain on muscles in your lower back. It may be tempting to lie down when you ache, but any exercise that helps you strengthen these deep transversus abdominis muscles will ease the pain or discomfort. Consider antenatal Pilates classes, which specifically target your "core stability" – strengthening these core muscles so that your back remains as steady and supported as possible – or try the exercises shown opposite. These gentle stretching and strengthening movements will decrease muscle spasms, release back tension, and improve your spinal flexibility.

Any exercise that helps **strengthen the transversus abdominis muscles** will ease pain and discomfort.

TRANSVERSUS ABDOMINIS MUSCLES

This "core" of deep abdominal muscles lies beneath the outer muscles (such as rectus abdominis, or the "six pack"). They wrap around the spine and help to stabilize your trunk and lower back. The stronger the tranversus abdominis muscles are, the more support they give.

Linea alba This is a fibrous band running down the midline of the abdomen connecting the abdominal muscles.

External abdominal obliques These are located on the sides and front of the abdomen.

Internal abdominal obliques These sit under the external obliques.

Pelvis

Muscular corset Layers of abdominal muscles are situated at the front of the tummy and wrap around the sides of the body to support the spine.

Q How do I ease the symptoms of water retention?

There are a couple of options you can try if you are experiencing water retention, or oedema, in your ankles, feet, and hands, or if your joints are feeling stiff. One of the best choices is to walk around for a while every so often during the day to get your circulation going (avoid sitting or standing still for long periods), or go for a daily walk outdoors, or swim. Swimming has the added benefit of cooling your body down in hot weather; becoming too hot can cause water retention. Elevating your feet can help, too. Use a footstool if you work at a desk, or elevate your feet properly for a while: sit back in a chair, raise your feet right up, and rotate your ankles several times in each direction to get the blood flowing.

Complementary therapies

Massage can be very beneficial in helping to dissipate fluid and reduce tension. For a home massage, gently massage your feet, ankles, and lower legs with a lotion or cooling gel; use upward strokes working towards your knees. If you are heavily pregnant, you may find it easier to ask your partner to do this. When massaging your hands, press firmly from your nails to the base of your fingers. Reflexology and acupuncture can also help; your practitioner may be able to show you acupressure points to use in between visits.

Water retention often occurs during the last three months of pregnancy due in part to the extra blood – up to 50 per cent more than usual – that you produce. It also occurs if you are dehydrated, as your body tries to retain as much fluid as possible, so drink plenty of water.

When you exercise, ensure that you wear clothing that gives you a **full range of movement** and choose suitable footwear that will **support** your ankles and feet. Keep drinking plenty of water and take regular rest breaks.

Q What simple exercises can I try at home?

Recommended by midwives, these exercises are easy to do at home. However, check with your midwife first that they are safe in your specific case. Stop if you feel any discomfort or dizziness.

HAND STRETCHES

Try these simple stretches if you feel pain, tingling, or numbness in your hands.

» **Shake your hands for one minute** as if air-drying them after just washing them.

» **For a deep stretch,** hold out one arm, keep your elbow straight, and drop your wrist so your fingers face the floor. Using your other hand, apply gentle pressure to the back of your hand to gently stretch your wrist and fingers for 20 seconds. Repeat with the other hand.

» **Put your hands together in a prayer position**. Spread your fingers, then pull your palms as far apart as possible while keeping your fingertips together. Repeat several times.

FOOT STRETCHES

Relieve foot cramps and ease any arch strain, or even plantar fasciitis, with this exercise.

» **Foot roll** Stand in bare feet on a non-slip surface. Roll a tennis ball or golf ball around under the base of one foot for two minutes to gently massage all the muscles. Repeat with the other foot.

BACK STRETCHES

Keep your spine flexible by warming up and strengthening the muscles around it. Kneeling on all fours also helps to relieve tension in your spine.

1 **Kneel on the floor,** then lean forwards and support your weight on your straightened arms (don't lock your elbows), so that you're on all fours. Keep your hands, knees, and feet in line with each other. Keep your back horizontal. Relax your neck and inhale.

2 **Slowly draw up your abdominal muscles** as you exhale, tuck your pelvis under, and lengthen the base of your spine gently so your back is arched like that of a cat. Keep your elbows gently straight, but not locked. Inhale and release to straighten your back again; take care not to hollow out your back.

3 **Repeat the arching movement ten times** altogether. When you've finished, sit back on your heels and breathe deeply a few times to relax. Get up slowly so you don't feel dizzy.

SPINE STRETCHES

As your baby grows heavier, it's beneficial to align and stretch your spine every day. Try these two simple exercises to relax and refresh you.

1 **Stand with your feet** hip-width apart just in front of a wall. Bend your knees slightly and rest the length of your spine against the wall. Breathe deeply.

2 **When you're ready,** breathe out and pull your tummy button towards your spine. Your pelvis should tilt up and away from the wall slightly, so that your lower back presses into the wall. Hold briefly, then inhale and release. Repeat ten times.

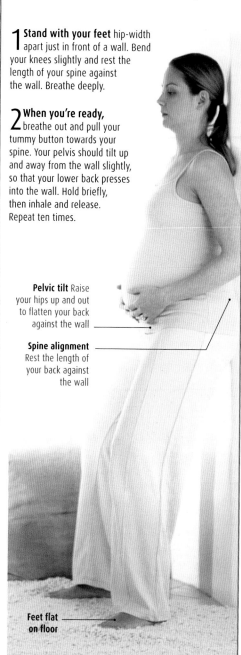

Pelvic tilt Raise your hips up and out to flatten your back against the wall

Spine alignment Rest the length of your back against the wall

Feet flat on floor

Ease discomfort and stabilize your back using these **stretching** and **strengthening** techniques.

Q I've heard I need to exercise my pelvic floor. Where is my pelvic floor and why is it important to my pregnancy?

Your pelvic floor is a group of strong, layered muscles that stretches like a double sling, or a hammock, from your pubic bone to your tailbone. This sling supports your abdomen and holds in your reproductive and pelvic organs. During pregnancy, the muscles support the growing weight of your uterus and baby; during labour, they help guide your baby out of your body.

Some muscles of your body, such as your heart, are involuntary, but most are voluntary, which means you can consciously tighten and release them. You do this with your pelvic floor muscles when you "hold on" if you need to go to the loo (the double sling of muscle has holes in it that correspond to your urethra, rectum, and vagina).

How the pelvic floor muscles work

During pregnancy, your pelvic floor muscles are loosened by the hormone relaxin, and then stretched and weakened by the weight of your growing baby bearing down on them. Having strong pelvic floor

muscles is crucial: an already weak pelvic floor can mean that during pregnancy and afterwards you can leak urine when you cough, sneeze, laugh, jump, or run – a condition known as stress incontinence. Also, during labour your pelvic floor forces your baby to turn in the cavity of your pelvis. He is then able to fit into the birth canal so you can push him out during second-stage labour. A weak pelvic floor may make this process less efficient. A surge of relaxin loosens your pelvic floor further to enable the baby to move through the birth canal: the pelvic floor muscles near the front of your body are forced downwards and those near the back are forced upwards, creating an opening for your baby.

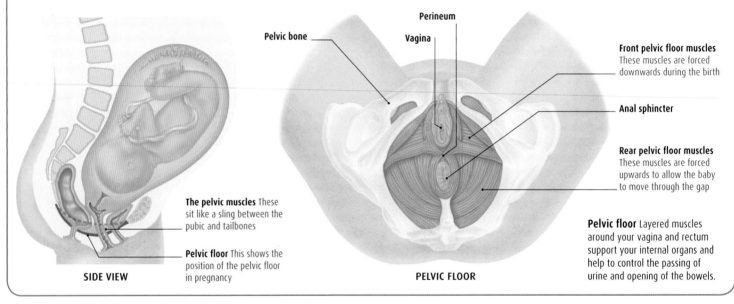

Perineum

Pelvic bone

Vagina

Front pelvic floor muscles These muscles are forced downwards during the birth

Anal sphincter

Rear pelvic floor muscles These muscles are forced upwards to allow the baby to move through the gap

The pelvic muscles These sit like a sling between the pubic and tailbones

Pelvic floor This shows the position of the pelvic floor in pregnancy

SIDE VIEW

PELVIC FLOOR

Pelvic floor Layered muscles around your vagina and rectum support your internal organs and help to control the passing of urine and opening of the bowels.

Q Are the pelvic floor muscles permanently stretched after labour? What's a prolapse?

After labour, your pelvic floor muscles should "ping" back into place relatively quickly, keeping your organs neatly tucked in as they were before. If the muscles are damaged during labour, however, you may suffer a "prolapse", when your abdominal organs bear down into your vagina. Often, it's not until later in life that any damage becomes apparent and a prolapse occurs. So it's important to practise pelvic floor exercises throughout pregnancy and afterwards, aiming to reverse the damage and give the muscles back as much strength as possible.

Q I have a toddler who still expects to be carried. Will I harm the baby – or myself – if I lift him?

As long as your midwife hasn't told you to the contrary, careful lifting is fine – it poses no threat to the safety of your unborn baby. Your back and pelvic floor, though, can be a different matter. It's vital that you protect your back by lifting carefully, whether you are picking up your toddler or lifting and carrying shopping bags or heavy objects.

To lift safely, plant your feet shoulder-width apart and flat on the floor. Bend down from your knees (not your waist), tucking your buttocks under and keeping your back straight.

Wrap your arms around your toddler, asking him to lock on with his legs, or hold the shopping bags or heavy object firmly. Push up with your thighs (use one arm to hoist yourself up against something if you need to), rather than straining your back. Once you're standing, adjust your toddler's position so it's comfortable for you – his legs straddling the bump, for example, or on one or other of your hips (if you carry your toddler to the side, swap sides each time to balance out the strain). If you carry several shopping bags, make sure that you distribute the weight evenly between both hands. Lifting also strains your pelvic floor, so always engage your pelvic floor muscles before lifting anything, and practise your Kegel exercises frequently (see opposite).

Q How do I do pelvic floor exercises? Is there a way to be sure I'm doing them correctly?

Pelvic floor exercises or Kegels – named after US gynaecologist Arnold Kegel – are the exercises that keep the pelvic floor muscles toned so that they are strong enough to assist the second stage of labour (see opposite).

It's important to perform Kegel exercises daily while you are pregnant, as the pelvic floor muscles work with your deep transverse abdominal and back muscles to stablize your spine, support your baby, and help prevent stress incontinence. However, don't over-exercise your pelvic floor when you do this internal movement – more than 100 squeezes a day could make it difficult for the muscles to relax during the birth, which then makes it harder for the baby to make his way out.

Firstly, find out what your pelvic floor muscles feel like: imagine you are drawing up water into your vagina. Another way to find the muscles is to stop yourself urinating towards the end of your flow (don't do this in the middle as it could lead to a urine infection). The muscles you tighten to do either of these actions are your pelvic floors. The movement is completely internal and not visible to other people.

Benefits of pelvic floor exercises

Do them anytime, anywhere, in any position. Practise them when you boil the kettle, wait in a queue, or to the rhythm of a song. If you only do a few at a time, the cumulative effects will be worth every one, and may even help to improve your sex life. If you suffer from stress incontinence, you should notice a difference in around six weeks.

DO A SIMPLE PELVIC FLOOR EXERCISE

Here is a simple routine you can follow. Aim to do the whole sequence three times a day. You might find it helps to lift starting with the rear muscles and then moving forwards to the front, before holding and then releasing.

If you find it hard to know whether you are locating the right muscles, it can help to try doing the exercises in different positions. Below are some options that will help you to focus all your attention on the correct area and relax the rest of your body.

1 SQUEEZE THE MUSCLES
Sit comfortably in a chair with your feet flat on the floor and your back straight. Keep your body and your face relaxed. Pull up and squeeze your pelvic floor muscles as tightly as they will go and hold for ten seconds. Release the muscles.

2 SLOW SQUEEZE AND RELEASE
Repeat the squeeze 9–20 times, holding each for ten seconds. Do not use your abdomen or buttock muscles. Make sure you rest the muscles for ten seconds between contractions.

3 QUICK SQUEEZE AND RELEASE
Finally, do a set of quick squeezes. Following the natural rhythm of your breath, lift the muscles as you inhale. Exhale and release and briefly relax the muscles. Repeat ten times.

Birthing ball or firm bean bag Place the ball against a wall and sit up straight with your knees apart. Place your hands lightly on your lower abdomen. Relax your face and body.

Kneeling on floor head down Kneel down on the floor, then get down gently onto all fours, place your elbows on the floor, and rest your head on your hands. Focus on the sense of space around your pelvic floor.

Astride a chair Sit upright on a chair with your knees wide apart and your feet at an angle that allows for maximum stability. Rest your hands on the front of the chair seat. Relax your face and body and focus on your pelvic area.

Q Will I have to give up running? I want to stay fit and feel my best throughout my pregnancy.

You can keep up some sports, such as running, for as long as feels comfortable and is medically safe; then swap to low- or no-impact sports later on so you can continue exercising.

Low-impact exercise This exerts minimal stress on your weight-bearing joints.

As long as you are a seasoned runner, continuing to run during your first trimester and into your second trimester is fine if you feel well and comfortable. You may find that the increasing weight of the baby and your changing centre of gravity mean that you won't want to run as far or as fast as before, and you may tire more quickly. Avoid running on bumpy or icy ground in case you fall. After 12 weeks of pregnancy, check with your doctor or midwife how long it is safe for you to continue.

With any high-impact sport, you should follow a few rules while pregnant. Warm up and cool down gently and don't overstretch: unlike muscles, which regain their shape after the birth, ligaments will not recover if stretched excessively. Exercise moderately below your usual fitness levels; you should be able to talk easily while you exercise – so avoid pushing yourself too hard. If you overheat, the fetus may suffer, particularly in the first trimester when it can't regulate its own temperature. If you are out of breath for a period it may reduce the amount of oxygen the fetus receives. It's especially important to rehydrate properly afterwards, as dehydration can lead to complications including premature contractions.

Do not attempt any high-impact, high-risk, or contact sports if you exercised intermittently before becoming pregnant, or are new to exercise.

Did you know...

Exercise has the happy consequence of causing the brain's transmitters to release endorphins into the brain and nervous system. These hormones have a number of physiological functions, including triggering a positive feeling and reducing stress, helping to boost your mood.

WHICH SPORTS TO ENJOY AND FOR HOW LONG

Exercise is a wonderful way to maintain your energy levels and feel good, but you may need to exercise within a different set of parameters as you move through each trimester.

SPORT	PROS & CONS	FIRST & SECOND TRIMESTER
Swimming	Strengthens your heart and lungs and tones your muscles while supporting all your weight and keeping your body temperature stable.	Ideal for all levels of fitness. Sign up for water aerobics classes if available.
Badminton	A low-impact aerobic sport that promotes cardiovascular health.	As with most raquet sports, unless you are a regular player, don't play while pregnant. Try other low-impact alternatives.
Cycling	Gives you a cardio workout while supporting your weight so there is less stress on your body.	Start slowly and don't overexert yourself. Cool down with gentle stretches afterwards.
Golf	Low-impact golf works core muscles, helps to improve stability, and improves cardiovascular health if you walk the course.	Continue if you already play golf regularly, but stretch well first, adjust your game to "slow and easy", and take care not to lose your balance.
Gym	Has a variety of equipment and exercise classes to give you a cardio workout and strength training (use light weights only).	Exercise at a moderate intensity on machinery. Sign up for antenatal exercise classes.
Hiking & climbing	Hiking improves your strength and cardiovascular health. Climbing is not advised.	Consult your doctor or midwife first before going hiking, then choose even terrain and ensure you have supportive hiking boots and hiking poles.
Pilates	Focuses on core muscles – abdominal, pelvic floor, and back – to promote good posture, stability, and strength without straining other joints.	Ideal for all levels of fitness, but speak to your instructor first if you are new to Pilates. Choose a pregnancy class.
Walking & power walking	Strengthens your heart and lungs, tones your muscles, and is safe for your body.	Walk for 30 minutes three times a week if you are a beginner. If you are fit, focus on power walking – walking at a brisk pace – to raise your heart rate.
Yoga	Gives you techniques to help you breathe, move, stretch, and relax while pregnant. Also strengthens your muscles. Avoid hot yoga.	Ideal for all levels of fitness. Speak to your instructor first if you are new to yoga.
Dancing	Gives you a good cardio workout, but can stress the joints. Always keep one foot on the ground and avoid spinning, leaping, jumping, and so on.	Continue if you already dance regularly, but exercise below your usual fitness levels.
Running	Elevates your heart rate and works your muscles, but can cause stress to your joints.	Continue if you run regularly, but listen to your body during your second trimester in particular.
Tennis	Gives you a cardio workout, but rapid changes in direction can stress your joints and cause falls.	Unless you are a fit and very experienced player, don't play while pregnant. Try low-impact alternatives.

KEY

	No impact
	Low impact
	High impact

THIRD TRIMESTER	WHEN TO STOP
Listen to your body and slow down if need be.	You can continue swimming until the birth.
Change to a recumbent bike if you feel uncomfortable.	Stop if you feel too tired or get dizzy.
Try other alternatives unless your GP or midwife says it's safe to continue.	Stop when you feel too tired and heavy.
Find out which equipment is safe to use. Continue antenatal classes.	Stop if you feel too tired or get dizzy or light-headed.
Check with your GP or midwife that it's safe to continue hiking.	Stop if you feel too tired or get dizzy or light-headed.
Focus on relaxation and breathing techniques.	Continue with gentle Pilates until the birth.
Listen to your body and slow down if you feel tired.	Continue walking until the birth.
Don't lie flat on your back after 16 weeks or you may feel faint.	Continue with gentle yoga until the birth.
Try low-impact options unless your GP or midwife says it's safe to continue.	Stop if you feel too tired or get dizzy or light-headed.
Try low-impact options unless your GP says to continue.	Stop if you feel too tired or get dizzy.

Q Will having sex affect the baby at all?

There is no medical evidence to suggest that having sex if your pregnancy is straightforward will harm your baby in any way – it's perfectly safe for you to enjoy sex in each trimester. Neither is there is any risk of miscarriage or premature birth when you have penetrative sex. Once you become pregnant, your baby is well protected: your cervix is sealed with a thick mucus plug, and as the fetus grows the amniotic fluid around it helps to cushion it from any pressure. If you have complications, however, such as heavy vaginal bleeding or your waters break, you are advised not to have sex and should seek medical attention straight away.

Increased libido

Making love during your first trimester shouldn't feel any different physically, but if you are nauseous or chronically tired, you may have a low libido. If you've had a previous miscarriage or assisted conception, you and/or your partner may feel nervous about having sex. Reassure each other and cuddle to maintain your intimacy until you want to make love.

During the second trimester, your body changes shape noticeably, which can make some women feel less sexually attractive. However, you should have more energy, feel more relaxed about the baby's safety, and find your libido has returned: the increase in blood volume in your body can heighten sensations, and help you reach orgasm more readily. If you feel your baby moving after sex, it may be due to the adrenaline release you receive at orgasm.

During your third trimester, you may have Braxton Hick's contractions if you reach orgasm and these can last from a few minutes to half an hour afterwards, which is normal. However, if the contractions continue for longer and you are concerned, contact your midwife.

Q I can't stop thinking about the birth. How will I handle labour, and motherhood?

It's hard not to leap ahead and think about the future, but as your body changes and the baby grows your emotional mindset will evolve. Your hormones are already responding to the new life inside you and gradually preparing and

Taking up an **antenatal exercise class** provides more than just physical rewards: it's a great way to meet other, like-minded **mums-to-be** to share your experiences and enjoy making some new friends.

enabling your body to give birth, but it can be hard for your thought processes to fall in line with your natural instincts. Your wellbeing is of paramount importance so that you are in the best possible shape physically and mentally to give birth and care for a baby. For now it's good to focus on the present and how best you can look after yourself and the fetus. Keeping fit, eating healthily, and avoiding stress, anxiety, and fear are key. Try to relax and unwind as much as possible, talk to your midwife or GP about any concerns you still have and, as much as you can, be aware of the miracle of pregnancy and how your baby is growing.

Q I'm still in shock about being pregnant. Will I ever get excited and enjoy my pregnancy?

If you feel that you can't shake off your state of shock, be reassured. The first few weeks are an unusual time as you battle to cope with the onset of early pregnancy symptoms, wonder about the future, and yet see no real evidence of a baby. Sometimes negative feelings arise partly as a result of having to keep it all a secret for a while. As you open up about your news, and start to feel physically better, the shock should dissipate. Do positive things to make your experience of pregnancy as enjoyable as possible: pamper yourself with relaxing baths and massages, sleep in when you can, organize events to look forward to, and enjoy closer bonds with family members and friends and enjoy their excitement and good wishes, for example. If the feelings of shock or fear don't subside, talk to your doctor or midwife to ensure you don't have the condition tokophobia, a fear of pregnancy and childbirth.

If you want **extra support** through your pregnancy, try out a few of the online **social media forums** for expectant mums – you'll be joining a wonderfully empowering and reassuring **support network** that you may want to continue with after your baby is born.

Q I'm going to be a single parent. Will I be able to cope and how can I prepare properly?

All new mums worry about being able to cope, and those concerns are often heightened if you feel you have no one to share them with. But you aren't alone. Firstly, discuss how you feel with trusted friends and family, and with your midwife, and ask them for reassurance.

Then, even before your baby is born, start building your support network. Identify a birthing partner and share your birth plan with him or her. Talk to the people you are closest to about who can be around to help you in the first few weeks after the birth – to do some practical essentials such as the shopping or cleaning, but also to provide some companionship and to look after the baby occasionally, so you have time to yourself (your wellbeing is important for your baby, too). You may want to make a list of what chores you normally do so that your "support team" know what to do and can divide up the tasks.

Ask your midwife if she can put you in touch with other single mums-to-be, or look online for single parent groups in your area. Find out what help your local authority can give you. Never be afraid to ask for help, nor to accept offers of it.

Finally, well before your due date, get organized: prepare and wash clothes and bedding for your baby, and cook yourself some nutritious meals and freeze them – stews, pies, and bakes that you can eat with just a fork in one hand are best. Leave yourself as little as possible to do after the birth so you can spend the time fully engaged with your baby.

Q How expensive is having a baby going to be? I'm not sure I'll be able to afford it.

You may never feel financially ready to welcome a newborn into your life, but your baby needn't be a money drain if you take a realistic approach.

Although every parent wants the best for their child, it is vital not to have sky-high expectations about what your baby needs, or insist on the best. You may have a clear vision of the life you want to give your child and be anxious that you won't be able to fulfil this desire, but all your new baby really wants is to be close to you and be warm, dry, and fed. There's no need to buy every piece of baby equipment brand new. Babies quickly grow out of clothes and equipment, so it's usually easy to find good-quality second-hand items via local nearly new sales or online forums. You might also be pleasantly surprised by how many gifts you receive – and by the money you save staying in.

It's true, however, that having a baby will impact on your income if you intend to continue working and have to take childcare costs into consideration, and as your baby develops into a child and then a teenager, supporting him will become more expensive. If this is a concern it's worth taking advantage of the time you have now to make a clear financial plan. Discuss your household finances with your partner so you are both aware of the issues and responsiblities ahead and there are no misunderstandings.

You may want to discuss the idea of **setting up a joint "baby" account** and start saving for your child's future.

FINANCIAL CHECKLIST

Get your finances in order as soon as possible so that you have the right systems in place and feel in control of your money by the time your baby arrives.

HOUSEHOLD BUDGET

Look at your monthly outgoings Pinpoint where you can save money – perhaps gym memberships and subscriptions that you rarely use, for example, or unessential purchases. If you and your partner have separate bank accounts, work out how to share the bills and seek out the most cost-effective way to pay them. You may want to discuss the idea of setting up a "baby" account.

ENTITLEMENTS & CREDITS

Check out entitlements and tax credits You may be aware of entitlements such as free dental treatment while you are pregnant, but as a parent you may also qualify for benefits such as a tax-free childcare scheme if you go back to work, for example.

BABY EQUIPMENT

Make a list of baby equipment Include essential items only, and think before you buy - a bulky, unwieldy pram may prove too unpractical, or a nappy disposal bin may never get used. Ask friends and family if they have items you can borrow, or buy secondhand; you may just need to buy a few new items like muslins, a changing mat, and a cot mattress. If you buy new, shop around first.

Q Will my relationship with my partner change forever with a baby around? How do we adapt?

There is no doubt that having a baby around will change the current dynamic of your relationship, but that in itself can have positive rewards.

It's normal to feel concerned about the impending changes ahead and worry that you may lose something of the precious intimacy you currently enjoy. Whether you have planned this baby or not – and even if you feel a sense of contentment about creating a family – your relationship with your partner will inevitably need to evolve as you become parents.

It's worth defining the feelings you have about a change in your relationship and becoming parents. If your relationship is strong, take heart from the fact that you already understand the process of getting to know each other, learning about each other's qualities and character so you can relate to one another and support and nurture each other in life.

Talk to each other

It's important that you find time to talk about issues on your minds. These may include worries about spending less time with each other after the birth, and maybe more time with your in-laws; the changes in your roles and how to manage household tasks; moving from two wages to one (even if it's only temporary) and the sense of dependence or pressure this may bring; and personal expectations about how you want to parent your baby.

If you worry about becoming parents, be reassured that it's not as difficult as you think. You will adapt to your roles, but give yourselves time. Researchers have estimated that it takes new parents at least four months to establish a routine and feel confident with their baby.

Keep **communicating** openly and **showing respect** to each other as you prepare for, and then **parent**, your child.

DISCUSSION POINTS

Talk through your expectations of life as a family so you understand each other's hopes and feelings and know how to keep your relationship a priority once you become parents.

Parenting styles
You may have different ideas of what constitutes "normal" family life – chat through them now.

Work pressures
Brainstorm ideas about how you can both try to create a good work/life balance.

Tiredness
Discuss possibilities for each of you to take turns in having regular "time out" for yourself to relax or rest.

Time alone together
Sex and intimacy and effective communication are important discussion points.

Responsibilities
Delegate chores between yourselves so you have a clear understanding of who will do what and when.

Support
Talk about whether you can afford – and want – to have some extra support at home after the birth.

Q I feel stressed. Will the baby be affected?

It's perfectly natural to feel anxious about how you will cope with life – and a baby. There probably isn't a woman who hasn't felt worried, anxious, inadequate, or even fearful at some point during her first (or subsequent) pregnancy. Bringing a new life into the world is a magical time, but it's also one filled with unpredictability and change. And if you work or lead a busy life, the prospect of trying to process all you need to do before the birth can sometimes feel incredibly pressured.

If you feel stressed, your body produces higher levels of the hormone cortisol. Research is still being conducted as to whether prolonged bouts of cortisol affect your unborn baby: some studies have shown that the effects of chronic stress on a fetus can be minimal; others that constant stress may put your baby at risk. We all experience stress at various times, but it's important that you don't let it overwhelm you. Try to live in the moment, learn to delegate and don't attempt to do everything yourself, rest when you can, and exercise moderately – it's a great way to release stress.

If your stress has turned into anxiety and you feel you can't cope, have no appetite, you're worried about going out, you cry much of the time, and feel lethargic and uninterested in life, you may have antenatal depression (AND). Although less well known than postnatal depression (see p.263), it probably affects more women than we realize simply because mums-to-be often feel ashamed of and are afraid to mention their negative feelings. If you're at all concerned, talk to your healthcare provider, as well as your family and/or friends.

Q I am excited about our baby, but my partner isn't. How can I get my partner more enthused?

It seems obvious, but make an effort to involve your partner in as many ways as possible. Encourage your partner to stroke the bump often, for example, and talk to your baby: around 24 weeks gestation the fetus can hear what's going on outside the uterus. Also consider whether what you see as lack of enthusiasm may in fact be anxiety about your partner's responsibilities, so ask your partner how they are feeling. Finally, while pregnancy is a living part of you, for your partner there's probably something a bit unreal about it. Hang in there; for many partners, full and enthusiastic engagement happens only when finally they hold their baby in their arms.

{ Q How can I prepare myself for labour and birth?

Approaches to childbirth have changed dramatically over recent decades: nowadays it is considered perfectly acceptable to try different techniques and positions in labour to help you manage pain and stay focused yet relaxed for a positive, calm birth. Practising different techniques while you are still pregnant can help you feel in control when the time comes.

Physical preparation

Thanks to the pioneering efforts of some childbirth experts (see opposite), it is no longer standard procedure to be confined to a bed during labour. Moving around and staying in an upright position may help to shorten the length of your labour. So it's worth practising safe squats, for example, while pregnant to strengthen your legs and thighs in preparation for giving birth standing up. "Labour breathing" is another effective way of helping you to manage the pain of each contraction and keep a positive, relaxed attitude. Practise labour breathing regularly in pregnancy so you feel familiar with the technique once in labour.

Mental preparation

As your body goes into labour, your brain triggers the release of the hormone oxytocin, which increases the contractions of the uterus to ease labour along, and endorphins, which help you feel calmer and can alleviate pain. Staying as relaxed as possible during labour will let these body chemicals work effectively; if you feel scared or fearful, adrenaline, a stress hormone, will flood your body and limit their effects. For some women, techniques such as hypnobirthing, audio-analgesia, visualization (see pp.228–29), meditation, and relaxation will enable an easier labour and birth as well as offering a sense of spiritual wellbeing.

PATTERNED BREATHING

Consciously changing your breathing patterns as labour progresses helps to force oxygen into your bloodstream so you can stay calm and relaxed enough to handle the pain. Remember, breathing out properly is all-important.

1 Late first stage of labour During this early stage take deep, slow, even breaths at the start and end of a contraction, and light breaths during its peak.

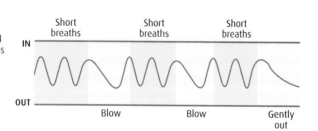

Deep, even breaths   Light breaths   Deep, even breaths
IN
OUT

2 Transition stage As the contractions become intense, and to avoid pushing too early, take shorter breaths in groups of two to three, blowing out each time (see right). Breathe out gently when the contraction ends.

Short breaths   Short breaths   Short breaths
IN
OUT
Blow   Blow   Gently out

3 Second stage of labour Take and hold a deep breath while pushing down smoothly. After each push, take deep, even breaths.

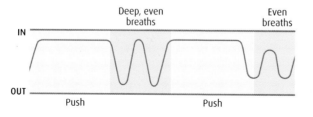

Deep, even breaths   Even breaths
IN
OUT
Push   Push

 ### Breathing tips

» Start practising as early in pregnancy as you like, so that you are familiar with all three stages of breathing when you eventually go into labour.
» Inhale calmly through your nose and concentrate on relaxing your muscles. Focus on your out-breath: blow out slowly through your mouth and imagine you are exhaling the pain of a contraction. Everyone's pain threshold is different: don't be afraid to ask for medical pain relief if you feel you need it.

Breathing out properly Hold one hand about 30cm (12in) away from your mouth and join your thumb and index finger. You are exhaling properly if you can feel your out-breath cooling your fingers. This may help especially with more intense contractions.

TYPES OF PREPARATION

If you are interested in practising one or more of these approaches, look out for dedicated birth preparation classes in your area.

 ### Mind

» Hypnobirthing is a form of self-hypnosis where you consciously take calm control of your birthing experience with breathing and relaxation techniques. You remain fully aware and focused throughout (you are not in some kind of hypnotic "sleep").

» Audio-analgesia uses a combination of music and white noise to help you control and dull the sensation of pain.

 ### Spirit

» Relaxation, meditation, and mindfulness can clear your mind of thoughts and block out what is going on around you while you remain calm, aware, and centred (below). Find a warm, quiet space. Lie down. Gently stretch out your arms, legs, shoulders, wrists, shoulders, and neck. Get comfortable, close your eyes, breathe regularly, and focus on an object or a view you love.

 ### Body

» Squatting opens out your pelvis to ease the baby's passage through the birth canal. Stand up straight with the back of a sturdy dining chair facing you. With your feet hip-width apart, toes pointing slightly outwards, and hands on the chair back, bend your knees until you're in a sitting position. Push your weight into your heels. Push up from your thighs. Repeat five times.

Clear your mind and still your emotions Concentrate only on the present moment and the rise and fall of your hands on your chest

Breathe evenly Keep a regular rhythm. Breathe in through your nose and blow out through your mouth

Sit crossed-legged Choose a soft surface on the floor and sit with your back upright. Relax your inner thighs to help to open your pelvic girdle

Calm your body Breathe in deeply to boost the amount of oxygen you inhale. Relax all your muscles with each inhalation

Cross your hands over your chest Focus on the rhythm of your breathing

CHILDBIRTH PIONEERS

You might find the writings of some of the different childbirth philosophers and practitioners inspirational when considering the type of birth you want.

» **Dr Ferdinand Lamaze** investigated effective relaxation and breathing techniques, now known as "Lamaze breathing".

» **Frederick Leboyer** seeks to reduce the trauma of birth, saying that babies should be born into calm, softly lit surroundings and placed on the mother's skin before the cord is cut. He is also an advocate of water births.

» **Sheila Kitzinger** enabled women to reclaim some control over the way they want to give birth. She campaigned for the avoidance of unnecessary obstetric intervention where appropriate so that giving birth is a powerful, positive experience.

» **Michel Odent** endorses active childbirth techniques, so reducing the need for pain relief and the number of assisted deliveries and Caesarean sections.

Learning to relax Try focusing your awareness on your natural breathing rhythm to link your emotions and thoughts to your physical sensations. The more relaxed you are, the less tension, and therefore pain, you will experience.

Q What exercises can I do immediately after having my baby?

You may be desperate to lose any excess pregnancy weight and tone up again after the birth of your baby, but you must take things gently until the six-week check, when your GP should give you the all-clear.

Childbirth has a profound effect on your body and it takes a while to recover your pre-pregnancy strength and resilience. Although it's good to be active again as soon as possible after the birth, the general advice is that for the first six weeks you should not attempt to return to – or improve on – your pre-pregnancy fitness levels. Your transverse abdominal muscles (see opposite) may still be stretched apart, and levels of relaxin are still high in your body, so your joints will remain loose for a while yet; you may inflict serious long-term damage to your ligaments if you try any high-impact exercise. Your lochia (vaginal bleeding) may get heavier or turn bright red if you do exercise too hard too soon after giving birth – a warning sign that you need to dial down your activities again. If you want to swim, leave seven clear days without vaginal bleeding beforehand so you don't pick up an infection (and avoid it if you have had stitches or a Caesarean section). Anything other than gentle exercise and pelvic floor exercises is off-limits until

at least after your six-week check. To get your circulation going, take a gentle walk every day, and gradually build your stamina. Remember to keep your back straight as you push the pram.

Pelvic floor and stretch exercises

Focusing on your pelvic floor exercises again after the birth is essential to retone the muscles as soon as possible, so practise them throughout the day, sitting, standing, kneeling, or lying down as often as you remember (see pp.66–67). If you can't feel the muscles, try practising first on a birthing ball. Now that you don't have to limit the number of pull ups you do in order to be able to consciously relax the muscles during labour, do as many repetitions as you can manage – the more the better. You can also start gently exercising and stretching (see below) to begin toning major muscles, boost your recovery from the labour and birth, and help you get rid of any aches and stiffness.

GENTLE EXERCISES FOR THE FIRST SIX WEEKS

You can do these gentle exercises to tone your lower stomach muscles and stretch out your body after the birth, even if you have had a Caesarean section. Start with just a few repetitions if you can manage them in the early days, and gradually build up your strength over six weeks with more repetitions.

Lower back Press the small of your back into the floor

Pelvic tilt Lie on the floor and support your head and shoulders with a cushion. Relax your arms at your sides and press your back into the floor. Keep your knees bent and your feet flat on the floor. As you exhale, press the small of your back into the floor for 10 seconds. Then release and relax. Repeat this 3–4 times initially, building up to 12 and then 24 repeats.

Legs Extend one leg at a time down to the floor

Leg slides Lie on your back with your head and shoulders supported, knees bent with feet flat, and arms at your sides. Exhale and slide one leg down until it is flat on the floor. Repeat with the other leg. Inhale and slowly bring one leg back up. Repeat with the other leg. Repeat the exercise 3–4 times. Increase gradually over the weeks until you can do 12 or more leg slides comfortably.

Arms Extend your arm along the floor for a full stretch

Keep one leg bent and extend the other right out along the floor

Spine alignment Lie on your back with your head and shoulders supported and knees bent with feet flat on the floor, and the small of your back pressed into the floor. Exhale and extend your right leg down so it is flat on the floor. Breathe in, then as you exhale stretch your right arm along the floor behind your head. On your next exhale, stretch from heel to fingertips. Repeat on the other side.

Resting pose Stretch out your arms and rest your forearms on the floor

Extended Child's Pose Get down onto all fours, then sit back on your heels, separate your knees, extend your arms out in front of you, and rest your forehead and your forearms on the floor. Your belly should rest between your thighs. Hold for 2 breaths or as long as it feels comfortable. This pose will enable you to elongate your back fully and release any tension in your hips.

Q I thought I'd get my stomach back quickly, but it's so wobbly! Will it ever recover?

Your stretched transverse abdominals and uterus mean that your belly won't recover its pre-pregnancy shape immediately. But fear not – the muscles will gradually recover and contract after the birth. The time it takes will be different for each person. Breastfeeding will help speed up the contraction of the uterus, as the hormone oxytocin, which is released when your baby latches on, contracts both the smooth muscles of the milk sacs in your breasts and the smooth muscle cells in your uterus walls.

You can start with some simple exercises to regain your waistline, but you must perform a simple check first on your abdominal muscles (see right). Once you feel a gap of just one finger-width between your transverse abdominals, begin with a simple head and shoulder lift. After your six-week check, move on to doing abdominal crunches and sit-ups.

Q How soon is it safe to start having sex after the birth?

Traditional advice recommends no sex until the six-week check, although there is no danger to your health if you have sex sooner. When you resume your sex life is a very individual issue, and something you should both take gently. If you feel ready to have sex again as soon as two to three weeks after the birth, that's fine. Penetrative sex may feel a little dry and painful though, so use a lubricant. However, don't feel pressured to resume your sex life until you feel ready. Exhaustion, soreness, and your physical recovery can all take its toll on your libido in the days, weeks, and even months following the birth. Take things slowly with your partner, discuss what you both want, and enjoy kissing and hugging until you are ready for sex. And don't worry if sex feels like it's out of the picture for the foreseeable future: a study conducted by the *British Journal of Obstetrics and Gynaecology* in 2013 found that only 41 per cent of first-time mothers had had vaginal intercourse by the time their baby was six weeks old. The most important thing to be aware of is that you are potentially fertile again, even if you are breastfeeding, so take precautions and use contraception.

Q How do I get back into shape after the six-week check?

Your aim to regain your former level of fitness, or improve your fitness if you were previously quite sedentary, should be gradual, and you shouldn't start high-impact activity too soon. Let your body be your guide.

Once you have the all-clear at six weeks, you can build your fitness levels again. However, before you hit the gym in a flurry, do a simple test. Lie on your back, place your hands behind your neck to support it, and slowly lift your head. As you hold that position, place a finger just above your belly button and press down gently to feel the gap between the muscles. If the gap is just one finger-width, you can start exercising normally; workout moderately for 30 minutes or more a day for three to six months and then gradually work up to high-impact sports. If it is wider – two or more finger-widths – don't resume regular exercise yet.

TRANSVERSE ABDOMINAL MUSCLE CHANGES

The natural changes that occur to your muscles in pregnancy need time to revert to normal before you can begin exercising again.

Linea alba — Abdominals

Pre-pregnancy The muscles are aligned at the front on either side of the linea alba.

Linea alba — Stretched muscles

During pregnancy The muscles stretch and usually split apart to allow the fetus to grow.

Contracting muscles — Closing gap

Postnatal The stretched muscles take time to close up again. You must wait until the gap has almost closed before resuming normal exercise.

Q I still have backache. Why hasn't it gone away now I've had my baby?

You need to continue to protect your back to prevent backache from bad posture and injury from lifting and carrying. Your loose ligaments, which still haven't tightened up yet, account for some of the pain. But constantly bending down to lift a baby can strain your back muscles. When you pick him or anything else up, bend from your knees, keep your back flat, hold him close to you, and lift up by straightening your legs. Check your posture, too, and keep your back straight and your shoulders back. Ideally your baby should be the heaviest thing you lift for at least the first six weeks after the birth.

In the early weeks after the birth, **resting** when you can and slowing down are two of the most **positive things** you can do, so **don't feel guilty.** Concentrate on your recovery and your baby, exercise gently, eat healthily, and your **energy levels will gradually return.**

Antenatal care

Antenatal care appointments steer you through your pregnancy journey. This chapter explains where your care will take place, who your **healthcare professionals** will be, and what is likely to happen at your **antenatal appointments**, from your booking in appointment through to your final visit just before you give birth. Find out about all the **tests and scans** on offer and start thinking about your **birth choices** and who you would like to be your birth partner.

The care that you receive during your pregnancy will be a mixture of **routine checks** and **personalized care** that works to look after the **health** of you and your baby. Your appointments are also an opportunity to **ask questions** that will inform your choices when you **plan and prepare** for the day your baby will arrive.

Your care explained

What your antenatal care involves

Once you've absorbed the news of finding out you are pregnant, you'll probably start to focus on the practicalities of what happens now. Should you go to see your doctor? How do you get yourself into the system of antenatal care? Who will look after your health and the health of your unborn baby?

For most women, there will be a standard number of regular appointments to check their progress; for others there can be extra appointments if their healthcare professionals need to keep a closer eye on them and their baby as they progress through pregnancy. You'll be offered routine blood and urine tests and your blood pressure will be checked. Advice on lifestyle and wellbeing will also be offered by your midwife. You can opt to be screened for infections and complications that could affect you or your baby, and there are scans and tests to assess your baby's health (see pp.92–103).

Antenatal appointments are a great opportunity to seek advice about the many changes you are experiencing, as well as to connect with your pregnancy, and with your baby (you'll find out how much she's growing and you might get to hear her heart beating). You can even go to birth preparation classes if you want to learn more about what happens during labour and birth, and how to care for your new baby afterwards.

Your birth, your choices

The healthcare team will lead your care so that you have a pregnancy that is as healthy and safe as possible, but they should take into account your needs and preferences. There will be some decisions about which tests you do and don't want, how and where you'd like to give birth, and whom you'd like with you when you do.

When planning your birth you might consider: Are you more comfortable with the idea of a home birth or a hospital birth? How would you describe your pain threshold? Does the idea of giving birth in water appeal or fill you with dread? What about giving birth standing up, sitting in a birthing chair, or lying down? Your answers to these questions might change over the course of your pregnancy – and that's fine, too. Mapping out your wishlists is a good way of honing in on specific aspects of your pregnancy, but don't let yourself get too frustrated if things don't always go to plan. Nature sometimes has different ideas, which is all part of the adventure.

Q What should I do when I first find out that I am pregnant?

Make an appointment at your doctor's surgery, or you can self-refer to a midwifery unit and book directly with a midwife. Your healthcare professional will schedule your first appointment with your community-based midwife, known as the booking appointment, for when you are 8–12 weeks pregnant.

You may be asked when the first day of your last menstrual period (LMP) was, in order to calculate an estimated date of delivery (EDD), or due date. Give your healthcare professional a rough idea if you don't know this date for certain; you'll be offered an ultrasound scan at around 12 weeks pregnant to assess the due date more accurately (see p.94).

You will need to tell your GP about the history of any previous pregnancies (including terminations), any health issues you have, and any relevant family medical history for both you and the baby's father. If you're taking medications, have them with you, so he or she can tell you if it's safe to continue taking them. Be prepared to say how long it has taken you to get pregnant (if you've been trying), and if you had fertility treatment. In the latter case, you will have an early scan to confirm the pregnancy and make sure all is well (see p.93).

You can be asked about your diet, alcohol consumption, and any smoking or drug use. It's important to be honest in your answers as this appointment is an opportunity to ensure that you get the best available care for yourself and your baby. Everything you tell your care team is confidential – even if you are under the age of 16.

Finally, you will be given information on nutrient supplements to take (including folic acid and vitamin D), food safety, nutrition, and the various screening tests available to you in pregnancy.

> You can ask your doctor about **any concerns** you have in the early weeks of pregnancy before you meet your midwife, whether about your health or that of your baby.

Q Who will look after my health, and that of my baby, during pregnancy?

If you have a straightforward pregnancy, your regular check-ups will be carried out at your doctor's surgery by a midwife (or doctor, depending on your area) rather than at a hospital. In most cases you will have one primary contact.

Your community midwife (the person who does your booking appointment) is usually your primary carer throughout. He or she will take your blood samples, conduct your urine tests, measure your blood pressure, and check the growth and wellbeing of your baby. He or she will also book your scans and be a regular point of contact for support and advice.

If your pregnancy is not straightforward, (if you have a multiple pregnancy, have pre-existing conditions or risk factors, or if any clinical factors develop during your pregnancy), you may be referred to a specialist for additional care.

When the time comes to have your baby, if you choose to have your baby at home, your community midwife may be the person who supports you during the birth, too – this is known as continuous care. If you go into hospital to have your baby, you will usually be cared for by hospital midwives.

You might meet the following healthcare professionals during your pregnancy:

» Your doctor is the first person to see when you become pregnant. You should continue to consult him or her during pregnancy about other health problems and medication.

» A community midwife conducts your antenatal appointments and monitors you throughout your pregnancy, and when you first come home after the birth. He or she is a point of contact for all your concerns.

» A sonographer is a midwife or radiographer trained to use and take readings from an ultrasound scanner in order to monitor the intrauterine health of your baby.

» An obstetrician is a doctor who specializes in pregnancy and birth. You'll see an obstetrician if your GP or midwife has a concern about your pregnancy or if you're carrying multiples, and sometimes as a matter of routine during your labour.

Q Can I check I've understood?

Q Can you explain it again?

Q Is there a leaflet I can take home?

You can always ask questions Quiz any healthcare professional you meet. There is often a lot of new information to absorb; asking the three questions suggested above can help to make things clearer.

» A gynaecologist is a doctor specializing in women's health. You may see a gynaecologist in the Early Pregnancy Unit (see p.94) if your midwife has a concern about your anatomy or reproductive health, for example, if you have cervical insufficiency (see p.147) or fibroids (see p.146). You may also see a gynaecologist if there are concerns in the third trimester.

» An anaesthetist is a doctor who specializes in pain relief and anaesthesia. You'll see an anaesthetist if you ask for an epidural in labour, or if you have a Caesarean section.

» A hospital midwife is one of a team of midwives who work within a hospital setting or birth centre during labour and birth. They also look after any women who have to be hospitalized during pregnancy.

Q What will happen at my booking appointment with the midwife?

The booking appointment is a chance to identify your needs (such as additional care for pre-existing conditions, extra monitoring for risk factors, or support for personal circumstances), discuss your options for screening tests, and do a health check. You and your midwife have a lot to discuss, so allow a couple of hours for the booking appointment. He or she will:

>> **Discuss your general medical history.** Give your midwife details of any illnesses or operations you've had, and about any medications you're taking.

>> **Ask you questions to get to know you**, your circumstances, and your family history.

>> **Take a history of your gynaecological health**, including your menstrual cycle, use of birth control, and details of any previous pregnancies (including your labours and your babies' health and weight at birth).

>> **Ask about your pregnancy symptoms** (tiredness, nausea, and so on) and whether you've had any bleeding.

>> **Ask about how you're feeling emotionally**. It's normal to feel anxious – even terrified and confused! – so don't be worried about saying so.

>> **Do a basic health check** to check for general wellbeing, including taking your BMI (see p.51) and blood pressure, and doing a urine test to check for infections. Your midwife may take blood samples if you opt for screening tests.

>> **Advise you about optional screening tests for your baby**, such as screening for spina bifida and Down's syndrome (see p.95-9).

>> **Give you information** about nutrition and diet, exercises (including pelvic floor exercises), your baby's development, antenatal classes, planning your labour and place of birth, and maternity benefits.

You will be given your own **antenatal notes**, which you need to bring along to every check-up that you have.

 ## How often will I have follow-up appointments?

In a straightforward first pregnancy, you will have follow-up appointments at 16, 25, 28, 31, 34, 36, 38, 40, and 41 weeks. If you opt for them, there will also be two ultrasound scans – one at 8 to 14 weeks (dating scan), and another at 18 to 22 weeks (anomaly scan).

If this is not your first pregnancy, there will be fewer follow-ups, usually at 16, 28, 34, 36, 38 and 41 weeks. You will still be offered two ultrasound scans if your pregnancy is free of complications.

Every antenatal appointment will involve a urine test and a blood pressure check. Your midwife will measure your bump (from 24 weeks) to check your baby's growth, and also feel your tummy to establish the position of your baby (from 36 weeks).

You'll be able to talk through any scan or screening test results, and implications where necessary. Over the course of your appointments, your midwife will discuss with you such topics as labour expectations, the use of vitamin K for your baby after birth, post-natal depression, and breastfeeding.

Q I've been to see my GP to tell him I'm pregnant, but he didn't do any tests. Is that normal?

It's perfectly normal. If you've had a positive home pregnancy test, the GP will accept it as confirmation of your pregnancy since they are so reliable now. Finding out you have conceived, whether it's planned, unexpected, long-awaited, or quick, can feel instantly life-changing for you, but unless your GP suspects anything is amiss after talking with you, antenatal tests won't begin until your booking appointment. Take it as a good sign that you don't need tests right away. For now, remember to ask your GP any questions you have and gather information.

Q I have a nine-month-old baby and I'm pregnant again. Are there risks?

It's important that you see your doctor as soon as you know you are pregnant because your body can take at least a year to recover before safely undertaking pregnancy again. Problems are, of course, relatively rare, but it's important that you are carefully monitored from the start and advised about how best to cope with both the demands on your body and looking after a small baby during the tiring early stages of pregnancy. Pregnancies that occur in quick succession raise the risk of placental abruption (see p.147), low birthweight for your baby, and your own nutritional deficiency.

Q My midwife has said that our relationship is confidential. Can I really trust him or her?

It's important that you and your midwife develop a mutually trusting relationship that enables him or her to provide you with the most appropriate advice and care. However, your midwife's responsibility for your health and your baby's health means that he or she may sometimes have to share medical details relevant to your pregnancy with doctors or other medical professionals, such as informing your obstetrician if you have a sexually transmitted disease, a dependency (for example, on drugs or alcohol), or you feel especially anxious or depressed.

Q Can I use a private midwife and keep my rights to NHS care?

Yes. Having a private midwife does not change your right to antenatal care, tests, and scans on the NHS, and your private midwife can work alongside an NHS community midwife. A private midwife can work well if you want to ensure continuity of care, and he or she often can carry out more complicated procedures when not limited by NHS rules of practice. However, if you have a hospital birth, it may be led by hospital midwives, though your private midwife can support you. Choose someone who is registered with the Royal College of Midwives.

Q What blood tests are taken at my antenatal appointments?

A range of tests can check for blood type, infections, genetic diseases, and anaemia. Your midwife may take samples for the following:

» **Your blood type and rhesus status** Tested once in early pregnancy. Your blood type (A, B, AB, or O) will be recorded in your notes in case for any reason you need a transfusion during delivery. If you are rhesus negative (see p.82) you will need one or two additional injections.

» **Hepatitis B** Tested once, in early pregnancy. This viral infection can cause liver damage in the baby, and the baby needs treatment at birth.

» **Anaemia** Tested at the booking appointment and at 28 weeks. A full blood count can suggest anaemia if your haemoglobin levels are low. It also tests levels of blood folate and vitamin B_{12}, blood platelets, and white cell count (to check you aren't fighting an infection).

» **Rubella immunity** Tested once in early pregnancy. The rubella virus can cause serious congenital abnormalities in babies (see p.139). If you're not immune, you can't be vaccinated in pregnancy so your midwife will advise on how to minimize your risk of exposure in pregnancy.

» **HIV and syphilis** Tested once in early pregnancy. These diseases pose a significant risk to your baby if you don't know about them – but your baby can be protected if you do. You have the right to refuse an HIV/AIDS test.

» **Sickle cell disease and thalassaemia** Tested once in early pregnancy. This is a test for genetic blood disorders that can be passed to the baby. Usually offered to those at risk of being carriers.

» **Other tests** If you're at high risk, you may have blood tests for hepatitis C, vitamin D deficiency, toxoplasmosis, and for chickenpox immunity if you're not sure of your history.

Q Will I be screened for Group B streptococcus (or GBS)?

There is no screening for GBS because it affects a very small percentage of babies in the UK. If you're worried, ask your midwife for a screening test, or have one done privately. You'll have two swabs, one vaginal and one rectal, at between 35 and 37 weeks pregnant. If you carry the infection, you may be offered intravenous antibiotics during your labour; or the baby will be given antibiotics as soon as he is born.

Q Why do I need to provide a urine sample at each appointment?

Your midwife tests urine for protein (high levels indicate high blood pressure, pre-eclampsia, urinary tract infection, or kidney disease). You can bring a sample with you (ask for a sterile pot), or provide one at appointments.

If you are aged 25 or under, you will be offered a urine test for chlamydia, too.

Q Will I need a whooping cough vaccine? Why?

You will be offered a whooping cough vaccine between 28 and 38 weeks. Cases of whooping cough have gone up in recent years. Babies are routinely vaccinated against the virus at two months, but before this time they're vulnerable to infection. If you are vaccinated in pregnancy the immunity crosses the placenta and protects your baby in the weeks after birth.

Q Why is my blood pressure measured at every check-up? What are they looking for?

Pregnancy-induced hypertension (high blood pressure) (see p.144) can restrict the flow of blood to your baby, interfering with his growth. Your midwife will take your blood pressure throughout your pregnancy in order to be vigilant.

If your blood pressure rises too much, it also carries risks for you (the same risks as high blood pressure in non-pregnant people). It can also be a symptom of pre-eclampsia (see p.144), along with protein in your urine. Average pregnancy blood pressure is actually a little lower than normal non-pregnancy blood pressure for most of pregnancy, because hormones dilate your arteries to cope with the extra blood volume your pregnant body creates to grow your baby. By the end of pregnancy, you have about an extra litre (1 ¾ pint) of blood pumping around your body.

Blood pressure readings These have an upper number (systolic) that denotes the pressure in your arteries when your heart pumps, and a lower number (diastolic) for the pressure between pumps when your heart rests.

Q Why am I being tested for rhesus status? What is it?

As well as having a blood group (A, B, AB, and O), all blood is either rhesus positive or rhesus negative.

A blood test early in pregnancy checks rhesus status. About 15 per cent of people have rhesus negative blood. If your blood is rhesus negative and your baby's blood is rhesus positive, you may develop antibodies (defensive cells) if the baby's blood leaks into your blood. This contact can happen for example during a miscarriage or termination, at birth, or if you fall on your tummy. It doesn't usually affect first babies, but once you have developed antibodies, these can attack a subsequent rhesus-positive baby, causing anaemia in the baby. In a first pregnancy, you'll be offered anti-D serum injections to prevent antibodies developing if you're Rhesus negative. If your blood already has antibodies, extra scans will monitor the baby, and treatment may be needed.

Fetal blood is rhesus positive

Mother's blood is rhesus negative

Fetal blood enters mother's bloodstream

Antibodies cross placenta

Antibody

1 In a first pregnancy, a rhesus-positive baby's blood will not cause issues unless it leaks into the rhesus-negative mother's body.

2 During childbirth the mother's rhesus negative blood creates antibodies in reaction to the "foreign" blood.

3 In a subsequent pregnancy, the antibodies can destroy a rhesus positive baby's blood cells, causing anaemia in utero and jaundice after birth.

Q How will my midwife know if my baby is growing properly?

Your baby's growth is usually monitored by the growth of your uterus from its highest point (fundus) to the top of the pubic bone (symphsis pubis). This is called the "symphysis fundal height" (SFH) and, interestingly, the measurement in centimetres often corresponds to your baby's gestational age in weeks. Your midwife will check your fundal height at every appointment from 24 weeks until birth, using a tape measure placed over your tummmy as you lie on your back. The fundal height is recorded on a centile chart that plots this measurement against your baby's gestational age. At your next appointment a new fundal height measurement will indicate whether or not your baby is growing as expected. Before you are 24 weeks pregnant, your dating and anomaly scans (see p.95 and pp.100-01) indicate how your baby is growing, and your midwife might listen to your baby's heartbeat at your check-ups. Towards the end of pregnancy, your midwife will palpate your tummy (see right) to check your baby's position and growth.

Q Do I need to go to antenatal classes? How do I choose them if I do?

Whether or not you attend classes is entirely up to you. However, there are great benefits if you do – including learning about your pregnancy, labour, and birth, and how to look after your newborn baby. You will also meet other mums- and dads-to-be in your area due at the same time, which can be a great support when you are a new parent.

Your midwife will give you details of local antenatal classes – both those run by your community midwives and private classes run by organizations such as the National Childbirth Trust (NCT). You can attend either course, or both if you wish. Most antenatal courses begin at around eight to 10 weeks before the baby is due (at 30 to 32 weeks pregnant). If you are expecting twins or more, you should book your classes to begin when you are around 24 weeks pregnant, because your babies are more likely to be born early. Classes usually run for between three and six weeks, with one class every week, and each class lasting up to two hours.

Antenatal classes are very popular, so it is a good idea to put your name down when you are 13 to 15 weeks pregnant to get a place.

Antenatal classes You are encouraged to bring along your birth partner, so that he or she can learn some specific techniques to relax you during labour.

Q Is it safe to use complementary therapies in pregnancy?

There are certain complementary therapies, or aspects of them, that are not safe for you or your baby during pregnancy. Your midwife is trained to support you in your decisions about your care and will guide you on what is appropriate and what's not, based on medical evidence. Avoid buying over-the-counter remedies, and consult a practitioner qualified in antenatal care before using any oil or herb.

» Chiropractic: useful for back and joint pain. Always look for a practitioner with a qualification in antenatal care.

» Acupressure, acupuncture, and shiatsu: can help with nausea and sickness in early pregnancy. Always go to a practitioner qualified in antenatal care.

» Bach flower remedies: can help with stress and anxiety. Clinical studies consider Bach Flower Remedies to have a "psychophysiological" effect only – that is, feeling that you're taking control of an issue is the effective part of the treatment, rather than any active ingredient in the treatment itself.

» Osteopathy: useful for back and joint pain. Always choose an osteopath trained to treat pregnant women.

» Homeopathy: can help with nausea and sickness, and fatigue. It is a matter of continuing medical debate as to how and why homeopathy works – but it seems to. Use it only under close, qualified supervision.

» Hypnotherapy: can help you manage labour pain. See a practitioner who can teach you self-help techniques to keep you relaxed and focused during your labour and birth.

» Moxibustion: reported to help turn a breech baby. Moxibustion is a form of traditional Chinese Medicine – choose only a qualified practitioner trained in antenatal care.

» Massage: useful for stress, anxiety, back and joint pain. Find a masseuse trained in antenatal care. You shouldn't lie on your back in the third trimester – instead lie on your side or try a foot, facial, or hand massage. Avoid essential oils.

Q What's my midwife feeling for when she presses on my tummy?

Your midwife's pressing, stroking, and pushing movements across, above, and below your bump are known as "palpation". He or she will do this primarily to determine the position of your baby from around 36 weeks onwards.

By palpating your tummy, your midwife will be able to tell when your baby has moved into the head-down position ready for birth, when your baby's head has "engaged" (moved downwards into your pelvic area), whether your baby is curled over, head to chest (the ideal position for birth), or is more extended, and the position of the baby's spine compared with your spine. As you lie on your back, your midwife will use both hands to smoothly and firmly feel all over your tummy with the pads of his or her fingers. Try to stay relaxed throughout the procedure, as this makes the palpation more accurate. Let your midwife know if anything causes you any discomfort.

Fundal palpation This manoeuvre checks what part of your baby's body is at the top of your uterus. At 36 weeks, it's hoped to be your baby's bottom.

Lateral palpation Your midwife's hands move to the side of your abdomen so that he or she can check the position of your baby's spine.

Pelvic palpation This helps your midwife determine what part of your baby is in your pelvis. It's the most important manoeuvre in the palpation sequence.

Pawlick's grip This is a form of pelvic palpation and it tells your midwife whether your baby's head faces downwards and is engaged in your pelvis.

Q My mother is a twin. Should I tell my care team about that?

Yes, do say if your mother has a family history of non-identical twins. In some cases, you may go for a scan as early as five weeks to see if you are carrying more than one baby. However, about 20 to 30 per cent of twin embryos seen early on become single pregnancies before the next scan – known as "vanishing twin syndrome". Specialists are not sure what causes it but there are no ill effects on the remaining embryo.

Q Will my symptoms be twice as bad if I'm carrying twins?

Some pregnancy symptoms may be more severe (but not twice as bad) than if you were carrying a singleton, but thankfully this is not the case for everyone. Nausea can be worse because you'll have higher hCG levels than in a single pregnancy. You may also put on more weight, and more quickly; in later pregnancy this can put added strain on your back. You might be more breathless as your babies grow and push against your diaphragm. You are also more likely to experience swelling, heartburn, constipation, and indigestion.

When it comes to labour and birth, having twins (or more) should not take much longer than if, under the same circumstances, you were to give birth to only one baby. Very rarely, "deferred labour" of the second baby can occur: the first baby is born, then labour stops and there is a significant gap (a day or more) before the second baby arrives. Your hospital would offer you lots of support and careful monitoring until the second baby was born.

Q Are my twins identical or non-identical?

You're not the only one who is curious to know the answer – your medical team will want to find out whether your twins are identical, and more importantly whether they share a placenta or even an amniotic sac.

Placenta ⎯
Smaller twin ⎯

Placentas

SHARED PLACENTA **SEPARATE PLACENTAS**

Identicality often becomes obvious as twin babies grow older.

You will usually find out if you are carrying multiple babies at your dating scan, when you are between 8 and 14 weeks pregnant. At this scan, the sonographer will assess what type of placenta the babies have (chorionicity) and what type of amniotic sac (amnionicity), as this is critical for their care.

Chorionicity and amnionicity

All non-identical twins have separate placentas (dichorionic) and amniotic sacs because they come from two different eggs that each attach separately to the uterus (see p.33). Sometimes the two placentas can fuse, but they are still considered dichorionic. Identical twins may or may not have separate placentas and amniotic sacs, depending on how early the initial fertilized egg (zygote) divided. A split within three to four days of fertilization creates a placenta and

Mono- and dichorionic identical twins A shared placenta may cause unequal blood circulation, thereby restricting the growth of one twin. Babies with separate placentas, and separate blood circulation, are more likely to grow to equal size.

amniotic sac for each twin (one-third of cases); a split during days four to eight forms one shared placenta (monochorionic – the majority of identical twins) and two amniotic sacs (diamniotic); after eight days, the babies will share both a placenta and an amniotic sac (monochorionic and monoamniotic).

Twin-to-twin transfusion syndrome

A shared placenta can result in "twin-to-twin transfusion syndrome" (TTTS), when one baby "donates" blood to the other, but fails to thrive properly itself. Furthermore, the extra blood can put a strain on the receiving twin's heart. This condition occurs in about 15 per cent of identical twin pregnancies. If you've monochorionic twins, you may have scans every two to three weeks from 16 weeks to keep a close eye on how the babies are growing. Recent obstetric advances have improved the survival rates of twins with TTTS, with laser surgery helping to ensure a better flow of blood between the babies.

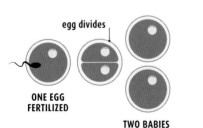

egg divides

ONE EGG FERTILIZED

TWO BABIES

TWO EGGS FERTILIZED **TWO BABIES**

Identical twins (monozygotic) When a single egg that is fertilized by a single sperm splits in two, it forms twins that share the same DNA: identical. They are always the same sex.

Non-identical twins (dizygotic) If two eggs are fertilized by two different sperm, your twins will have different DNA: non-identical. They may be the same sex or different sexes.

Q I'm carrying twins. Will my antenatal care be different from someone carrying a single baby?

You'll be more closely monitored than a woman carrying just one baby. You won't necessarily have complications, but since there is higher risk with multiple pregnancies you will have more antenatal appointments and ultrasound scans than for a single pregnancy. Your check-ups may be in hospital with an obstetrician and a midwife rather than a midwife alone. You may even be assigned a midwife who specializes in multiple births to offer you support and advice.

Q I wanted to have a home birth. Can I still do that if I'm carrying twins?

Multiple births generally happen in hospital because there is a greater risk of complications during labour, and thus they need larger medical teams. It's more likely that your babies will be in a difficult position for birth, for example, or suffer a cord prolapse (when the umbilical cord starts to protrude from your uterus ahead of the baby). It's also more likely that one or both of your babies will have low birthweight, which requires specialist care in a hospital immediately after they are born.

Q I feel a bit daunted about having twins. Is there someone I can talk to?

Your midwife can put you in touch with local twin (and greater multiple) support groups and other recent mothers of twins. Try to gather as much information and reassurance as you can – and also any practical tips about how best to look after yourself and your babies in pregnancy and after the birth. Organisations such as Twins UK and TAMBA (see pp.338–39) are a good source of information and advice for parents of twins. You should also be able to start antenatal classes earlier than women carrying singletons, usually around 24 weeks, rather than the usual 30 or 32 weeks. Encourage your partner to come to these classes, too – although the role of a partner can never be underestimated for any mother and baby, when it comes to multiple births, the practical and emotional support of your partner will be more significant than ever.

Q Is it possible to have a vaginal birth if I'm carrying multiples?

If you are having three or more babies, you will be recommended a Caesarean section as the safest option. With twins, a vaginal birth is possible if your pregnancy is uncomplicated and the babies are in good positions at labour.

Towards the end of pregnancy, multiple babies have less space in the uterus and the placenta(s) can become less efficient. For these reasons, unless the babies arrive prematurely, you'll have a scheduled early C-section for triplets or more; twin pregnancies are offered induction at 37 weeks plus for monochorionic twins, and 38 weeks plus for dichorionic twins (see opposite and pp.224–25). You could be offered an elective C-section for a twin pregnancy if there are known complications such as a shared placenta or amniotic sac, one or both of your babies are especially small, the placenta is low-lying, you have had a previous C-section, or if you've had complications such as pre-eclampsia. If your pregnancy has been a healthy one, you may be able to have a natural birth. Your options will depend on how the twin who is closest to the birth canal (the "presenting" twin) is positioned in your uterus.

BOTH CEPHALIC

ONE BREECH

ONE TRANSVERSE

BOTH BREECH

Both cephalic (head down) When both babies are head down, there is a good chance of successful vaginal birth for both. Around 45 per cent of twins present in this position.

One breech (bottom first) About 25 per cent of twins present with the first baby head down, and the second breech. In this case, vaginal birth of the first twin is possible. If the presenting twin is breech, a Caesarean section is advised.

One transverse (horizontal) Babies who lie transverse can turn, so if the presenting twin is head down, vaginal birth may be possible. If the presenting baby is breech, a Caesarean section is more likely.

Both breech When both babies are bottom first, in most cases you will be offered a Caesarean section because the babies are less likely to turn.

Women pregnant with multiples are at a slightly increased risk of pre-eclampsia, **anaemia**, low-lying placenta, and **mid-term bleeding.** For all these reasons, your **antenatal** healthcare professionals will be **extra-vigilant** throughout your pregnancy.

{Q Is it possible to choose where I have my baby?

It's possible to choose a location as long as your healthcare provider says that you can and your local area has the facilities. The main choices are to give birth in a hospital, at home, in a birthing centre or unit (a dedicated building, sometimes attached to a hospital) or in a free-standing midwifery unit. Studies show that for low-risk pregnancies, home births are as safe as hospital ones.

Visit each venue

In order to make an informed decision, it's advisable to take a tour of all the places you can give birth at. When visiting a venue bring a notepad with you to jot down answers to your questions. Don't be afraid to trust your instincts. If you're considering a home birth meet with your healthcare professionals to discuss this option. Your midwife will give you a list of what you will need to have for a home birth.

What to ask at every venue

- Who will manage my birth plan?
- How easy is it to park and how far away is the parking?
- If I felt unable to travel once I went into labour, would one of your midwives be able to come to me at home or would I need to go to hospital or the unit?
- Do you have birthing balls, mats, and chairs available in every birthing suite?
- Can I give birth in water?
- How many birth partners can I have?
- Can I bring my other children?
- Can my partner stay with me overnight after the baby has been born?
- How soon will I be able to go home?
- What pain relief will be available to me when I'm in labour?
- Other than my birth partner, who will be in the room with me?
- Will the baby stay with me all the time?
- What help will I have with starting to breastfeed?

Monitoring equipment This includes a sphygmomanometer (to measure your blood pressure) and an electronic fetal monitor (to measure your baby's heartbeat and the strength of uterine contractions).

A bed for your baby This is ready and waiting. There is also a resuscitator in the room just in case the baby needs to be kept warm or given oxygen.

Hospital birth room This contains a range of medical equipment. On a trolley in the room there will be a delivery pack, surgical scissors, a haemostat, umbilical clamp, and instrumental equipment such as a speculum and amniotic hook. There may also be piped gas outlets in the wall as a source of "gas and air" pain relief, as well as oxygen.

A birthing bed This can be raised and lowered electronically. There are leg stirrups at the end of the bed to raise your legs if a forceps delivery or stitches are needed. There may be a bed pan, urinary catheter, and sick bowl.

Chairs and comfort aids There is usually a chair for you or your birth partner to rest in. There might also be a birthing pool and an exercise ball.

THE PROS AND CONS OF WHERE TO HAVE YOUR BABY

Remember it's never too late to change your mind and if your circumstances change you may have to rethink your decision. This table sets out some of the points to consider when you are deciding where to have your baby.

 Hospital

 Instant specialist medical attention if necessary.
» All forms of pain relief available.
» All technical gadgets and gizmos to react quickly in a changing labour situation.
» Baby unit (NICU) usually available if your baby needs medical attention immediately after birth.

 Lack of continuous care
» The midwife you see during your pregnancy will not be the one who supports you in labour.
» There may be changes of shifts during your labour, so you may see several hospital midwives before you have your baby.
» Increased likelihood of having to spend a night on the postnatal ward after your baby is born.

 Birthing centre

 Midwife-led care in a low-tech envirnoment attached to a hospital.
» Although the unit is independently run, full medical care is close by.
» More relaxed birthing environment.
» More opportunity to let your labour run its course without intervention.
» Lower rates of assisted birth (use of forceps or ventouse).
» May lead to a shorter labour.
» Fewer Caesarean sections.
» Greater chance that your birth partner can stay overnight.

 40 per cent of women giving birth to their first baby have to go into hospital anyway (and about 10 per cent for second or subsequent babies), although there is more immediate access to full medical care.

 Home

 Continuous care.
» Your community midwife is likely to be the person who supports you in labour.
» You won't have to endure travelling during labour.
» Statistically reduced risk of assisted birth.
» You're at home with your baby right from the start.

 40 per cent of women giving birth to their first baby have to go into hospital anyway (and about 10 per cent for second or subsequent babies).
» No access to pain relief (you may hire a TENS unit, or your midwife may have a portable gas-and-air machine).
» Your birth partner may not be allowed to come in the ambulance with you if you have to go to hospital.

■ Will someone show me how to change a nappy, top and tail, and bath the baby?
■ What happens if I decide to bottle-feed – do I have to bring the bottles and formula with me?
■ Can we buy snacks and drinks here during labour, or should we bring them with us?
■ What facilities do you have for playing music in the birthing room?

What to ask at hospital
■ Will I be moved to a ward after I've had the baby?
■ Is an anaesthetist always available if I want an epidural?

■ What are the visiting hours and do they apply to my partner? What are the visiting hours for siblings?
■ Are there any single rooms and, if so, how are they allocated? Do we have to pay for them?

What to ask at a birthing unit
■ How quickly could I get to hospital if I needed to, and would I need to go in an ambulance?
■ For what reasons would I need to go into hospital and which hospital would I go to?
■ Is a medical doctor able to come to the unit in an emergency?

 Did you know...

In the 1930s, about 80 per cent of babies were born at home. This figure fell to around 30 per cent in the 1960s, and is now less than 3 per cent. In a healthy pregnancy it's fine to have a home birth. Free-standing midwifery units, available in some areas, offer a similar experience to home births, providing a relaxing birth environment. However, as with home births, if you have a complication in labour, you'll need to transfer to hospital.

Q What is a birth plan? Do I need one and, if so, when should I write it?

A birth plan is your opportunity to put down on paper your preferences for labour and birth. You don't have to have one, but it's a good idea to at least think through what you would like. You can create it at any time.

A birth plan is a means of thinking through what's important to you about the process of having your baby and to highlight any queries you might have for your healthcare professional. It can include anything and everything from what music you'd like to have playing to the type of pain relief you'd prefer. You can start writing a birth plan as soon as you like, and amend it and add to it as your pregnancy progresses, gathering wisdom and ideas from midwives, medical staff, family, friends, and other mums-to-be. It is worth remembering though that labour does not always go according to plan; you need to be flexible in the event that you or your baby need medical assistance at any time that means you may need to deviate from your birth plan.

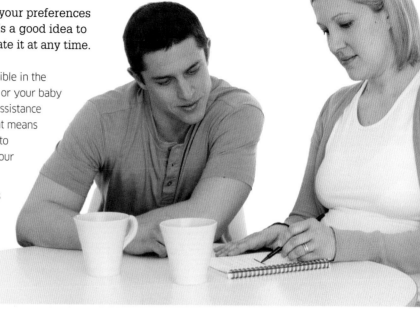

Your preferences
Run through your wishes with your partner.

STRUCTURING YOUR BIRTH PLAN

Use the following headings and ideas as a guide to writing your birth plan. Remember that it can be more or less detailed than this.

 » My birth environment: Where you want to labour and give birth; what music (if any) you want playing; any other ways in which you want to set the right mood.

 » Emotional support and your personal care: Who you want with you and how you want them to support you; whether you want your birth partner near your head, or at the birth end; what snacks and drinks you'd like.

» Positions and props: My preferred position for birth, whether or not you want to move around during labour, and whether or not you want to use a ball or chair and so on.

 » Pain relief and physical care: Whether you're happy to have pain relief and if so, what kind; if there are any forms of pain relief you want to avoid; whether or not you are happy to have an episiotomy if your midwife thinks it would ease your labour.

 » Caring for my baby during birth: Whether you want to stay upright and mobile while your midwife is checking your baby's heart rate; if you have any objections to your baby's heart rate being monitored continuously.

 » Assisted birth: If you are given a choice, whether or not you have a preference for forceps or ventouse; whether you are happy to be given drugs to increase the strength of your contractions.

 » The moment of birth: Whether or not you'd like your baby placed on your tummy; who holds your baby first; whether you or your partner would like to announce the sex; who will cut the umbilical cord, and if you'd like to delay cord-cutting.

 » My placenta: Whether you want to deliver the placenta naturally, or you want medication to speed along delivery of the placenta; whether you'd like to see your placenta, or even keep it.

 » Caring for my newborn: Your wishes for feeding and skin-to-skin contact; who holds the baby while you deliver the placenta or have any stitches.

 » Telling the world: Who you'd like told first about the birth and even in what order; whether there are certain people you'd like to tell yourself, or whether you're happy to let your birth partner spread the news to everyone.

 » Emergencies: If you're having a home birth, which hospital you want to go to (if you have a choice) in an emergency; if you're having your baby at an independent midwifery unit, where you'd like to be transferred if you have an emergency.

 » Special requirements: Whether English is your first language; if you need a sign language interpreter; if you have special dietary requirements; if you or your partner has special needs; if you would like certain religious customs to be observed.

Write your **birth plan** using broad headings – see the box below for **some ideas**. Make the plan as **detailed** or as **vague** as you want. Read about the birth and all the options available to help you think ahead to what you might want. It's important to make sure you feel **confident** and **fully informed** about all of your choices beforehand.

» Caesarean sections: Who you want with you in theatre; what music (if any) you want playing in theatre; whether you would like the screen lowered at the moment your baby is born so that you can see the obstetrician lift the baby out; if you would like silence among the medical staff as your baby is lifted out so that yours can be the first voice your baby hears; who you would like to cuddle your baby if you have to have a general anaesthetic, and whether you are happy for your birth partner to tell anyone else about the birth and baby before you've woken up from the anaesthetic. Also, if you've had a general anaesthetic, whether you'd like your baby to be bottle-fed from the breast milk bank, or to have formula if he needs feeding before you wake up. Whether you would like a video or photographs taken of your baby as he's lifted out of your uterus; whether you'd like to have skin-to-skin contact and to try to breastfeed while your uterus and abdomen are being stitched, or you're happy for your partner to hold your baby until you're settled in the post-op room.

Q My partner has some ideas for the birth plan, but I don't agree with them all. Should I try to fit them in?

Your birth plan is about your care during your labour, so ultimately it should reflect your wishes. However, parenting is something that you are going to do together, so if there are things he feels strongly about that matter less to you, then in the spirit of this new and exciting joint venture, make sure you give his views consideration. When it comes to anything that might happen to your body your wishes and the advice of your healthcare professionals always comes first.

Q Will I need to have my birth plan with me while I'm in labour? What if I'm too distracted to remember what's in it?

Your midwife will put a copy of your birth plan in your antenatal notes so that it is available to whoever is caring for you at the time of your labour. It's also a good idea to give a copy to your birth partner, who can represent your wishes if you aren't able to articulate them yourself. Do brief your birth partner, though, that although you might have said you want to avoid an assisted birth, for example, if the situation dictates that this is the safest way for your baby to be born and you understand why, your midwife's advice is paramount.

Q What does VBAC stand for and is it something I should consider?

VBAC stands for "vaginal birth after Caesarean section" and it means exactly what it says: if you had a C-section for your last birth, you might be able to have a vaginal birth instead this time. Assuming that you are able to have a VBAC, whether or not you want one is entirely a matter of personal choice and practicality. For example, you will recover more quickly from a vaginal birth than from a C-section, which can make it easier to look after your other children with a newborn in tow, too. A VBAC can have fewer complications than a second C-section, but this is not always the case.

Q Are there any reasons that I wouldn't be able to have a VBAC?

You will be able to have a VBAC as long as your previous Caesarean section was straightforward, and for pregnancy rather than anatomical reasons. So, if you had a complication during labour that made C-section a safer way to deliver your baby, there's no reason why you wouldn't be able to have a VBAC this time. However, if you weren't able to give birth vaginally because, for example, you have a small pelvis that makes it hard for your baby to get through, you will probably have to have a second C-section. If the cut in your uterus was a standard horizontal incision, you should be fine for a VBAC, but cuts elsewhere into your uterus will need to be considered on a case-by-case basis.

Q What's the likelihood that I'll end up having another C-section, even if I start out with the hope of a VBAC?

Assuming you had a straightforward, non-anatomical-related previous Caesarean section (see above), there is a 70 to 85 per cent success rate for VBAC. Specifically relating to your previous C-section, the main obstacle to success is that there's around a 0.5 per cent chance that you develop a tear along your scar line during your contractions. The risk of a tear occurring during VBAC rises to 1 per cent if you have had two previous C-sections; there is little data on the risks after three or more C-sections. It's often a case of waiting to see what happens.

70–85% Most hospitals record VBAC success rates of 70 to 85 per cent.

Q What should I look for in a birth partner?

Ideally the person you have by your side during labour and birth will be incredibly patient, cool under pressure, and extremely caring. Here's a list of the qualities your perfect birth partner would possess:

» **A sense of calm:** a natural ability to stop you from getting worried or stressed.

» **Confidence:** to support your wishes and to support your medical team if they offer advice that will speed your birth and is in the interests of the best health for you and your baby, even if that's at odds with your birth plan.

» **Being able to respond:** and take comments or wishes from you without judging them - or taking offence.

» **Reasonable lack of squeamishness:** at the sight of blood or sick.

» **Empathy:** someone who can respond to your mood without even being asked to, and in the right way.

» **A firm respect for medical care:** knowing when to step aside to let the medical team work with you unimpeded and unchallenged.

» **Someone without any time restrictions:** a person who can give you all of his or her attention, unselfishly and unequivocally throughout your labour, however long it may take.

» **Someone who will talk through any decisions:** while you're in labour, he or she can give you sensible, sound advice with the interests of you and your baby in mind.

Back massage Your birth partner should be willing and able to give you a gentle massage during the early stages of labour. You can practise together before labour begins.

Q What is a doula and how can they help with my labour and birth?

From the Greek word for "caregiver", a doula is a birthing companion whom you choose to help prepare you for labour and birth, stay with you throughout birth, and, sometimes, help after the birth. This can be in practical ways (with household chores, for example) and by giving advice on babycare and breastfeeding. Some doulas offer only antenatal care and birth support, and others specialize in postnatal care. Some will do both. Research in the UK suggests that C-section rates fall by as much as 50 per cent for women who have a doula as a birth partner, and that labour may be up to two hours shorter. If you employ a doula as a birth partner, she can also support your partner if you wish – talking him through what's happening, reassuring him, and guiding him on how best to help you.

Q Will I still need a midwife if I have a doula?

Yes, as doulas work alongside midwives and do not replace a midwife's role, but rather provide extra support and continuity of care. A doula isn't necessarily medically trained, though she will have completed a doula course that means she can support pregnancy in safe, medically recognized ways. If you wish to use a doula, you will need to hire one privately. Look for a doula who has a qualification that is accredited by the governing body in your country (such as Doula UK or Doulas of North America).

Today more **fathers** than ever attend the births of **their babies**. However, a close family member or friend, a **private midwife**, or **a doula** are also all good choices to **support** you, or both you and your partner through **labour and birth**.

Q I have more than one person in mind as a birth partner. Am I allowed to have two?

Most hospitals will allow two birth partners to be present in the delivery room with you (you may be able to have more, as long as none of them interferes with the medical staff). Talk to both of your potential birth partners and ensure they each understand that the other will be there. Check, in particular, that your partner is happy about the arrangement – this is an intimate occasion and he or she may feel strongly that it's something that needs to happen only between the two of you. It can be good to assign roles to each person attending – perhaps you can ask one birth partner to be there to support you emotionally, while the other one takes a more practical role, ensuring you have enough snacks and drinks and creating the right ambience in the room for you. Be clear about whom, if anyone, you want to be at the birthing end of the event. The last thing you want is for each of them to start jostling to get the best view.

Q Can I have my older children present at my home birth?

Talk to your community midwife in advance of your labour and establish what the rules are for accommodating other children. If your older children are with you, it's a good idea to assign someone else to look after them for snacks and general entertainment (remember, labour can be a long process). That person may be your partner or another adult who has come to help. Your children shouldn't be a distraction for you or source of worry. They shouldn't get in the way or interfere with the procedure. Also, consider your children's ages and personalities and whether or not you think they will be able to cope with seeing their mum go through labour and birth. Even an easy birth can be traumatic for young children to witness. Talk through with them what's going to happen, and tell them that giving birth hurts the mummy, but it's safe pain and goes away as soon as the baby is born. Use words suitable for your children's level of understanding and encourage lots of questions. If you decide, on reflection, that it might be too much for them, ask a close friend or a grandparent to occupy them nearby

Q Is the baby's dad less likely to bond with the baby in the long term if he isn't at the birth?

Studies show that his presence at the birth doesn't make a difference to a dad's ability to bond with his baby.

As long as he is fully engaged in the newborn's care once he or she has arrived in the world, a dad will definitely bond with his baby in the long term. Bonding is an intense attachment between parents and their baby. Bonding with a baby takes time and is a process that takes place as a mum or dad gets to know and looks after a newborn baby. It gives a parent the desire to nurture and care for their baby. The only measurable difference is that fathers who are present at the birth tend to be more confident handling the baby; fathers who feel really positive about watching the birth tend to be more willing to take care of the baby independently of the mother (which gives you the opportunity to have a break every now and then).

Doting dad Make sure dad is just as involved as you with nappy changing and outfit changes from the start. Encourage him to have skin-to-skin contact and make sure he gets to hold your new bundle of joy.

(in the garden if it's nice weather or in another room in your home) and invite them in only once (even as soon as) the baby has been born. It will be an unforgettable experience for everyone involved.

Q My partner doesn't think he'll be able to cope with seeing me in pain during labour. What can be done to help?

Many men confess that the hardest part of being with their partners as they give birth is seeing them go through pain and feeling helpless to do anything about it. The person you have with you during labour and birth needs to be calm, composed, and authoritative (with you and perhaps with the hospital staff); sometimes making decisions for you based on your birth plan. If your partner thinks he's likely to panic or faint, perhaps he may indeed be better waiting outside the delivery room until after your baby is born. You have several options:

» **Separate birth partner** Choose someone whom you trust entirely as a birth partner and who can support you fully to stay in the delivery room from start to finish, calling your partner in only when the baby is born.

» **The early part** Have your partner in the room with you, but have someone else available to come in as soon as your partner finds it's getting too much for him to be present.

» **Time limit** Ask your partner to stay with you for as long as he can stand it, and then to step out and let the hospital's midwives support you until the baby is born.

» **Stay throughout** Ask your partner to stay the whole time, but tell him that it's fine if he stays at your head end (in which case it's unlikely that he'll see anything too gory) and turns away if he wants to during any stressful moments. Practise breathing techniques together so that you can both use them to relax during labour – for you to cope with the pain, and for him to cope with you being in pain.

During your pregnancy, you will be offered a series of **scans and tests** to monitor the **growth** and **development** of your baby, and to ensure that your own body is coping well with your pregnancy. **Scans** provide a wonderful opportunity to **"meet" your baby** and various **tests** check for abnormalities.

Scans and tests

What you might expect to happen

The blood, urine, and blood pressure tests that are routinely offered throughout your pregnancy are there to keep a close eye on you and your baby. The aim of these tests is to identify warning signs before they turn into problems. For example, if a blood test shows low levels of haemoglobin, this can indicate low iron levels, a sign of anaemia; and high-blood pressure and/or protein in the urine are symptoms of pre-eclampsia.

You will also be offered ultrasound scans, which use sound waves to visualize your baby in the uterus. They are painless and carry no known risks to you or your baby. Apart from enabling you to see your baby, they also give a good assessment of how he is growing and developing, even down to checking the structure of his heart. They also indicate any issues that you might have, such as fibroids or a weak cervix. You will usually be offered a minimum of two scans, one between 8 and 14 weeks which is known as the dating scan, and a second at around 18 to 22 weeks called the anomaly scan.

During your pregnancy you will also be given the option of having antenatal tests that check for various genetic or chromosomal abnormalities such as Down's syndrome. Some of these assess your risk of carrying a baby with an abnormality and involve a blood test combined with measuring the fluid at the back of the neck

known as the nuchal translucency via ultrasound scan. If there is any concern that your baby might have a congenital abnormality of any kind, you'll be offered further tests that are more invasive, such as chorionic villus sampling or an amniocentesis. These scans and tests enable the healthcare professionals to gain as clear a picture as possible of your baby before he is born.

You will always have a choice as to whether you consent to the scan or test in question; none of them is compulsory. However, all the tests are there to ensure that the appropriate care is given to you and your baby. Feel free to discuss any concerns you have with your midwife before an investigation takes place. He or she will be able to talk you through the details and risks of all the procedures so that you can make an informed decision.

Your timeline of care

On the opposite page is a timeline of tests and scans that you can expect during the course of your pregnancy. Unless there is a specific reason (such as a family history of twins) for having an early scan, the tests and scans usually begin with the booking appointment (see p.80). Some of these are scans and tests that every pregnant woman will be offered; others are exceptional, depending upon your circumstances. All of the tests are to monitor the health and wellbeing of you and your baby.

Q When might I be offered the different scans and tests?

The table below sets out the expected pattern of scans and tests during the course of your pregnancy. Some of these investigations are offered to all pregnant women, others are for those in certain situations.

TIME LINE OF TESTS AND SCANS

WEEKS PREGNANT	TEST/SCAN	WHAT IS IT FOR?
4–5	Scan if family history of twins	Check growth and heartbeats
8–14 *	The dating scan	Measure growth and estimates delivery date
11–14 *	Nuchal translucency scan	Assesses risk of abnormalities
10–20	Blood tests	Assess risk of abnormalities
11–15	Chorionic villus sampling (CVS)	Diagnostic test for abnormalities
18–22	Fetal anomaly scan	Diagnostic test for abnormalities
from 14	Amniocentesis	Diagnostic test for abnormalities
22–23	Repeat of anomaly scan	Take detailed fetal measurements
18–24	Cordocentesis	Diagnostic test for abnormalities
28–40	Scan or scans	Check growth and development

* The nuchal translucency scan may be combined with the dating scan if the latter is done around 11 to 14 weeks.

Q I've never had an ultrasound before. What does it involve?

During an abdominal ultrasound appointment, you will be asked to lie down on a raised bed. The room will be dark so that the images show up clearly on the screen – rather like dimming the lights in the cinema. The sonographer will apply gel to your stomach and then move a handheld scanner over your abdomen. Don't worry if he or she has to press hard from time to time to get the right position. A sonographer is a medical professional, who may also be a radiographer (a person who takes X-rays), with training in skeletal anatomy, or a midwife with specialist training in antenatal ultrasound. He or she will make assessments of your baby's health according to certain statistics (the length of the baby's spine and femur, head circumference, abdominal circumference and so on) and what observations he or she can make from the images on the screen. If your ultrasound suggests there may be a problem, the sonographer will most likely ask for a second opinion there and then. If the two opinions concur, they will talk you through their concerns and tell you what will happen next. Most likely, they will pass on the information to an obstetrician, who will give you an appointment within a few days to explain the potential diagnosis and discuss any options for further tests with you. Try not to worry, though – most scans are happy occasions without cause for any concern (see p.101).

Q Is an ultrasound scan safe for my baby? Are there any risks?

As far as it's possible to tell, it is perfectly safe for you and your baby. The ultrasound is performed using a handheld device that uses sound waves to build a picture of your baby. Unlike X-rays (which use radiowaves), sound waves have no link to increased risk of childhood cancer or congenital abnormality in babies. The "beams" of sound penetrate your amniotic fluid and bounce off your baby's tiny body to create a moving image. Some people worry that sound waves will raise your core temperature, but actually the temperature rise from using an ultrasound is usually no more than 1°C (1.8°F), which is well below any level for concern.

Q I've got an early scan appointment because I've been bleeding. Do I need to rest until my scan?

It's estimated that 10 per cent of women experience some spotting or bleeding in the very earliest stages of pregnancy and most of them go on to have full-term, healthy babies.

While you're waiting for your scan appointment, avoid heavy lifting and sexual intercourse and try to rest as much as possible, but don't fret about doing so – as long as your normal day is unstrenuous, there's no reason to imagine that it will make your bleeding worse, and you can carry on as usual. Keep well hydrated and try to eat normally (even if you don't feel like eating). If your bleeding worsens, call your doctor and ask for advice. He or she may ask you to go to your local accident and emergency department so that you are seen

Six-week scan The embryo will only be between 5–9mm (¼–⅜in) long at this stage of pregnancy.

straightaway. If your scan shows that things are normal, you'll be sent home. Usually the bleeding will stop within 10 days, but if it doesn't, call the hospital. If the scan shows that something is wrong, your sonographer will advise you what to do next.

Q Can I take someone with me to my scans, and can we have a picture?

Most antenatal units and hospitals recommend that you have someone with you to enjoy the experience of seeing your baby, but also so that you have support if something is not as you'd hoped or expected. It can be useful to have someone there to ask questions. Your partner, or a close family member or friend are the obvious choices. Sonographers are usually very happy to give you a photograph taken from the scan. There may be a small charge for this – check at the reception desk beforehand.

Early scans at **six to seven weeks** are usually done **transvaginally**. Vaginal scans give a clearer picture at this stage than transabdominal ones and also use **sound waves.**

Q What's an EPU? My GP mentioned it if I need to have an early scan.

An EPU is an Early Pregnancy Unit (sometimes known as an Early Pregnancy Assessment Unit or Early Pregnancy Assessment Centre; EPAU and EPAC respectively). It is a specialist unit in a hospital dedicated to detecting and treating concerns in early pregnancy. If you need to have an early scan and your local hospital has one of these units, this is probably where you'll go. Not all hospitals have an EPU, in which case early scans are performed in the regular antenatal hospital clinic. There are often strict criteria for referral (from your doctor) to the EPU, including how far along your pregnancy is ("early" usually means within the first trimester, but not usually earlier than seven weeks along), whether or not you've had a positive pregnancy test recently, and the nature of your concern. EPUs can be reluctant to scan women to assess the viability of their pregnancy if there's no immediate cause to suspect that the pregnancy is anything but viable. Straightforward referrals include a family history of twins, having period like bleeding, or spotting that has lasted over a week.

Q I've been having fertility treatment. When will I have my first scan?

Systems differ depending on the clinic. You may have a scan as early as three weeks pregnant to locate the embryo sac in your uterus. Other clinics wait until you have a positive pregnancy test result and offer you a scan at around six weeks pregnant (about four weeks after collecting your eggs), because it's around this time that the scan can detect your baby's heartbeat. If it appears that your treatment has been successful, you'll have another scan two weeks or so later (around eight weeks pregnant) to check that the embryo is growing as expected. You will probably then be discharged from your assisted conception clinic and asked to make an appointment with your doctor so you can join the usual system of antenatal care.

Q I don't want to wait for my 12-week scan to see my baby. Can I pay to have a private scan?

Absolutely. Private hospitals will perform ultrasound scans from as early as seven weeks gestation (before this, there is very little an ultrasound scan can show). Most sonographers will begin by giving you an abdominal ultrasound (using the handheld scanner over your growing baby), but at such an early stage in pregnancy, it's possible that he or she may switch to using a vaginal ultrasound to get a better picture of your baby. In this case, a long, thin sonograph device is inserted into your vagina to get closer to your uterus.

Q Why might I be recommended an early scan?

If you struggled to get pregnant, have a history of recurrent miscarriages or a multiple pregnancy, are at risk of an ectopic pregnancy, have an incompetent cervix, or have had some vaginal bleeding, or uterine pain unrelated to your last menstrual period, your doctor may refer you for a scan at around seven weeks pregnant. Similarly if you already know that you suffer from fibroids or you're suspected to be carrying twins or multiples, your doctor will want to check that everything is as it should be.

Q What happens at the dating scan?

The scan at 8 to 14 weeks, also known as the dating scan, confirms your estimated delivery date, ensuring that you get the right antenatal screening tests at the right time.

You may be asked to drink water before the scan as a full bladder makes the ultrasound images clearer. During the scan, the sonographer will determine the exact gestational age of your baby and estimate your estimated delivery date. At this stage all babies develop at the same rate, regardless of their future size. The measurements taken at this scan are used to ensure that your baby is growing normally. Two key measurements are taken: the crown–rump length (the length from the top of the baby's head to the base of the spine), and the diameter from one bone across to the other on each side of your baby's head. The heart rate will also be measured and the position of the placenta will be checked.

This may be your first glimpse of your baby and it is a particularly exciting moment if she is moving around. You can ask to take a photograph home from your scan to share with others; you may have to pay for it.

White areas Hard tissues such as bone show up as white on the image.

Black areas These identify the fluids such as the amniotic fluid that the baby lies in.

Grey areas Soft tissues appear grey and speckled on the image.

Dating scan This is the first of your routine ultrasound scans. This will indicate how your baby is growing and developing.

Having the scan The sonographer will move a small hand held transducer or probe over your skin to get a view of your baby (below).

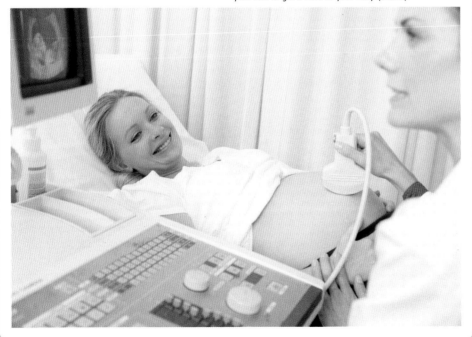

Q What tests are available to check for abnormalities?

There are various tests that can be performed at different stages of your pregnancy to check for abnormalities. Some provide information on the risk of your baby being affected by an abnormality. These involve a scan and blood tests. If these tests indicate that your risk is high, you will be offered further diagnostic tests, which allow specific conditions to be confirmed. Knowing for certain can help parents decide how to proceed, but these tests are invasive and do carry a 1 per cent chance of miscarriage.

Q What is the combined test and when is it done?

To give you the most accurate risk calculation of various abnormalities, including Down's syndrome, you should be offered the combined test, which involves a blood test and the nuchal translucency scan. The blood samples are measured for levels of beta-human chorionic gonadotropin hormone (beta-hCG), which are usually higher in the blood of a mother carrying a Down's syndrome baby, and pregnancy-associated plasma protein (PAPP-A), levels of which are usually lower. The blood samples are usually sent away for analysis, so it can take up to two weeks to receive the results. The blood samples must be taken between 10 and 14 weeks of pregnancy.

Q What are the quadruple and triple tests and when are they done?

You may be offered a quadruple test if you are between 14 and 20 weeks pregnant, when the combined test would no longer produce a reliable result. The quadruple test measures blood levels of beta-hCG, alpha fetoprotein (AFP; a protein produced by the fetus), unconjugated oestriol (uE3; a form of oestrogen that shows a lower level in Down's babies) and the hormone inhibin-A. The blood levels are analyzed in light of your age and how old the fetus is to produce a calculated risk. The triple – or Bart's – is the same as the quadruple test but does not look at levels of inhibin-A.

Q What's the nuchal translucency (NT) scan?

This is a scan used to estimate the risk of Down's syndrome. Although it cannot tell you for certain whether your baby will have Down's, it will inform you if he is at high risk. All women are offered the NT scan.

Your baby's nuchal translucency is the pool of fatty fluid beneath the skin at the back of the baby's neck. A sonographer can measure the thickness of the nuchal translucency during an ultrasound scan at around 11–14 weeks' gestation. After your scan, this measurement is considered in relation to your own age, the baby's length from crown to rump, and the results from the combined blood test (see p.95). Analyzed together, these results can tell you what risk your baby has of being born with Down's syndrome.

Comparing the nuchal measurement, your age, and your blood test results has an accuracy of more than 90 per cent. Don't worry if your hospital doesn't offer a combined test – a nuchal translucency test combined with your baby's measurements and your age is still a good indicator of risk. If your risk is high, remember that the test is not a diagnosis. You'll be offered diagnostic tests (choronic villus sampling or amniocentesis, see opposite) that will give you a definitive result.

Nuchal fluid While all babies have some fluid at the back of their necks, babies with Down's syndrome or other genetic disorders have more. The test for this might be done at your 12-week dating scan.

UNDERSTANDING THE NUCHAL TRANSLUCENCY RESULT

The thicker your baby's nuchal translucency, the greater the risk of your baby having Down's syndrome. It is important to note that the measurement is only one part of the test and should be assessed alongside blood test results and your age.

The result is expressed as a ratio. For example, you might be given the result 1:1,500, which means your baby has a one in 1,500 chance of being born with Down's (or, expressed as a percentage, this means a risk of 0.07 per cent). A ratio of 1:150 or greater is considered high risk, although even then it's still more likely that you won't have a Down's baby, (expressed as a percentage 1 in 150

is only a 0.67 per cent chance). It's also worth remembering that even if you fall into the low-risk category, there is still a chance (albeit a very slim one) of your baby being born with Down's syndrome. If you have a low risk of having a baby with Down's syndrome you'll be given the results of the scan within a fortnight. If your risk is high, you'll normally get your results within a

week, and often within two or three days, so that you have as much time as possible to consider whether you would like further diagnostic tests such as an amniocentesis. Whether or not you take these tests is entirely your choice.

When making your decision, bear in mind that some physical indicators of Down's syndrome can become apparent at later scans in your pregnancy, and in these cases your sonographer will tell you what he or she has discovered and what it means in terms of your baby's health.

Low risk If the measurement is under 2mm (¹⁄₁₆in) at 11 weeks or under 3mm (⅛in) at 14 weeks, your baby is unlikely to have Down's syndrome.

 Normal nuchal fold

High risk If the nuchal fold measures more than 3mm (⅛in), there is an increased risk of your baby being affected by Down's syndrome.

Larger nuchal fold

Q I've been offered a chorionic villus sampling (CVS) test. What's a chorionic villus?

The term chorionic refers to your placenta, which is covered in tiny finger-like fronds known as villi (singular, villus). These fronds increase the surface area of your placenta, maximizing the transfer of nutrients to your baby's body and waste out of it. The villi contain genetic material that is identical to your baby's, so the CVS test harvests some villi to analyze your baby's genetic make-up.

Q What are the risks associated with invasive tests?

Any invasive procedure carries with it a risk of infection, so be aware of any swelling, heat, or redness at the puncture site on your abdomen, if relevant, and if you develop a raised temperature. Both CVS and amniocentesis have a small increased risk of miscarriage above the normal risk of miscarriage at this gestation – around 1 per cent each – with a slight increased risk for a CVS if performed earlier than 10 weeks and amniocentesis performed earlier

than 15 weeks. Some figures show that in general the miscarriage risk with CVS is slightly higher than it is with amniocentesis, particularly if your baby is small for his gestational age. Most miscarriages relating to these procedures occur within 72 hours of the test, but may occur up to two weeks later. Some people worry that those babies whose mothers have undergone CVS are at risk of being born without some of their fingers or toes. This risk is believed to exist only when CVS is performed at less than nine weeks pregnant. Your doctor should make you aware of all the risks before you consent to tests, and it is up to you as to whether or not to proceed.

Q What diagnostic tests are available? Can they detect all fetal abnormalities?

CVS, amniocentesis, and cordocentesis, are diagnostic tests that will confirm whether or not your baby has specific abnormalities. As these tests are invasive, it is vital to know which one is right for you and what they involve.

Performed between 11 and 15 weeks, CVS can detect some chromosomal abnormalities, genetic abnormalities (such as in cystic fibrosis), musculo-skeletal disorders (such as muscular dystrophy), blood disorders (such as sickle cell anaemia, haemophilia or thalassaemia) and nervous system disorders (such as Tay Sachs disease). It can't tell you if your baby has a neural tube defect such as spina bifida. This is usually diagnosed through your anomaly scan (see p.100), and it can be detected through amniocentesis.

CVS, AMNIOCENTESIS, CORDOCENTESIS, OR NIPT

The table below lists the diagnostic procedures, the window of time in which they are performed during your pregnancy and the general conditions that they are testing for. Before undergoing any of these procedures talk to your healthcare providers about the pros and cons.

PROCEDURE	WHEN	TESTING FOR
CVS (Invasive)	11–15 weeks	Chromosomal and genetic conditions, blood disorders, nervous system and musculoskeletal disorders.
Amniocentesis (Invasive)	from 14 weeks	Chromosomal and genetic conditions, blood disorders, neural tube defects, and musculoskeletal disorders.
Cordocentesis (Invasive)	18–24 weeks	Chromosomal and genetic conditions, blood disorders, neural tube defects, and musculoskeletal disorders.
NIPT (Non-invasive)	from 10 weeks	Chromosomal and genetic conditions. CVS and amniocentesis may be offered after this test.

Allow yourself time to **think about** which test you will have, if any, as this is an **important decision** and you need to be **prepared** as much as possible for the result.

Q Is there a safer non-invasive alternative to CVS or amniocentesis?

Non-invasive parental testing (NIPT) is a blood test that analyzes tiny amounts of fetal DNA in the mother's blood. It is a simple test and the sample is sent away for analysis. Early indications are that NIPT is around 99 per cent accurate in the identification of babies who have chomosomal abnormalities. Many private antenatal clinics in the UK will offer the test from 10 weeks pregnant, and it's starting to be available on the NHS for high-risk groups of women. The results take up to two weeks to come back. However, it's worth knowing that present statistics reveal that up to 5 per cent of blood samples won't contain enough of the baby's DNA for proper analysis.

Q Did you know...

Midwives and doctors use the following generalized statistics as a measure of how age might affect your risk of having a baby with Down's syndrome. The risks are:

Age 20 the risk is **1 : 1500**
Age 30 the risk is **1 : 800**
Age 35 the risk is **1 : 270**
Age 40 the risk is **1 : 100**
Age **45** the risk is greater than **1 : 50**

Q What's the procedure for CVS and how long will it take?

Chorionic villus sampling (CVS) is carried out at 11 to 15 weeks to check your baby for certain disorders and abnormalities. The test is offered in pregnancies where a screening test shows there is a high risk of the baby having a condition.

Your doctor will remove the villi sample either by inserting a syringe needle through your abdomen into your placenta, or by inserting a tube via your vagina and entering your uterus through your cervix. In the latter case, a small amount of suction is passed through the tube to remove some villi from the placenta. The procedure your doctor uses will depend upon the position of your baby and the placenta.

You will be asked to go to your appointment with a full bladder, as you will need to have an ultrasound scan first to establish the position of the placenta in your uterus, and then to guide the doctor as he or she takes the villi

sample (although in some circumstances your placenta may be positioned in such a way that you need to empty your bladder before the test continues). Including preparation, the whole procedure should take no more than 30 minutes, of which removing the villi will take only 5 to 10 minutes. The villi are then sent for testing. Your doctor will check your baby's movement and heartbeat after the procedure to make as sure as possible that all remains well.

Syringe and needle

Scanner

Having the test A minute sample is taken from the placenta using a syringe with a long needle.

Bladder | Vagina | Cervix with mucus plug

Before you decide to have the test, the possible **risks** will be **discussed** with you and your partner.

Q What's the procedure for amniocentesis and how long will it take?

Syringe and needle

Scanner

Amniotic sac

Bladder | Vagina | Cervix with mucus plug

Having the test Guided by the ultrasound probe, a needle is inserted to remove a small amount of amniotic fluid.

Offered to pregnant women from 14 weeks, this is another invasive diagnostic test. As with any diagnostic test, careful consideration needs to be given as to whether you need it and the result you might be given.

At the start of the procedure, your doctor will use an ultrasound scan to determine the position of your baby, your placenta, and the umbilical cord. He or she will then insert a needle with a syringe attached into your abdomen, through the wall of your uterus, and into your amniotic sac. The aim will be to draw out around 20ml (¾fl oz) of fluid with the syringe. Amniotic fluid contains cells from your baby's skin, and these cells contain

DNA, which reveal details about your baby's genetic make-up. The fluid is then sent away for testing.

As with CVS, you'll need a full bladder so that your doctor can get a good ultrasound picture. (If you're more than 20 weeks pregnant, you may be asked to have an empty bladder.) Once the procedure is over, the doctor will also check your baby's movements.

The whole procedure should take 20 to 30 minutes. If your doctor doesn't draw enough in the first instance (this happens in around 8 per cent of cases), he or she will reinsert the needle and take some more fluid.

Q I have heard of the cordocentesis test. Should I be having it?

Like CVS and amniocentesis, this test detects chromosomal abnormalities. It can be performed after 18 weeks of pregnancy and is most commonly carried out if the other tests have not provided a reliable diagnosis. It is conducted in the same way as an amniocentesis, but with this test a tiny sample of the umbilical cord is taken. The results are usually available within three days. Careful consideration needs to be given before any of the diagnostic tests.

Q Will I be able to drive after I've had an invasive procedure? Can I go straight back to work?

Whether you've had CVS or an amniocentesis, it's a good idea to have someone drive you home afterwards. Although there are no risks involved with driving, you may feel wobbly and experience some stomach cramping for a few hours, which can make driving uncomfortable. You'll be asked to rest for 24 hours, which means you should certainly take the following day off work, and then to take it easy for the next few days. Whether or not you take more time off depends upon your job: you should avoid doing any strenuous activity and any heavy lifting.

Q How quickly will I get the test results? How will they be given to me?

Processes differ from hospital to hospital, but in many cases you will be offered the option of having the results of the three main chromosomal abnormality tests (Down's, Edwards', and Patau's syndromes, see box right) within two to three working days – this is called the Rapid Test, and you may have to pay for it. The results of a full chromosomal analysis (known as full karotyping) and genetic and blood analysis will usually take two to three weeks. You'll be given the option of finding out the results on the telephone or face to face (in both cases your obstetrician will write to you afterwards confirming what he or she has told you). Remember that you have had these tests because you are considered at "high risk" of

your baby being born with genetic abnormalities, which means you may be faced with difficult news about your baby's health. However you choose to receive the results, make sure someone is with you to support you if necessary.

Q What happens if my test confirms that my baby has a genetic or chromosomal abnormality?

Once you have absorbed the initial diagnosis, your doctor will arrange another appointment for you to talk through the options in more detail if you need to. Make sure you understand the results in lay terms – keep asking for clarification until you do. Some of the main things to consider are: whether the condition can be treated while your baby is still in the

uterus, or when she is born; what type of special needs your baby might have and to what extent; and will the condition be life-limiting, and, if so, what is the baby's life expectancy. There is no doubt that these are questions no prospective parent wants to ask. Make a list and take someone with you to the appointment who can support you and be a second set of ears to hear what you're being told. Depending upon the diagnosis, you may be offered a termination, although ending a pregnancy is a huge and emotional decision. Take your time. You won't have to make a decision there and then. Your hospital will offer you specialist counselling to help you to come to terms with the situation before you do. Accept the offer if you think talking to an independent person will help you. In the end, though, no one but you can make the decision about what is right for your family. Surround yourself with people who will love and support you through your decision.

Q I know that Trisomy 21 is another term for Down's syndrome, but what are Trisomy 13 and Trisomy 18?

Chromosomal abnormalities occur when there are either too few or too many of a specific chromosome. There are hundreds that are incompatible with life, meaning the pregnancy might end or the baby might survive for only a short time after birth.

All three of these conditions relate to chromosomal abnormalities. Healthy humans have 23 pairs of chromosomes, each numbered 1 to 23. Occasionally, a baby develops with an extra chromosome on one of the pairs, making a group of three (trisomy). Trisomy 21 (Down's syndrome) means that there is an extra chromosome 21. Trisomy 18 indicates an extra chromosome 18, resulting in Edwards' syndrome; Trisomy 13 results in Patau's syndrome. Edwards' and Patau's syndrome are both extremely rare but life-limiting conditions, in which the baby is born with severe neurological and physical abnormalities. In either case babies aren't expected to live for more than a few days after birth. Both CVS and amniocentesis can detect whether or not your baby has any of these extra chromosomes.

Chromosome 21 In this intance there are three copies of this chromosome.

Chromosomal abnormalities When an abnormality is found, it can be an error in the number or structure of the chromosomes or a problem with a gene. This can be caused by various factors.

{Q What is the anomaly scan?

Between 18 and 22 weeks pregnant you'll be offered a mid-term (or mid-pregnancy) ultrasound scan. It is also known as the anomaly scan. This is the first point in your pregnancy when a sonographer can make a detailed assessment of your unborn baby's health. A series of measurements are taken and physical features are checked to ensure there are no defects.

Seeing your baby

This is an exciting, but also potentially anxious time for prospective parents – the image you see of your baby on the ultrasound screen will, possibly for the first time, really look like a baby now. Even without specialist training, you'll be able to make out his eyes, ears, nose, fingers, vertebrae, and even perhaps some fingers and toes. At the same time, you will hear whether your baby is developing healthily. If you're worried, remember that most anomaly scans turn out to be happy, reassuring occasions. Only very rarely are parents faced with news that dramatically affects the care a baby might need after birth, or a difficult decision about whether or not to continue with the pregnancy at all.

Chin   Lung   Liver

Neck   Spine   Diaphragm   Blood vessels

Heart ventricles and atriums   Leg

Your baby's heart The four chambers of the heart are checked to see if they are roughly the same size as each other, making sure the valves between them are working. If any problem is detected, you will be referred on to a heart specialist for more detailed checks on your baby.

Your baby's leg A measurement is taken of your baby's femur (thigh bone), which gives a good indication as to how he is growing. Your baby's feet, toes, hands, and fingers will also be examined, checking that the digits are present – although they won't be counted now.

Taking a look The sonographer will need to change the position of the handheld sonograph as the ultrasound takes place – getting a good look at your baby from all angles.

Bowel

Looking at your baby's scan At the 20-week scan the sonographer will look closely at the structure of your baby's organs, and will also study external features, such as your baby's facial features.

Your baby's vertebrae and spinal cord All the bones along the length of your baby's spine will be checked to see that they are properly aligned and that the spinal cord is fully enclosed in skin to eliminate the possibility of a neural tube defect such as spina bifida.

POSSIBLE ANOMALIES

The table below details specific checks your baby will be given. It's important to remember that the anomalies are all very rare. The chance that problems are detected – the pick-up rate – is affected by factors such as obesity, scar tissue from a previous C-section or operation, and the baby's position.

CONDITION	DESCRIPTION	PROGNOSIS	PICK-UP RATE
Neural tube defects (occur in six out of 10,000 births)	Anencephaly and spina bifida are neural tube conditions in which the skull, spine, and/or brain don't develop fully.	There is no treatment for anencephaly and the baby will die before or shortly after birth. Spina bifida can be a limiting condition, but with considerable support, children can go on to lead active lives.	98 per cent for anencephaly; 90 per cent for spina bifida
Hole in the abdominal wall (occurs in 4–5 out of 10,000 births)	This can result in gastroschisis or exomphalos where part of the intestine and possibly the liver develops outside the baby's body.	Both conditions are potentially treatable with surgery as soon as the baby is born. Some babies with exomphalos also have heart defects.	98 per cent for gastroschisis; 80 per cent for exomphalos
Diaphragmatic hernia (occurs in 4 out of 10,000 births)	A hole in the baby's diaphragm means that his lungs aren't able to develop properly.	Around 50 per cent of babies with this will die as soon as they are born, because their lungs are simply too underdeveloped even for emergency surgery at birth.	60 per cent
Cleft lip and cleft palate (occurs in 1 out of 1000 births)	Your baby's lips grow in two parts, sometimes including the palate inside the mouth. If the parts don't join together properly, or at all, the baby will develop a cleft lip and palate.	Neither cleft lip nor palate are life-threatening. Your baby will have surgery usually within six months after birth, to knit the two parts together, often with little scarring.	75 per cent
Major heart defects (occur in 3–4 out of 1000 births)	Enlarged heart chambers, valves that allow a two-way flow of blood and holes in the heart are some of the congenital heart problems that are classed as major defects.	Only once a specialist has diagnosed the nature of the baby's heart problem can any real indication be given of his likely prognosis.	50 per cent
Lack of kidneys (occurs in 1 in 10,000 births)	Medically known as bilateral renal agenesis, this means that the baby has developed without any kidneys, and possibly a bladder.	Sadly, we need our kidneys to survive so babies with this condition die as soon as or before they are born.	84 per cent
Lethal skeletal dysplasia (occurs in 1 in 10,000 births)	With this, the baby's bones don't develop fully, making the trunk of the body very short, as well as giving the baby short limbs.	The short trunk means that the baby's lungs don't develop fully, making it very hard for a baby to survive after birth.	90 per cent

Q I'm 26 weeks pregnant and my midwife is worried about the size of my baby. What will happen?

When a baby's growth slows or ceases in the uterus, this is known as intrauterine growth restriction (IUGR), which can be the result of a variety of factors. If your midwife is concerned about your baby's growth, he or she will arrange extra scans to see what the problem is and how it can be treated.

The size of a developing baby is measured according to centile graphs (you'll have these to keep track of your baby's length and weight once she is born, too). From 24 weeks onwards, these graphs can plot the average growth rate of a baby according to the height of the mother's fundus. This is the measurement your midwife makes during your antenatal appointments using a tape measure and is taken from the highest point of your bump under your breastbone, over the top of the bump to your pubic bone.

If this measurement falls beneath the tenth centile when you are between 26 and 28 weeks pregnant, your midwife will probably send you for additional scans so that your baby's skull diameter and abdominal circumference can be checked directly over a given amount of time (and these measurements plotted on relevant centile graphs that appear in your notes). The height of your fundus is influenced not

An ultrasound scan If your baby's growth appears to be slowing down you may be offered more than one scan to assess progress more accurately.

only by your baby's size, but also by the amount of amniotic fluid you have – too little or too much fluid can also, rarely, be cause for concern. Having these growth scans is a precaution intended to reassure you and your medical team that all is well.

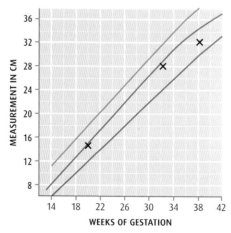

Growth graphs The graph on the left shows that a baby's head is growing steadily. The graph on the right indicates that the growth of the abdomen is showing decline possibly due to blood and nutrients being pumped to the heart and brain.

KEY

| — 90th percentile | ✕ Test results |
| — 50th percentile | ▬ 10th percentile |

Q What sort of situations mean that I will need to have additional scans and checks?

Some pregnancies require extra monitoring to ensure that the baby is growing well. Sometimes this is because of issues identified at the start of pregnancy, and extra scans and checks can be planned. Other problems arise during the course of pregnancy. The following conditions mean that extra checks may be planned at your booking appointment:
» Complications in a previous pregnancy, such as a small baby or a stillbirth.
» A pre-existing medical condition, such as diabetes or a heart condition.

Situations that develop during pregnancy that may require additional monitoring include:
» Being pregnant with multiples, which you are most likely to find out about at your dating ultrasound scan.
» Developing gestational diabetes.
» If you are rhesus negative and you have developed anti-D antibodies.

The following situations mean that you may need extra scan(s) towards the end of pregnancy to check your baby's wellbeing:
» If your waters break before your due date.
» Having too much or too little amniotic fluid.
» Being two weeks past your due date.
» If your baby stops her normal movements.

Q My midwife mentioned a doppler scan. Why might I need this?

If you have complications in your pregnancy, or a scan confirms that there is a problem with your baby's growth you may be offered a **Doppler scan.** This specialized scan measures blood flow in the umbilical artery and uterus and determines the placental health. You may have more than one Doppler scan during your pregnancy to monitor your baby's growth over a period of time. If there are concerns about your baby's movements, a type of Doppler scan known as a cardiotocograph may be done that traces your baby's heartbeat, and depending on the results, an early induction of labour may be advised. Cardiotocographs are typically done in the third trimester, but can be done earlier.

Q At what stage can I have a 3D scan of my baby?

3D scans can be done at any stage of your pregnancy. They show still pictures of your baby in three dimensions. 4D scans show moving 3D images of your baby, with time being the fourth dimension. With these scans you will see your baby's skin rather than her insides.

In the UK, NHS antenatal care usually offers only a 2D image of your baby. However, there are many private clinics that will offer 3D (and even 4D – with sound) scans, if you're happy to pay for them. Ask your doctor's surgery or midwife for recommendations of reputable private antenatal clinics near you. Some women worry that creating the 3D image must mean using rays that could be harmful to the baby, but a 3D (or 4D) scan is no more dangerous than one that is 2D – the sound waves are just put together from more angles to create the 3D image. If you are carrying more than one baby this type of scan is really useful as it can show whether fetuses share a placenta or amniotic sac and can provide valuable information about the state of a pregnancy.

3D scan A 3D photo allows parents-to-be to see what their unborn baby looks like.

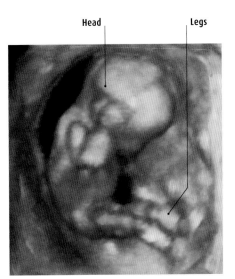

14 weeks By 12 weeks a fetus is fully formed, and it may be possible to tell the gender of a baby at 14 weeks. If you want to see the whole of your baby on a 3D scan photo, then make sure you have a scan earlier on in your pregnancy. Space gets tighter as the weeks go by.

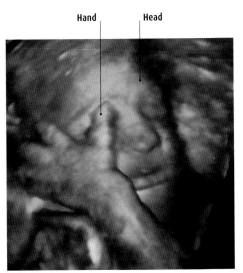

Close up 3D scans reveal a vast range of expressions on the face of a fetus, for example, frowning and smiling. Sometimes a fetus can be seen opening its mouth. This 38-week-old fetus is rubbing her eyes.

Triplets In this amazing 3D image of triplets, each fetus has its own sac. In between the sacs a small amount of placenta is seen as a V-shape. This indicates that each fetus not only has its own sac, but also its own placenta.

All about you

Your body will undergo **incredible changes** over the next nine months. Some of these will affect the way you live your life, and this can feel both bewildering and exciting as you watch your bump grow. Learn about the **lifestyle adjustments** you will need to make and read about the physical and **emotional changes** you are likely to experience. Find out how to deal with **common complaints** and any complications that might arise.

People often tell you that when you're pregnant **your life** will take on new meaning – but you may also be **wondering** how life will change on a more **day-to-day** basis now that you're expecting. There's a lot you can do to give you and your baby the **best possible chance** of enjoying a healthy, safe, and manageable pregnancy.

Lifestyle changes

The world around you

Now you are pregnant you may be more conscious than ever before of how the environment we live and work in has a direct impact on our health and wellbeing, and you may wonder how it affects your developing baby's health and wellbeing, too. In this chapter we'll look at some of the questions you might have about the environment you live in and the chemicals you come into contact with and how you can minimize their effects (if there are any) on your own and your unborn baby's health. We consider the effects of air pollution if you live in a city and exposure to toxic heavy metals, and what to do if you have lead water pipes in your house.

The world of work

How pregnancy affects your working life will obviously depend significantly on the type of work that you do. In the UK expectant mothers have specific rights designed to protect them and their unborn baby. In this section we look at any aspects of your job that might be hazardous to your unborn baby or particularly debilitating for you so that you can ensure your employer takes steps to protect

you. We cover the rules for when you must inform your employer that you're pregnant. And we'll also investigate what pregnancy rights you have, in terms of time off for appointments and then later, for caring for your newborn – both for you and your partner.

Lifestyle matters

We'll look at issues such as pets, the cosmetics you use, and leisure activities such as gardening. We'll answer some of the most commonly asked questions to guide you on where to make changes in your lifestyle. We'll put your mind at ease where you might have concerns. We all need our rest and probably no one needs it more than an expectant mother. Perhaps you want to take a holiday abroad before your baby is born – how late can you fly? What happens if you need vaccinations? How can you make car travel comfortable? What holiday insurance cover should you get? Finally, we'll take a look at sleep – more precious now than it might ever have been. How can you make sure that you get all the rest you need when being pregnant? We suggest the best time to sleep and how to limit naps to your body's natural sleep cycle.

Q Is it safe to have sex now that I'm pregnant, or could it harm the baby or even break my waters?

It is safe to have sex in a straightforward pregnancy. It won't harm your baby as he is well cushioned in his amniotic sac and research has shown that it's highly unlikely that penetration can rupture your membranes and cause your waters to break.

The biggest challenge to having intercourse when you're pregnant is accommodating your growing abdomen, but there's no health reason why you should stop having sex. In fact, later in pregnancy, the uterine contractions of an orgasm can help prepare you for birth. Many couples enjoy the freedom of having sex without using any contraception or without having to give thought to the consequences. However, remember that you can still contract sexually transmitted diseases, so if this is a concern do use a condom.

Although sex is safe for your baby, it might not be all that comfortable for you, due to breast tenderness, cramping, nausea or increased tiredness. You might find gentle lovemaking more comfortable and you may need to adapt or experiment with different positions at various stages of your pregnancy. Many couples report that a side position works best of all, either facing or in spooning position with your partner behind you.

Many women experience swings in their sex drive during pregnancy. You may feel more sensitive due to the increased blood flow to the breasts and vagina, and the rise in progesterone and oestrogen in your body, which can increase your libido. Your changing body might be incredibly exciting to your partner, or he might be too fearful of hurting the baby to relax. If you don't want to have sex, find other ways of being intimate with your partner. Communication and touching are essential for keeping you close and connected as a couple. For many couples the knowledge that they have created a life together helps to enhance their lovemaking.

Take time to rest together By having a cuddle you can feel connected with your partner. Take a nap together or just have a lazy afternoon relaxing.

WHEN TO AVOID SEX

There are a few cases where it is best to avoid penetrative sex and your GP or midwife may advise it for some medical situations. If you have any signs of infection, such as an unusual discharge, itchiness, or pain when you have sex, consult your GP or midwife.

» **Bleeding:** If you've had any heavy bleeding during pregnancy, there may be an increase in the risk of further bleeding.

» **Previous miscarriages** or premature births.

» **Waters have broken:** Once this happens, sex could introduce infection.

» **Cervical insufficiency** (see p.147)

» **Placenta praevia** (see p.147)

Q Did you know...

Later in pregnancy, an orgasm can set off Braxton Hicks contractions (see p.201). Don't worry – this is a fairly common occurrence but if you're uncomfortable, try slow, deep breathing or relaxation techniques until they pass.

Q I'm worried about radiation harming my baby. Can I still use my mobile phone or microwave?

There is no evidence to suggest you should stop using your mobile phone or microwave during pregnancy. Studies into the long-term effects of mobiles on our health (whether we're pregnant or not) are still in their infancy, so for the time being, it's impossible to be definitive about possible hazards. Mobiles send out radio waves, just like (and no more dangerous than) the waves that come from your computer or your television set. People worry more about phones because we hold them against our heads while we're using them. If you keep yours in a pocket close to your abdomen when you're not using it, on present evidence there's no danger to your baby. But if you're worried, carry your mobile in your handbag or breast pocket and when you talk, use speakerphone and hold the mobile away from your body.

Modern microwave ovens are built to strict guidelines that ensure any radiation "leakage" falls well below levels known to harm humans. If you're pregnant and you use a microwave, make sure it's up to modern safety standards. Stand back while the microwave is in operation.

Q Can I have a dental X-ray while I'm pregnant?

Most dental X-rays are too short, far enough away from your abdomen, and of low enough strength to be perfectly safe during pregnancy. However, do make sure you tell your dentist you're pregnant so that he or she can advise you. Similarly, most chest and limb X-rays are safe during pregnancy. In almost all cases, if your medical practitioner thinks you need to have an X-ray despite your pregnancy, it's because the benefits of doing so far outweigh the risks to you and your baby.

Q I live in a city. Will the air pollution harm my baby?

If you minimize your outdoor activities during peak pollution times then you will also lower the chances of pollution affecting your baby. You would have to be exposed to excessive amounts to cause serious harm to you or your baby.

In 2014, a study at the University of Florida concluded that women living in heavily polluted urban areas were more likely to suffer high blood pressure and resulting pre-eclampsia during pregnancy. Another study in Poland, which followed children from birth until the age of five, concluded that high pollution levels during fetal development and in the first years of life led to a small drop in the child's IQ. The Harvard School of Public Heath in the US has also recorded links between fine particulate pollution (emitted by fires, vehicles, and industrial smokestakes) and autism during the third trimester.

Although these findings seem alarming, we already know that air pollution is bad for our health, so, while we need much more research to be certain of the effects on a pregnant woman and her unborn baby, it makes sense to exercise caution whenever you can. Walk in the street at times of low traffic, avoiding rush hour, for example, and keep the windows at home closed at these times, too. If you can, invest in a home air purifier. Walk along quiet roads with traffic that keeps moving, or, ideally, through parks, rather than walking beside stationary traffic. And drink plenty of fluids to keep flushing out your system.

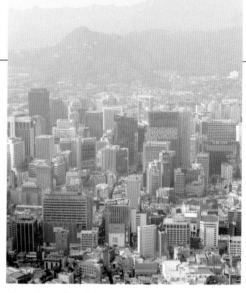

Living in a polluted city Try to keep your windows closed during peak pollution times and follow any instructions from health officials for residents.

AIR QUALITY CHART

An air quality index is used by many government agencies around the world to notify the public of pollution forecasts on a daily basis. Although each one varies slightly, they usually cover measurements of ground-level ozone, particulate matter, carbon monoxide, sulphur dioxide, and nitrogen dioxide. Check local news media for air quality forecasts and plan outdoor activities for days when particle and ozone levels are low. Pregnant women should always follow the advice for at-risk individuals.

AIR POLLUTION BAND	HEALTH ADVICE FOR AT-RISK INDIVIDUALS
Low	Enjoy your usual outdoor activities
Moderate	Consider reducing prolonged or heavy outdoor activity
High	Reduce or reschedule outdoor activities
Very High	Avoid all outdoor exertion

Q I've got cats. Is it safe for me to clean out their litter tray?

Ideally not. Cat faeces can carry the *toxoplasma gondii* parasite, which causes toxoplasmosis in humans. If you're pregnant and you become infected, it can cause miscarriage or stillbirth, brain damage, sight or hearing loss, or an enlarged spleen or liver in your baby. The earlier in your pregnancy you're infected, the less likely it is that you'll pass the parasite on to your baby, but if you do, the risks are greater. Later in your pregnancy you're more likely to pass on the infection, but the risks for complications are much lower.

Signs of toxoplasmosis infection in a baby only become clear over time, although babies may have a low birthweight, or show signs of jaundice or anaemia. Most women who own cats have had the infection, and as long as they were infected more than three months before conception, there's no risk to the baby.

It's best to err on the side of caution, so ask someone else to clean the litter tray. If that's not possible, wear rubber gloves and wash your hands immediately afterwards. The parasite is also found in soil and raw meat so it is vital to wash your hands after gardening or handling raw meat and wash fruit and vegetables before you eat them. If you think you are at risk of toxoplasmosis, ask your GP to test you.

Q I live in an old house that still has lead water pipes. Will drinking the water harm my baby?

For health reasons, even when you aren't pregnant, you should avoid contact with toxic "heavy" metals as much as possible. Lead in water can leach from your blood and bones and enter your unborn baby's system, and has been known to slow brain development in some children, both before and after birth. Some countries have local authority schemes that will subsidize (or even provide free) replacement of domestic lead water pipes. Talk to your council about schemes in your area and have the piping replaced if you can. Meanwhile, drink filtered water (a simple filter jug does a great job of removing impurities – including mercury and aluminium, as well as lead – from tap water) and use filtered water in cooking. If you prefer, use bottled mineral water, but make sure that it has the lowest available sodium levels.

Limit your exposure to toxic heavy metals by using **glass, stainless steel,** or **ceramic cookware** rather than pans and dishes made from aluminium or lead.

Q I usually dye my hair. Are there certain dyes that I shouldn't use?

If you want to be extra safe, you can switch to plant-based hair dyes, including henna. However, there are only very low levels of harmful chemicals in hair dyes, and dying your hair once every three months or so during pregnancy is generally considered safe for your baby. What is more likely to happen is that your skin, which is especially sensitive at this time, will have an adverse reaction to the dye, or that your hair will behave erratically – perhaps the colour won't take properly or your hair goes frizzy or brittle. If you're using a chemical dye, even if you've used it before, do a test patch on one small section of your hair first. You might also consider highlights rather than a full dye – highlights will limit the amount of contact your skin will have with the chemicals, minimizing the risk of an adverse skin reaction and reducing the quantity of chemicals that enter your bloodstream.

Q Can I still have a spray tan now that I'm pregnant?

Although there's no concrete evidence either way, in general it's better to avoid inhaling any chemicals, including those in a spray tan, while you're pregnant. Instead, use a tanning mousse or cream that contains the same tanning agents, but is applied directly to your body, removing the likelihood of you breathing in any chemicals. Also, cream and mousse tans only penetrate the upper layers of your skin, so there is limited risk to your baby.

60 million

people in the United States carry the **toxoplasma parasite**, but few show symptoms as the immune system stops the parasite from causing any illness.

Q I love gardening, but are there any hazards that might affect my growing baby?

There are several hazards in the garden, such as working with chemicals, exposure to toxoplasmosis in the soil and on unwashed fruit and vegetables, heavy lifting, and getting up from a kneeling position.

A little light gardening is an excellent way to get outdoors and enjoy nature when you are pregnant, but there are some potential dangers lurking out there in the garden. You need to protect yourself from exposure to toxins such as fertilizers and pesticides, and follow good work practices to avoid injury. Follow the advice here to be sure you and your baby stay safe.

 » Remember to kneel down and stand up safely; lower yourself and push up using your knees and thighs rather than your back or abdomen.

 » Always wear gardening gloves and try not to get soil on your hands; cats and other animals may have done their business in your garden.

 » Lift garden waste and heavy pots carefully, lowering yourself using your knees, instead of bending from your waist. Ask for help if something is too heavy for you to lift.

 » Wear a hat if it is warm and make sure to drink lots of water – gardening can be thirsty work. Try to do your gardening during the cooler part of the day.

 » Don't spray your plants with insecticide – leave that to someone else. If there's only you to do it, wear a mask that covers your mouth and nose.

 » Leave the really heavy work (such as mowing a large lawn or cutting back trees) for someone else and, whatever you're doing, if you feel dizzy or tired, stop.

 » Always wash your hands with antibacterial soap as soon as you've finished in the garden or allotment – even if you've been wearing gloves the whole time.

 » Wash vegetables and fruit thoroughly before eating them (even if you are picking them from your own garden) as the soil may contain animal faeces.

Q Where can I find out about my workplace maternity rights and rights for my baby's dad?

In the UK, the best place for up-to-date information about your maternity rights, your employer's responsibilities, and rights for the baby's father is the government's website. Working out when you can start your paid leave, how much leave you'll get, and how much you're likely to be paid can be mind-boggling, but the UK Government's website includes a handy calculator. Currently, you need to be employed continuously for 26 weeks up to the fifteenth week before your due date in order to qualify for statutory maternity leave and pay. If you need help deciphering the information, ask your HR department. They'll also be able to tell you whether your company offers additional benefits, such as extra paid leave. You could also ask your line manager. If you don't want to talk to someone at work, your local Citizens' Advice Bureau will be able to help you work out what rights you have.

Q When should I tell my employer that I'm pregnant?

Many women wait until they're 12 weeks pregnant before they share the news with anyone but immediate family. However, you may work in an environment that could be hazardous to your pregnancy. For example, if you're a dentist or doctor working with X-rays, or a hairdresser coming into contact with lots of chemicals, or if you're suffering from severe pregnancy sickness and it's stopping you from doing your job properly, it's a good idea to tell

Did you know...

As soon as you let your employer know you're pregnant, ask for a copy of your company's maternity policy and spend some time looking online to get to know your rights. Remember that there are certain deadlines for informing your employer of your intentions with regard to time off and returning to work.

Q What are my employer's responsibilities now that I'm pregnant?

The guidelines vary from country to country, but below are the main points that employers must take into account to ensure a safe pregnancy for a pregnant member of staff.

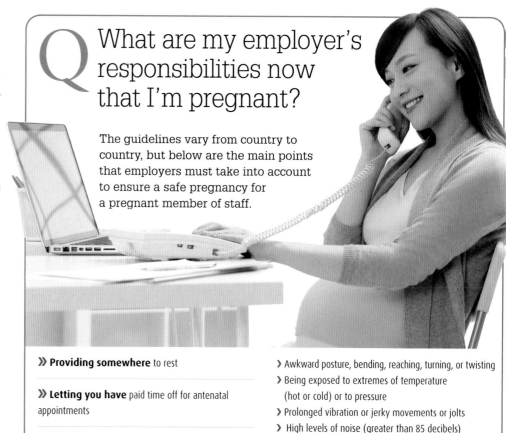

» **Providing somewhere** to rest

» **Letting you have** paid time off for antenatal appointments

» **Providing alternative work** at the same rate of pay if your job involves:
› Heavy lifting or other physical exertion
› Activities that require balance

› Awkward posture, bending, reaching, turning, or twisting
› Being exposed to extremes of temperature (hot or cold) or to pressure
› Prolonged vibration or jerky movements or jolts
› High levels of noise (greater than 85 decibels)
› Prolonged exposure to chemicals, radiation or other pollutants that might harm your baby
› Shift work, if your doctor thinks it's adversely affecting your pregnancy health

your employer sooner. In any event, you're obliged to let your employer know that you're pregnant not later than 15 weeks before your due date – and bear in mind that you won't be entitled to time off for antenatal appointments until your employer knows. To ensure you receive the full range of employment benefits, including maternity pay, you must provide your employer with proof of your pregnancy (a letter or a certificate – known as a MATB1 in the UK – signed by your healthcare professional).

Q Can my partner have paid time off to attend antenatal appointments with me?

UK law currently states that fathers can have two 6½-hour absences from work to attend antenatal appointments, but these are unpaid. Same-sex partners are entitled to attend two antenatal appointments (unpaid) and have all the same entitlements for time off after the

birth of the baby as heterosexual couples. Of course, your partner's employer may have its own policies, and they may be more generous than those the law provides. Some firms, for example, allow expectant fathers to attend all antenatal appointments and on full pay. If only statutory requirements apply in your case, then your partner could use his holiday entitlement (assuming he has any) to attend as long as he or she complies with the company's rules for annual leave.

Q My job is really high pressure. Is stress bad for my baby?

It is always a good idea to take steps to manage stress and anxiety. It is thought that the stress hormones cortisol and adrenaline can pass from you to your baby (studies have found both of these hormones in the amniotic fluid of stressed mothers). Some studies show that stress can increase the risk of premature birth, or of

52 weeks

is the amount of time (in the UK) that an **employed** woman is **entitled** to have off work after giving birth.

having a baby with birth defects or with a low birthweight. One study has also made a link between mothers who were stressed during pregnancy and introversion or hyperactivity in their children as they grow up. To help reduce stress levels, be sure to take your lunch break (rather than working through it), walk around the block to clear your head, and leave on time – at least for some of the week. You could also ask for extra help and delegate tasks where you can, in order to manage and streamline your workload effectively.

Q I want to go back to work after the baby is born – can I do that straight away?

In the UK mothers are not allowed to return to work for two weeks after the baby is born (or four weeks if you work in a factory). This is called the "recovery period" and is aimed at making sure you only go back to work after your body has had some time to recover from labour and birth.

Q I told my employer that I wanted to have six months off after birth, but now I'd like the full year. Is it a problem?

Not at all, as long as you give ample notice. UK law requires you to give your employer eight weeks' notice if you intend to change the date of your return to work. You are also entitled to have a small number of "keep in touch" (KIT) days, when you can go into work for a day or two at a time to keep yourself up-to-date with what's going on in your business. These are optional, paid days, and they don't affect your right to claim maternity pay.

Q How can I keep healthy during a long, exhausting day at the office?

It is likely that a typical eight-hour work day will affect you differently when you are pregnant, particularly during the most tiring first and last trimesters. Fortunately, a few minor adjustments in the way you work can help.

 » Use your lunch break to eat and rest, not run errands. Take time to sit in a park or café in order to switch off from any stress at work.

 » Set up your workstation correctly and adopt good posture. You may need to readjust the position of your chair and computer as your pregnancy progresses.

 » Take frequent, short breaks away from your desk. A short stroll every 45 minutes can help you avoid acidity and heartburn. Stretching helps aches forming.

 » Drink water and eat small healthy snacks, such as fruit and nuts, throughout the day. This will keep energy reserves high and combat any nausea.

 » Choose comfortable clothing and footwear. Wearing layers of natural, breathable fabrics will help you adjust to any fluctuations of body temperature.

» Stagger your commute by asking your employer if you can work slightly different hours to beat the rush hour – which can be challenging whether you are driving or using public transport.

 » Keep housework and cooking to a minimum in the evenings – this time is essential for relaxation so ask your partner or family members to help you out.

 » Go to bed early whenever you are able.

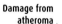

Q I want to take a holiday. What's the best time for me to go?

For most women, the best time is during their second trimester. This is when you're most likely to be enjoying your pregnancy, have increased energy, and feel sick less often. You're more likely to feel comfortable with the idea of travelling and leaving your creature comforts behind. During your first trimester you might feel nauseous and tired, and there is generally a greater risk of miscarrying your baby. During your third trimester you're likely to feel more uncomfortable during travel and most tired. On top of that, if anyone thinks there's a risk you might go into labour, you may have trouble arranging your travel to and from your destination as airlines might be reluctant to have you on board a flight.

Q What's the latest point in my pregnancy that I can fly?

There's generally nothing dangerous about flying during pregnancy, as long as you're in a pressurized air cabin (all large planes are pressurized, but small island-hoppers might not be). If you have high blood pressure, are very anaemic, or you've had a previous miscarriage, you may be advised to avoid flying. It's best to ask your midwife for advice that's right for you.

There's also the question of the airline's rules, which vary depending on the company. In general, they won't take you after around 32 weeks pregnant (some accept a slightly later date), or around 28 weeks if you're pregnant with twins or multiples (remember, these are the dates for your return). Some airlines will make an exception. If you're travelling during your third trimester, almost all will ask for a letter from your midwife to say that you can travel. Make sure you carry this letter with you if this applies to you: the airline has the right to refuse to let you board the plane if your due date or health are in doubt. They want to avoid having a pregnant woman in labour mid-flight.

Q Are there any types of holiday I should avoid while I'm pregnant?

Avoid any holiday that might put a lot of physical strain on your body, for example those involving activities that place you in danger of high impact, that restrict your oxygen intake, or that raise your core body temperature. This means that scuba diving holidays are temporarily off the agenda, as are skiing

Q Is there an increased risk of thrombosis for me during a "long-haul" flight?

Any flight longer than five hours is considered "long haul" for people at risk of thrombosis (blood clots) – which includes pregnant women.

During a long flight, blood can pool in your veins (usually in your legs) and cause clots. Before you book, check with your midwife that you're not at an especially high risk of developing thrombosis when you fly, for example if you suffer from diabetes, high blood pressure or high cholesterol. During any flight, whether or not it's long haul, call a member of the cabin crew straight away

if you feel dizzy – the oxygen circulating in the cabin can be a bit thin and you may need a boost from an oxygen mask. To minimize the risk of thrombosis when you're in the air, follow these tips (see right).

Formation of blood clots This begins when fatty deposits called atheromas form. The growing atheroma reduces blood flow and oxygen to the tissues and then ruptures, causing a clot to form.

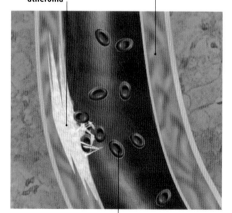

Damage from atheroma

Artery lining

Platelets (clotting agents)

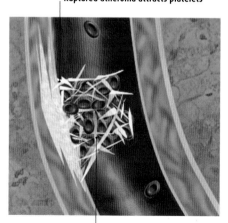

Ruptured atheroma attracts platelets

Blood clot blocking artery

» Wear support stockings or anti-compression flight socks to help keep your circulation flowing while you're airborne. Most chemists sell these.

» Walk up and down the aisle every 30 minutes if the seatbelt sign is off. Do gentle stretches if there is space to do so at the end of the aisle.

» Drink plenty of water during the flight. It will keep you hydrated and force you to take regular trips to the toilet (making you get up and move around).

» Ask for an aisle seat so you can stretch your legs (or, even better, pay for extra leg room if your airline offers it as an option).

» Point and flex your ankles from time to time while you're sitting. Move each foot round in a circular motion to help keep your circulation flowing.

» Wear loose clothes and shoes or sandals that will accommodate swollen feet. Take your shoes off while you're seated to make your feet less constricted.

Q I'm planning to drive rather than fly to my holiday destination. Can you give me advice on long car journeys?

Firstly, always wear your seatbelt: put the lap strap under your abdomen, across your thighs, and over the top of your abdomen. Adjust your seat a little or invest in a cushioning pad if the strap cuts into your neck.

If you're driving and find the driving seat a squeeze, tilt the steering wheel back if you can, or recline your seat slightly to give you more space. Never move your seat backward so much that you can't reach the pedals properly and always make sure you can still see over the top of the steering wheel. If you adjust your seat, don't forget to adjust your mirrors, too. Take frequent rest and toilet breaks. Sitting in the same

position for long periods of time can be uncomfortable during pregnancy. When you get out of the car, swing your legs out first, and try not to twist awkwardly. Push up from a seated position using your thighs rather than your back.

Comfort in the car Three-point seat belts with the straps placed above and below your baby bump will allow you to feel comfortable, while still being safe.

INCORRECT POSITION　　**CORRECT POSITION**

holidays – not only because of the altitude (you should not go more than 2000m/6500ft above sea level), but because of the risk for impact, too. Walking holidays on low, gently undulating foothills, or forest or seaside walks could be good for you, especially during your second trimester, but don't make each day's activity any more strenuous than your pregnant body can cope with. Take frequent rest stops. If you are going to a sunny climate or intending to be outside frequently, always practice good sun safety by wearing a high-SPF, broad-spectrum sunblock that doesn't contain oxybenzone (a chemical linked to low birth weights).

Q Is it safe to have holiday vaccinations while I'm pregnant?

Most vaccinations are made using small amounts of the disease you're vaccinating against, so in general it's better to avoid going to countries that require you to have immunizations. In addition, avoid malaria-risk countries. Although there are anti-malaria medications that are safe to take during pregnancy, malaria itself poses a high risk of death for

you and your baby. If you can't avoid travelling to a high-risk country, talk to your doctor well in advance about the immunizations you'll need and, if relevant, about anti-malaria tablets. On balance it's usually better to vaccinate than risk contracting disease, but you should always seek individualized medical advice.

Q Should I get special travel insurance that covers treatment for my pregnancy?

You won't necessarily need pregnancy-specific travel insurance, but check your policy to see what pregnancy issues are covered. Look for what will happen if you go into labour, have to cancel your holiday because of a pregnancy-related issue, or you need repatriating. Make sure your insurer knows that you're pregnant before you travel and that you are complying with any stipulations that keep your cover safe, such as carrying a letter or certificate from your midwife to say you're fit to travel. Some insurers won't cover you if you travel beyond a certain week of pregnancy, which may be different from the week the airline stipulates, and often insurers don't cover the neonatal period, for example, if your baby is born early and needs medical care.

Take your **pregnancy notes** when you go on holiday so that any doctor **treating** you knows your pregnancy **history** and can look after you safely.

{Q I'm so tired all the time. How can I get enough rest to feel refreshed?

Tiredness is inevitable in pregnancy. During the first trimester, it is caused largely by your body's effort to nourish your developing embryo, and a massive surge in progesterone. During the last trimester, it's the result of the general discomfort of carrying an ever-growing baby. However, there are techniques you can use to minimize tiredness.

Scale back

A busy social life is fantastic when you aren't pregnant, but during pregnancy you may need to be more selective about what you do. Try to cut back on events that are going to require very late bedtimes or long periods of time on your feet. Don't be afraid to cancel plans if you feel too tired to attend – your friends will understand. Work out what your social limits are and work within them. Scale back on your chores, too – consider getting the shopping delivered, for example.

Don't toss and turn

If you wake up in the night and can't get back to sleep, do something quiet but positive, rather than lying there ruminating. Keep a pen and paper beside your bed and write down a to-do list for the following day; read a few pages of a book; take a short walk to the bathroom and back. You could even listen to some soothing night music through headphones (quietly) to give your mind something else to focus on.

Support your legs
Place a cushion between them.

WAYS TO HELP YOU SLEEP

 Nap

Give your body (and brain) a chance to recuperate. If you're working, be unabashed about taking a nap at lunchtime (don't forget your employer is required to provide somewhere for you to rest). At the weekends, set an alarm for a 50-minute nap. This will give you five minutes to fall asleep, but should wake you during your lightest sleep stage (see top right for explanation on sleep cycles), so that you don't feel groggy.

 Rest

Even if you can't have a full nap during the daytime, make sure you make time to rest. That means sitting comfortably in a chair with your eyes closed. According to research, being fully at rest and with your eyes closed is almost as restful as sleep itself. If you're at work, put some earphones in and listen to some music that you find deeply relaxing, or even simply take earplugs to block out the white noise around you.

 Rehydration

Dehydration compounds the effects of feeling tired, making you feel even more drained and lethargic. It's really important that you keep up your fluid intake every day. You don't need to drink more than non-pregnant people, but you do need to make sure you drink enough, which is around 2.2 litres (3½ pints) of fluid a day.

 Food

Your body is best at sleeping when it is relaxed. If you have a light supper, not later than 8pm, by the time you go to bed a couple of hours later the hard work of digestion will be over and your body can concentrate on sleeping rather than digesting. See p.57 for advice on how to distribute your meals and snacks throughout the day.

STAGE OF SLEEP

Awake
REM
Stage 1
Stage 2
Stage 3
Stage 4

0 1 2 3 4 5 6 7 8 9

8-HOUR SLEEP CYCLE

SLEEP CYCLES

When you sleep, your body goes through "sleep cycles", each taking you through five stages, from light to dreaming to deep and back to light again. Each full cycle lasts around 90 minutes, although the time you spend within each stage varies depending on your overall level of tiredness. For a nap to be effective, you should aim for 50 minutes. If you're tired, you'll spend longer in deep, restorative sleep than any of the other stages, but by allowing yourself to come full circle into the light sleep that characterizes the end of a sleep cycle, you'll wake up feeling refreshed.

Did you know...

During each sleep cycle, we experience a period of REM or "dreaming sleep". Periods of REM sleep increase for pregnant women from about 25 weeks pregnant onwards, spiking at around 33 to 36 weeks. Your dreams aren't necessarily more vivid, but you are more aware of them.

Sleeping comfortably This will become more difficult as your baby grows. Use pillows and cushions to support your body while you get some rest.

Best practice

Sleep experts call the rituals and practicalities of sleeping our sleep hygiene. Good sleep hygiene is essential to good sleep. So, keep your bedroom dark and cool. Create a bedtime ritual so that your brain learns what the forerunners to sleep are and gets itself ready to switch off. Keep noise and activity levels low in the hour before bedtime – turn off the television, laptops, mobile phones, and tablets.

IMPROVE YOUR SLEEP POSITION

Sleeping with sore hip joints, nagging back pain, nasal congestion, heartburn, and a growing baby (not to mention other pregnancy niggles) is a challenge in itself. Try these sleeping positions to maximize your chances of a restful night:
» If you have heartburn or congestion, sleep on your left side. Raise the end of your mattress so that your chest and head are raised slightly.
» Avoid rolling onto your back, which in the second trimester onwards can restrict blood-flow to your baby – put a pillow behind your back to stop you rolling over, if necessary.

Pillow at your back
This stops you from rolling onto your back.

Sleep on your left side
This helps to avoid heartburn or congestion.

FASCINATING FACTS

As your bump grows, your body takes on many interesting changes, some of which are absolutely incredible.

23%

This is the amount of extra blood pumped into your uterus while you're pregnant.

30–50%

By 28 weeks your cardio output has increased by 30–50 per cent.

50cm (20in)

This is the average length that the umbilical cord will grow to during a woman's pregnancy.

45%

By week 16, your body will contain 45 per cent more blood than it did before you were pregnant.

37.5°C (99.5°F)

The temperature of the amniotic fluid that surrounds your baby.

50%

You breathe 50 per cent more deeply in pregnancy.

A CLOSER LOOK
Your growing bump

Being pregnant is amazing. Not only does your body change to meet the demands of growing a baby inside you, but also it all takes place in just 40 weeks. When you're pregnant your body creates a whole new organ, the placenta. Your heart and liver might grow in size to help meet the demands of your pregnancy and your uterus expands to accommodate your baby as she increases in size.

| MOTHER AT 12 WEEKS | MOTHER AT 20 WEEKS | MOTHER AT 28 WEEKS | MOTHER AT 40 WEEKS |

Growing bump As your uterus expands, so does your bump. The distance from the pubis to the top of the uterus is measured regularly from the second trimester of pregnancy. It's called the fundal height and is monitored as a marker of fetal growth. The measurement in centimetres usually matches the week of pregnancy that you're in.

1–4 **weeks** During the early weeks your baby is no bigger than the size of a grain of rice, so your uterus has only started on its growth spurt alongside your baby's. At four weeks, your uterus is pretty much the same size as before you were pregnant (about the size of a plum) and it measures between 6–10cm (2½ –4in) in length (not height as it's horizontal). **GRAIN OF RICE**

9–12 **weeks** At this stage your baby is about the size of a lime. You might notice that you need to pass urine more often as your growing uterus puts pressure on your bladder. Frequent urination can also be a sign of a urinary infection, so speak to your GP if it's painful when you pee. Your hands and feet may feel warmer because of the increased blood flow to your skin.

LIME

36-40 weeks

At the very end of your pregnancy your baby is on average 51.2cm (20⅛in) – similar to a medium-size watermelon. Your fundal height peaks at about 36 weeks and measures 36cm (14in). You might find that your bump is a bit of a burden at this stage as it makes simple tasks tricky.

WATERMELON

PUBIS

17-21 weeks

Your baby is roughly the size of a mango at this point of gestation. Your uterus has grown upwards and is now level with the height of your belly button. As your bump becomes more visible people might start to notice that you're pregnant, they might even want to touch your bump.

MANGO

27-30 weeks

Your baby is now about the size of a squash. Your fundal height at 30 weeks is 30cm (12in). The wall of the uterus is muscular and during pregnancy it enlarges to many times its original dimension. By 30 weeks it has tripled in size.

SQUASH

During pregnancy, your body goes through myriad **changes** that influence your emotional and physical **wellbeing.** There's more than just the **stretching** of your belly as the uterus grows; **you might notice** changes to skin, hair, feet, nails, and teeth, not to mention parts of the body you can't see.

Physical and emotional changes

How you change physically

Some of the physical changes that occur to your body during pregnancy might be ones that you are happy with; for example, you might enjoy having a fuller bust, more rounded hips, thick, glossy hair, and a translucent sheen to the skin. Other changes, though, such as stretch marks, may be less welcome and can feel like unpleasant side effects. You may also find that the arch of your foot drops and that you go up a shoe size, which may be a permanent change. Not all women experience all of these changes, but however you're affected, try to keep in mind that they're positive signs that your pregnancy is progressing. Almost without exception, changes to your skin, hair, and nails will reverse once your baby is born.

Understanding your hormones

All the changes that take place in your body during pregnancy are the result of messages that your hormones send to your brain. Pregnancy hormones affect you both physically – changing your body and helping your baby to develop – and emotionally, too. Pregnancy is known for triggering mood swings, and your hormones, combined with a heavy dash of tiredness and probably some anxiety, are to blame. If you have a partner, these moods may take a toll on him or her; make sure the two of you stay connected and find ways to both enjoy pregnancy. It is worthwhile learning about pregnancy hormones and how they affect your emotions. Then having a few strategies that help avoid arguments and allow you to express your feelings constructively will help to steer you through the emotional minefield of this amazing time.

The hidden changes

If the outward signs of pregnancy and the hormonal changes weren't enough to get to grips with, there are lots of internal changes taking place that you may not even notice, but which are essential for nourishing your baby and maintaining your pregnancy. As you'll see, being pregnant affects the functioning of all your internal organs – your heart and liver have to work harder, and your lungs have to adapt to increase their efficiency in a much-reduced space. Within your breasts, long before your baby is born, changes take place that turn them into perhaps the most efficient food source we know of.

Q I've heard about pregnancy hormones, but what are they and what do they do?

At the start of your pregnancy, there is a surge of two hormones, oestrogen and progesterone, which have an essential role in maintaining pregnancy. The rise of these hormones is the result of human chorionic gonadotrophin (hCG) signalling to the corpus luteum (the ruptured egg follicle) that pregnancy is underway.

At around six to nine weeks of pregnancy, the placenta takes over the production of oestrogen and progesterone for the rest of your pregnancy. Other key hormones during your pregnancy include relaxin, oxytocin, prolactin, and endorphins. These, along with androgens (the male sex hormones), are collectively known as sex steroid hormones. The right balance of hormones is essential for a successful pregnancy.

The body system that regulates all of your hormones is called the endocrine system. This includes various glands and organs throughout your body, including the thyroid, adrenal, and pituitary glands, and the hypothalamus, the pancreas, and the ovaries. All your body systems are affected by the action of your endocrine system.

hCG levels almost double every **48 hours** at the beginning of your pregnancy.

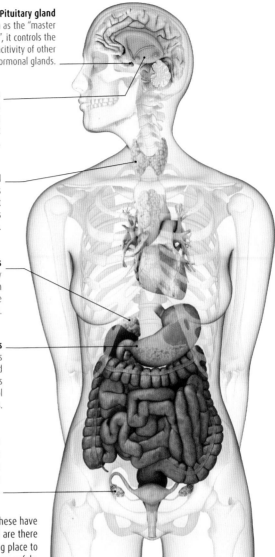

Pituitary gland
Known as the "master gland", it controls the acitivity of other hormonal glands.

Hypothalamus
Part of the brain, it is responsible for keeping the body in a constant and stable condition.

Thyroid
This gland secretes hormones that regulate the body's metabolic rate.

Adrenal glands
Hormones secreted by these glands act on body tissues to enable them to function.

Pancreas
The pancreas makes digestive juices and hormones such as insulin that control blood-sugar levels.

Ovaries
These produce eggs and the reproductive hormones progesterone and oestrogen.

Hormones during pregnancy These have powerful and varied functions and are there to regulate the many changes taking place to enable your baby to develop and be born safely.

OESTROGEN

Initially secreted by the ovaries, oestrogen prepares the lining of the uterus for a potential pregnancy. It also has the following key roles during your pregnancy:

» **Ensures the developing embryo** remains embedded in your uterus.

» **Dilates your blood vessels** so that blood can flow more easily and in greater quantity.

» **Stimulates the milk glands** in preparation for breastfeeding.

» **Improves bone health** while your body is under more pressure.

PROGESTERONE

This hormone plays a vital role in the early stages of pregnancy by preparing the body for fertilization and then establishing the placenta. It does the following:

» **Prepares the lining of the uterus** for implantation and encourages it to thicken.

» **Helps to regulate** the changes in your metabolism.

» **Thickens the "plug"** that forms in the cervix to avoid bacteria entering the uterus and causing infection.

» **Strengthens muscles** in the pelvic wall in preparation for labour.

OTHER HORMONES

Your pregnancy is also specifically influenced by the action of:

» **Oxytocin,** the "love" hormone that triggers labour and helps you to bond with your baby.

» **Endorphins,** the "feel-good" hormones that help to mitigate your experience of pain during labour.

» **Prolactin,** the hormone that stimulates your body to produce milk for your baby.

» **Relaxin,** the hormone that helps to loosen your muscles and ligaments to make space for your baby.

Q My mother had terrible varicose veins when she was pregnant. Will this happen to me?

Varicose veins are one of the most common side effects of pregnancy and they usually occur in the third trimester. If you do get them, your midwife can tell you how they can be treated after your baby is born.

A little under half of all pregnant women get varicose veins or haemorrhoids which are varicose veins in the anus (see p.132). You're more likely to suffer from them if a close member of your family has had them. They develop when progesterone levels in your body during pregnancy relax the walls of your blood vessels so they lose muscle tone. At the same time, your circulation is under greater strain from the increase in blood pumping around your body. Your veins are less taut and they also have more work to do. Aching in your legs is often the first sign that you might have varicose veins, as well as some itching around the affected veins.

If you think you might be at risk of varicose veins, your midwife can give you compression stockings, which help to keep your veins "tightened". It is a good idea to exercise regularly and to avoid excessive weight gain, as this can exacerbate them.

NORMAL VEIN   VARICOSED VEIN

Incompetent valve
Backflow of blood
Varicosities
Flow of blood
Valve

How varicose veins form
Valves in the vein walls stop your blood flowing back down your veins between pumps. During pregnancy, the valves, with only weakened vein walls to support them, can fail to work. Blood starts to pool, which makes the veins distended and swollen.

Relieving the symptoms Lie down and raise your legs so that they are higher than your hips. Avoid standing for long periods.

Q I had dreadful acne as a teenager and now it's back. Why is pregnancy doing this?

When you were a teenager the surge of hormones during puberty caused your body to create excess sebum – the skin's natural lubricating oil. Now that you're pregnant, the same thing is happening again. Follow a strict cleansing routine for the skin on your face, morning and night, using a gentle, hypo-allergenic cleanser. Avoid using a highly scented soap, which can dry out and irritate your skin. You can use an astringent if this has helped you in the past, but talk to your midwife before you do as many medicated astringents are not suitable for use during pregnancy.

Q What changes in my skin and nails should I expect?

You're likely to have a pregnancy glow from about the middle of your second trimester. It's partly because your blood volume increases, which means nutrients are carried more efficiently to all your organs, including your skin. Plumped-up cells – the result of increased fluid levels in your blood – can smooth out wrinkles and blemishes, while increases in the hormone progesterone can cause pinkness, making you look rosy. Hormone changes can make your body produce more sebum, which can give your skin a sheen. As well as making you look radiant, hormones can make your skin very dry and possibly itchy. Some women

sweat more, which can cause rashes. Make sure you drink plenty of water to keep hydrated and use an unperfumed moisturizer. Nails can become harder, more brittle, or softer.

25%
Up to a quarter of women have **itchy** or **sensitive skin** during pregnancy. Keep some calamine lotion on hand to soothe general rashes.

Q Are stretch marks inevitable? Why do we get them and is there anything I can do?

Stretch marks (or striae gravidarum) can appear on your abdomen, thighs, hips, arms, breasts, and buttocks. They tend to run in families, so if your mother, grandmother, or sisters had them, it's likely that you will too. There's very little you can do to prevent them, but you're not alone as 90 per cent of women get them.

They're caused when the collagen – the connective tissue in your skin – weakens, stretches, and tears as your bump grows. Hormonal changes make the problem worse.

A diet that's rich in skin-supporting nutrients (found in nuts and seeds, and fresh fruits and vegetables, which contain high levels of antioxidants), and not "eating for two" (see p.59) can help to minimize the effects. Try to gain weight steadily throughout your pregnancy (see chart, p.126) so that your skin has time to stretch. If you stay fit you may be able to limit the appearance of stretch marks. Keeping your skin supple with moisturizing creams will help it to ping back into shape after you've had your baby, but studies show that they have limited effect on stretch marks. This is because collagen works deep within the layers of your skin, so creams you put on top my not be enough.

Once you've had your baby, the stretch marks will gradually fade over time. In most women they will disappear altogether, or remain only as fine, silvery lines by the time a baby is six months old.

Q How common is it for skin pigmentation changes to occur and what exactly is the "butterfly mask"?

Chloasma, also known as the "butterfly mask" or melasma, gives you dark or pinkish patches over your cheeks, nose, eyes, and forehead – sometimes in a butterfly shape, hence the common name.

Butterfly effect Women with darker skin may be more susceptible than women with lighter skin.

Pregnant women are prone to this because the increased levels of oestrogen in their bodies make more melanin – the pigment that gives your skin, hair, and eyes their colour, and which protects your skin from the sun's harmful UV rays. Chloasma affects around half of all pregnant women, and is more common in those with darker or black skin, whose levels of melanin are already high. This side effect is completely harmless to your or your baby's physical health, but some women can be upset by it.

Being in the sun can make it worse, so stay in the shade and use a high-SPF, broad-spectrum sunblock that does not contain oxybenzone. You're probably already taking folic acid (see p.49), but if you aren't, or if you're past the 12 weeks' mark and have stopped taking it, talk to your midwife about a daily supplement; some studies show that being low in the mineral folate can make you more susceptible to chloasma. Finally, remember that it is almost always temporary; your skin should return to normal not long after you've given birth.

Cover up Exposure to the sun can make the mask more pronounced. Wear a hat to protect your face.

DARKENING SKIN

Increased levels of melanin in your skin are responsible for all manner of skin changes that may occur in pregnancy. These can include:

» **A greater number of freckles** on your face.

» **Darkening in moles**, birthmarks, and scars.

» **The line that may appear** from your navel to your pubic bone, known as the "linea nigra".

» **Your ability to tan** more easily.

» **Darker areolae** around your nipples.

Linea nigra This is situated where the left and right vertical abdominal muscles meet. Your growing bump causes them to separate and darken.

Q The palms of my hands are red and hot. Is this a recognized side effect of pregnancy?

Around 30 per cent of pregnant women get a condition called plantar erythema, which causes reddening in the palms, and in the fleshy pads underneath your thumbs and little fingers. It sometimes also appears on the soles of the feet. The condition is a result of higher oestrogen levels, which increase the amount of blood in your circulatory system. This in turn raises your body temperature and how warm your extremities feel and how red they appear. The condition is nothing to worry about and will go away after you've had your baby. If the reddening is bothering you, though, simply do what you can to keep your hands cool.

Q My hair is much thicker than it was before I got pregnant. Will it stay like this forever?

No, it won't. All that thick, glossy hair isn't just the result of increased levels of sebum (your body's natural oil) over your scalp. Higher levels of progesterone in the second and third trimesters of pregnancy mean that you don't shed hair in the way that you did when you weren't pregnant. However, when your hormone levels fall dramatically after the baby is born, you shed all the excess hair over a much shorter period of time, so it can appear as if clumps of hair are falling out daily. So, unfortunately, the locks you love now aren't for ever, but don't worry – after the birth, your hair is simply returning to its normal thickness.

Q I have tiny red and blue lines on my face and neck. Will they go away?

It's possible that you have some temporary "spider veins" appearing on your face, neck, shoulders and chest. They are simply where the very finest walls of your capillaries, near to the surface of your skin, have broken under the strain of the increased amount of blood in your circulation. They will usually disappear of their own accord once you've had the baby. Blue veins due to increased blood flow to breast tissue may become more noticeable.

Q I've heard that pregnant women are prone to tooth decay. Why is this, and how can I prevent it?

It's an old wives' tale that pregnancy rots your teeth. However, it is true that you're more susceptible to bleeding gums and gum disease, particularly if you had weakened gums before you got pregnant.

The weakening of the connective tissue that can lead to stretch marks can also make your gums softer and liable to tearing. Also, your saliva is now more acidic, which can exacerbate the effects. This can lead to infection and damaged teeth.

Reducing your sugar intake to protect your teeth and gums and good hygiene is essential. In the UK, dental treatment is free during pregnancy (and for 12 months afterwards), so take advantage of this perk and don't miss your check-ups. If you do need essential dental work, it is fine to have a local anaesthetic during the second trimester. There is no risk to your baby. Some dentists believe that because gum disease is linked with premature birth, it's better for the mother to have dental treatment when it's needed rather than waiting until after the baby's birth.

DENTAL CARE WHILE PREGNANT

The checklist below will ensure that you are clear about the things you need to do, what to tell your dentist, and procedures that should be avoided.

 » Maintain good hygiene using a soft toothbrush and floss regularly. Always brush after a meal, but be gentle, and use a non-alcohol-based mouthwash to help remove residual bacteria.

 » Tell your dentist that you are pregnant once you have booked in with your midwife. You should inform your dentist about any medication your are taking as some might affect the development of your child's teeth.

 » Tell your dentist if tenderness, bleeding, or gum swelling occurs at any time during your pregnancy.

 » Avoid dental treatment during the first trimester and the second half of the third trimester (the last six to eight weeks), as these are key times in the baby's growth anddevelopment.

 » Avoid dental X-rays during pregnancy if you can. If an X-ray is absolutely essential, your dentist will be extra vigilant to keep your baby safe, and most dental X-rays don't affect the abdomen.

 » Postpone all elective, non-essential dental procedures until after the delivery.

 » Avoid having an amalgam (silver) filling removed or put in during pregnancy, as a precautionary measure.

Q Pregnancy seems to have me elated one minute and devastated the next. Is this normal?

During your first trimester, the hormonal changes in your body are rapid and raging. It's a primeval response that ensures you maintain your pregnancy. These surges, primarily in the hormones oestrogen and progesterone, upset the chemical balance in your brain, causing neurotransmitters – your brain's chemical messengers – to switch on and off randomly. And that's what gives you the mood swings.

In many cases, your mood will settle by week 12. However, some women continue to experience severe highs and lows and may be diagnosed with antenatal depression. This is as common as postnatal depression and can be just as serious. As well as fluctuating hormones, there are other causes of antenatal depression such as anxiety about your pregnancy, feeling sick and tired, feeling low, previous depression, fear of something going wrong and isolation. If your mood swings are very extreme, or you suspect you may be suffering from depression (and almost 10 per cent of women are thought to experience this during pregnancy), speak to your healthcare professional, who will be able to get you the treatment you need.

Q What can I do to help myself manage my emotions?

There are many self-help techniques you can employ. Try some of these quick-fixes when you feel a negative mood – sadness or irritation – taking hold:

» Walk around the block or through a park, even if it's just for 10 minutes. Fresh air and a change of scenery are sometimes all you need to clear your head.

» Have a healthy snack as sugar lows exacerbate negative feelings or irritation so keep your energy levels stable.

» Write a letter explaining how you are feeling. Even if you never send it, it can help to put things into perspective.

» Knead some dough, make a cake, or make something that involves using some elbow grease. Physical exertion can help you to work through what's troubling you and may provide an outlet for your pent-up adrenaline.

Q I am so forgetful. Is there really such a thing as "baby brain"?

Anecdotal evidence suggests that forgetfulness and lack of concentration are natural side-effects of pregnancy. Scientists are still trying to find out if there is a physiological reason for this, with one recent study proposing that the emotional parts of the brain "plump up" during pregnancy and the more logical, functional parts wind down in order to maximize the mother's instinct for responding empathetically to her baby immediately after birth.

However, there are still questions about why physiological brain changes happen, if they do, with some studies pointing the blame at hormones. Experts tend to agree, though, that you are more tired, stressed, and distracted during pregnancy so the energy you have for clear thinking zooms in on important things (your health and that of your developing baby) rather than where you put the car keys. Just try to get as much rest as possible and be assured that there is no evidence to suggest that "baby brain" – physiological or anecdotal – lasts any longer than pregnancy itself, and the effects will reverse after birth.

Q My mood swings are causing rows with my partner. How can we learn to cope with them better?

First things first – get your partner on board. Learn about the hormonal changes of pregnancy together and try to rationalize your irrationality.

Your partner is less likely to take personally anything you throw at him if he knows what's happening in your body. Learning to support your mood swings, rather than dismissing or escalating them, is a key role for your partner, and should not be underestimated. Remember, too, that while the hormones are affecting your body, anxiety, nervousness, and excitement about impending parenthood are things that you both feel. Indeed, your partner may feel overwhelmed by the thought of an added responsibility.

Try counting to 10 when either of you is irritable and feels like snapping. It won't always work, but if enough seconds can elapse before you speak, your words are more likely to be constructive, conciliatory, or placatory.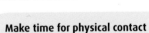

Make time for physical contact such as holding hands as you walk down the street. Even giving each other a hug at the end of a tiring day will give you a surge of endorphins and oxytocin – feel-good hormones that help to stabilize your moods.

 Find time to escape into your own personal space, if this suits the kind of person you are. Perhaps this happens naturally when you go to work, or maybe it means that one of you curls up with a book while the other takes a bath.

Make time for activities together that aren't related to the baby – give yourselves constant reminders of the good things about your relationship, so that when your mood swings you have a recent memory of why the two of you make a good team.

Q What happens to my amazing body during pregnancy?

Over the course of the nine months of your pregnancy, your body has to adapt and make space for your growing baby, to ensure your baby's growth and protection, and to prepare itself to give birth. Some of the changes you go through will be obvious – a growing abdomen and larger breasts, for example – but many will seem imperceptible to you, or you'll notice them only when they have a knock-on effect that makes you wonder what's going on. Here's an overview of all the amazing things your body is doing to adapt to pregnancy and nourish your baby.

NOSE

From early in your pregnancy you may notice that you have a heightened sense of smell. This may be due to more blood pumping round your body. However, some people believe it could be a protective mechanism – to keep you away from substances that could be harmful.

LUNGS

Your lungs move up and back as your pregnancy progresses. They are being pushed to their uppermost limits which can make you breathless. Your air intake increases to help to supply you and your baby with enough oxygen.

DIAPHRAGM

The increasing size of your uterus during pregnancy means that your diaphragm – the flat wall of muscle that controls your breathing and lies beneath your lungs – is pushed upwards, squashing your lungs in the process, but increasing your capacity for breathing deeply.

STOMACH

Your stomach may send signals to your brain for certain foods that you "must" have (cravings) and to avoid foods that make you feel ill (aversions). Some scientists believe that cravings encourage you to fill a nutritional gap, while aversions stop you consuming substances that could be harmful to your pregnancy.

INTESTINE

Increases in progesterone during pregnancy inhibit the the action that moves food along your digestive tract. Although this can cause constipation and heartburn, the slowing down means you can get the maximum nutritional benefit from food as it passes through you.

Did you know?

Before you are pregnant, your uterus is roughly the size of a plum. By the time you have reached six weeks, although you may not feel pregnant, your uterus will have grown to the size of an apple. During your whole pregnancy, your uterus will expand to become between 500 and 1000 times its normal size.

BEFORE PREGNANCY　　**SIX WEEKS**

CERVIX

During your pregnancy it remains strong, and tight. In labour, following hormonal changes triggered by the pressure of your baby's head, the cervix thins and widens. The cervix lets go of its "plug" and when it is fully dilated your baby is ready to be born.

UTERUS

The lining of your uterus - the endometrium - thickens to receive the embryo, and its muscular wall grows to accommodate the baby and to give you the strength to push the baby out when the time comes. Once you reach your third trimester, your uterus will start to produce "practice" contractions, known as Braxton Hicks. No one is sure why we have these, but it's assumed it's to prepare the uterus for the job it has to do during birth.

BRAIN

Some research suggests that the more emotional parts of your brain become dominant during pregnancy. This may occur to begin the bonding process with your baby – making you more emotionally attuned to your baby's needs.

LIVER

Your baby's waste passes through your system, which means that your liver has to work harder than usual to detoxify your own body. To accommodate the extra workload, it will often increase in size.

BREASTS

Your breasts prepare to produce milk from as early as seven weeks pregnant and in the following weeks you will notice them begin to grow. You might also notice that your areolae are darker, and that little bumps have appeared around your nipples; these are known as Montgomery's tubercles and these will secrete fluid to help entice your baby to your nipple. Towards the end of your pregnancy, your body will have created a highly sophisticated milk manufacturing and delivery system. Lobules within the breast get bigger and, even before you've had your baby, begin to make colostrum – a highly nutritious liquid that your baby drinks before your milk "comes in". Also, the delivery mechanism within your breast increases to make sure there are plenty of channels supplying milk to your nipples.

HEART

Your heart pumps harder throughout your pregnancy, increasing from around 65 beats per minute at the start of pregnancy to around 75 beats per minute by the time you are at full term. This is so that your body can meet your baby's increasing demands for nutrients and oxygen as she grows.

SPINE

As your pregnancy progresses, your centre of gravity changes. As your bump grows forwards, your centre of gravity shifts forwards, which means you have to "lean back" on your spine to correct your balance and stay upright. Your spine allows you to do this, but the unnatural posture may give you backache.

PELVIS

This is key to your baby's safety during pregnancy and at birth. At the start, the pelvic bones provide protection for your developing uterus. Then, during birth, your pelvis expands and contracts to push your baby through into the birth canal, even forcing her to turn during her descent.

VEINS AND ARTERIES

Your blood volume will increase by up to 45 per cent during your pregnancy and it gets better at clotting in preparation for when you give birth to your baby and when the placenta comes away from your uterus – the blood needs to clot quickly to minimize blood loss. Pregnancy hormones cause your blood vessels to dilate – that is, they open up to allow more blood to pass through them.

HIPS

Your body produces increasing amounts of the hormone relaxin, which loosens your ligaments. This can cause a few aches and pains during your pregnancy, but it allows your bones to move outwards enough to enable your baby to pass through your pelvis during birth. Your hips may also become more rounded as your body stores extra fat during pregnancy. This provides fuel for making milk.

Q I was overweight before I became pregnant. Should I try not to gain weight now?

Never restrict your calorie intake during pregnancy: your baby and you need a basic level of nourishment in order to remain healthy.

This is true whatever your weight before you discovered you were pregnant. However, that basic level of nourishment can be slightly different depending upon your weight at the start of your pregnancy.

To find out if your pre-pregnancy weight is within normal range, you can calculate your body mass index (BMI). You can do this up until about 8 weeks of pregnancy as you will not have put on a significant amount of weight by this time. Divide your weight in kilograms by your height in metres, then

divide it again. You don't need to consume extra calories during the first and second trimesters – the recommended 2000 per day is sufficient. In the third trimester you may need to eat 200–300 calories extra per day. Always discuss your calorie intake and weight with your midwife before doing any "counting", though; the most important thing is that you get enough calories and nutrients for your baby to grow properly. If you don't get enough, you can be facing a pregnancy that results in birth defects or other problems.

WEIGHT GAIN DURING PREGNANCY

The table below below shows the ideal weight gain during pregnancy for each of the four BMI categories - underweight, ideal weight, overweight, obese.

WEIGHT	BMI	WEIGHT GAIN	IDEAL WEEKLY WEIGHT GAIN
Underweight	less than 18.5	14–17kg (31–37½lb)	approx 1–1.2kg (2¼–3lb) every two weeks in the second and third trimesters
Ideal weight	18.5 to 24.9	11–16kg (24–35lb)	approx 800g–1kg (1¾–2¼lb) every two weeks in the second and third trimesters
Overweight	25 to 29.9	7–11.5kg (15½–25lb)	approx 500–800g (1–1¾lb) every two weeks in the second and third trimesters
Obese	30 or higher	4.5–9kg (10–20lb)	approx 300–600g (½–1¼lb) every two weeks in the second and third trimesters

Q A few years ago I was bulimic. Is this significant now that I'm pregnant?

During pregnancy, your baby receives all its nourishment from you. If your stores are depleted you can become malnourished and as a result risk having a baby with abnormally low birth weight and other possible problems. If you are suffering from an eating disorder such as bulimia or anorexia, or you are worried that a previous condition will return, you need to inform your healthcare professional. He or she can help you by providing emotional support throughout your pregnancy and also put a plan in place, should you need it, to help you have a healthy pregnancy.

Q How long will it take me to get back to my pre-pregnancy weight after the birth?

That entirely depends on how much weight you gain during your pregnancy, whether you breastfeed, and how much of a concerted effort

Learn to love your **"mummy tummy"**. Even when they lose their pregnancy weight, **some women never have the same figure** they had before they had their baby. Although this may cause wardrobe inconvenience, a different body shape – **curves** and angles in **different places** – it doesn't mean a body that is less attractive. In fact, it could be the start of a whole new image that you love even more than the last.

you make to lose weight after the birth. You'll feel extremely tired in the first few months of looking after a newborn, and you may not feel up to doing much exercise other than taking your baby out for a walk in the pushchair. But that's fine – gentle walking is wonderful exercise and there's no need to push yourself any harder than that. The most important thing is to try not to rush the process. Furthermore, making milk for your baby if you are breastfeeding uses a lot of energy, so you'll need to increase your calorie intake to keep going. In general terms, if getting back to your pre-pregnancy weight is a priority for you, think of your weight loss according to the old adage "nine months up, nine months down". Give yourself all that time to get back to where you want to be. Don't get frustrated if it takes you longer – some women take many years to regain their pre-pregnancy weight, often out of choice, waiting until they've completed their family so that they only have to think about weight-loss once. Of course, some women also slip straight back into their hotpants after birth. You're wonderfully lucky – and incredibly unusual – if that turns out to be the case for you.

Q How much of my weight gain is caused by my baby and how much of it is just me?

About a third of your pregnancy weight gain is your baby and the placenta, but that doesn't mean that two-thirds of it is you – or at least it's not "bad-for-you" you.

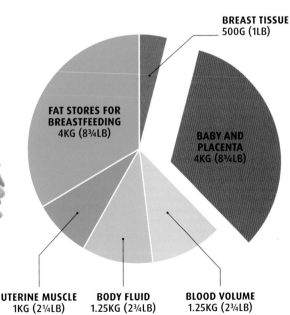

That two-thirds is made up of increased blood and fluid plumping up your cells; you also have more muscle around your uterus (it helps you to get the baby out), and the increase in progesterone and oestrogen mean that your breasts grow larger and therefore heavier even before you start making milk. You also have increased fat stores (usually around your hips) to prepare you for making milk and breastfeeding. All of these elements of your weight gain are positive, natural, and nothing to worry about. Try to welcome your curvier hips, larger breasts, and glorious skin. They are beautiful signs that your body is doing its job of nourishing your baby.

Growing bump As it grows you will notice other parts of your body changing, too. Try to enjoy this time.

WHERE THE "PREGNANCY WEIGHT" GOES

A woman who gains 12kg (26½lb) in weight during her pregnancy will have that gain distributed roughly like this:

BREAST TISSUE
500G (1LB)

FAT STORES FOR
BREASTFEEDING
4KG (8¾LB)

BABY AND
PLACENTA
4KG (8¾LB)

UTERINE MUSCLE
1KG (2¼LB)

BODY FLUID
1.25KG (2¾LB)

BLOOD VOLUME
1.25KG (2¾LB)

Key areas The increase in volume and weight supports and nourishes your growing baby.

Uterine muscle   Baby

Body fluid   Placenta

Change over the trimesters
Your baby and its placenta will grow; however, the fluid around your baby will reduce.

Pregnancy is a time of **blooming** and beauty, when your body is doing the most amazing thing possible – **creating** another human being. However, it also means that **your body** undergoes changes to **facilitate** the **growth** of the **baby**, and these can sometimes be less than desirable for you.

Common complaints

Common complaints in pregnancy

The complaints on the following pages highlight side effects that some women experience while pregnant. The common complaints experienced during pregnancy can be grouped into seven main types.

1. General symptoms that are as simple as tiredness, difficulty in sleeping, protruding navel, nasal problems, blurred vision, swollen feet and ankles, fluid retention (oedema), foot problems, and headaches.

2. Skin changes such as heat rash and extremely itchy skin.

3. Breast problems, including leaking fluid and clogged milk ducts.

4. Digestive problems such as nausea, vomiting, hyperemesis gravidarum, heartburn, indigestion, constipation, and increased flatulence.

5. Heart and circulation problems for example, dizziness, breathlessness, varicose veins, and haemorrhoids.

6. Aches and pains such as numbness in hands, lower abdominal pressure, abdominal pains, carpal tunnel syndrome, backpain, sciatica, and restless legs.

7. Urinary and vaginal problems which include thrush, vaginal discharge and bleeding, urinary tract infections, and the inability to urinate.

Coping with common complaints

This section offers explanations and advice for dealing with the range of complaints you may or may not experience during pregnancy. Some are worse than others and some can be embraced as a sign of your bump getting bigger and your baby growing in size (protruding navel). Try to look at the issues you might be encountering as a positive sign that your pregnancy is progressing.

Illness and medications during pregnancy

When you're pregnant your immune system is suppressed slightly so that you don't reject the baby. This means that you might be more likely to fall ill. If you are unwell during pregnancy it's important to know how to deal with an illness and which medications you can take. During the first trimester only paracetamol is considered safe. Once you're into your second trimester some other over-the-counter medications are all right, but you must always follow the advice from your healthcare professional.

{Q What pregnancy complaints might I come across?

You might be lucky and experience none or only some mild complaints during your pregnancy. Complaints can range from small things that are just plain annoying such as thrush, to more debilitating conditions, such as severe pregnancy sickness. Whatever you are experiencing, remember that it will soon pass. You will quickly forget the heartburn or indigestion that pregnancy brings once you're holding your newborn. However, if you are experiencing a complaint that is too difficult to deal with then ask a healthcare professional for advice.

Headaches

» What, when, and how often?
A heavy, pounding head is common in pregnancy – especially if you were prone to headaches during your periods. Headaches are most common in the early stages of pregnancy and usually don't follow any particular pattern or confine themselves to one part of the head. Later on they can be related to anxiety about birth and parenthood.

» What causes them?
Hormonal changes in your body are probably responsible, although feelings of stress about your pregnancy and tiredness can exacerbate the problem.

» What does it mean for my pregnancy?
Mild pregnancy headaches have no implications for your long-term health nor for the health of your baby: they're simply a side effect of what's going on in your changing body. However, if headaches are severe and long lasting, and/or occur later in pregnancy, they could be a sign of pre-eclampsia, and occasionally headaches in pregnancy indicate a stroke, so talk to your doctor if you're concerned.

» What can I do?
If your headache is bad, it's usually okay to take paracetamol. Stay hydrated, get lots of rest, and limit your caffeine intake. If paracetamol doesn't resolve a headache, consult a health professional.

Low iron/anaemia

» What, when, and how often?
Iron is the mineral that carries oxygen in your blood. It also helps to build and maintain muscles. The burden of pregnancy can cause your iron levels to drop in early pregnancy. When your iron levels are so low that you are deficient (measured as having less than 11g of iron per litre of blood), you have anaemia. This occurs in almost 25 per cent of pregnancies in the UK. Low iron levels make you feel lethargic and sometimes dizzy.

» What causes it?
A vegan or vegetarian diet can cause low iron levels, as meat and dairy products are the body's main sources. If you've had babies close together, your stores will be depleted at the start of your second pregnancy. If you're carrying more than one baby, you're likely to suffer too.

» What does it mean for my pregnancy?
Your body will prioritize the baby's iron (oxygen) requirements over yours, so you'll feel the symptoms of low iron before there's any danger to your baby.

You have a slightly increased risk of having a low birthweight baby or going into labour early.

» What can I do?
Your midwife may prescribe you with supplements. However, don't take supplements without medical supervision, as having too much iron in your blood can be toxic. Otherwise, try to get plenty of rest and eat lots of iron-rich foods as well as foods rich in vitamin C, which helps your body absorb iron.

RED MEAT

PUMPKIN SEEDS

Dizziness and breathlessness

» What, when, and how often?
Dizziness, dizzy spells, and breathlessness can occur frequently for women during pregnancy. If you experience frequent dizziness, if you've fainted or had a blackout, or if symptoms are accompanied by swelling in the legs, then inform your healthcare professional as soon as possible.

» What causes it?
In your first trimester dizziness can happen because there's not enough of a blood supply to fill your rapidly expanding circulatory system. In your second trimester it is likely to be caused by the pressure of your expanding uterus on your blood vessels. Dizziness can also be caused by low blood sugar, dehydration, or if you're feeling too hot. When you stand up too quickly it's caused by a quick change of blood flow away from the brain. Breathlessness is caused by your expanding uterus pushing everything upwards, leaving your lungs with less room to expand when you take a deep breath. High levels of progesterone also increase your breathing rate.

» What does it mean for my pregnancy?
If you faint or feel dizzy on a regular basis then it might be a sign of anaemia. Feeling dizzy every now and then isn't a cause for concern and won't affect your baby. It's completely normal to experience breathlessness and it doesn't harm you or your baby.

» What can I do?
Make sure you stay well-hydrated, get up slowly from lying down or a seated position, keep your blood sugar up, and avoid overheating. If you do feel like you're going to faint then try to increase the blood flow to your brain.

Overheating

» What, when, and how often?
Pregnant women often find they have hot hands and feet and are prone to their faces flushing.

» What causes it?
Increased blood supply to your skin and extremities, hormone changes, and the effort of carrying extra weight.

» What does it mean for my pregnancy?
Feeling hot is just part of being pregnant and isn't an indication of anything that can harm you or your baby.

» What can I do?
Wear loose cotton clothing, pop your feet or hands in a bowl of cold water, and try to keep your rooms cool.

Sickness and nausea

» What, when, and how often?

Appearing at around the fifth week of pregnancy, and usually at its worst around week 12, then disappearing by around week 20, nausea affects up to 80 per cent of women. It can occur at any time of day and cause vomiting. Mild forms cause pervading feelings of nausea. Hyperemesis gravidarum is a stronger form of the condition, but is not common.

» What causes them?

Sudden increased production of pregnancy hormones that upset the gut, as well as a slowing down of the passage of food and waste material through it.

» What does it mean for my pregnancy?

Sickness is generally a good sign that your body

is working hard to maintain your pregnancy. Hyperemesis gravidarum may, on rare occasions, lead to a baby having low birthweight due to it not getting enough nutrients from you, but overall, women who suffer with sickness are statistically less likely to have miscarriages or babies that are born prematurely.

» What can I do?

Snack little and often (see p.58), even if dry crackers are all you can keep down. Try not to have snacks that are high in refined sugar. Avoid strong-smelling and strong-tasting foods, and foods with a high fat content. Drink plenty of fluids and get plenty of rest. See your doctor if you're vomiting three or more times a day, or if you can't face eating anything at all.

Hyperemesis gravidarum

Hyperemesis gravidarum occurs in less than 2 per cent of pregnant women. It's a severe form of pregnancy sickness, characterized by frequent vomiting. If you are experiencing this condition and are unable to keep any food or drink down for more than 24 hours then you need to visit your healthcare provider. You will most likely have your urine tested to make sure you don't have an infection. You might also be referred for a scan to rule out any issues with your pregnancy. You will be weighed and if you have lost more than 10 per cent of your body weight then you are likely to experience complications with your pregnancy. Your doctor might send you to hospital if you are very dehydrated and you will stay there until you are well enough to go home. In hospital you will be given intravenous fluids, anti-sickness drugs, and possibly a vitamin supplement. The good news is that hyperemesis usually disappears when you are 13 weeks pregnant.

Nap time Try to take short naps or have periods of rest to help deal with the draining feeling that nausea and vomiting bring.

Heartburn and indigestion

» What, when, and how often?

Indigestion is the feeling that you have something permanently stuck in your windpipe, and may make you feel sick or as if you want to burp. Heartburn causes a burning sensation in your throat – it's usually a side effect of indigestion and often occurs after you've eaten. It is known medically as acid reflux. Around 80 per cent of pregnant women suffer from indigestion during pregnancy, and it's more likely to occur if this is a second or subsequent pregnancy.

» What causes them?

Everything in your abdomen is squashed as your baby grows, which means that your intestines get pushed upwards, making it harder for food to flow seamlessly

through your system. This, along with the slowed-down action of your intestine (caused by increased progesterone), means that your stomach acid remains in contact with the lining of your stomach for longer than it should, irritating it and causing the symptoms of indigestion. The relaxing of your muscles during pregnancy also relaxes a valve at the bottom of your oesophagus (gullet), that normally prevents stomach acid escaping back up to your throat.

» What does it mean for my pregnancy?

There is nothing sinister about indigestion during pregnancy and it poses no risks to you or your baby.

» What can I do?

Avoid spicy or highly flavoured foods, and eat little and often so that your stomach has as little to deal with at a time as possible. If your indigestion is affecting your life (perhaps you constantly feel sick or you're burping), you may be able to take antacids to help settle things, but you will need to consult your healthcare professional first.

Try propping yourself up with cushions at night or if you're having a nap during the day. This helps to prevent the acids in your stomach coming up into your throat.

Flatulence

» What, when, and how often?

Unfortunately, pregnancy can increase the likelihood that you'll need to expel wind from your anus – flatulence. it affects almost all pregnant women at some time during their pregnancy.

» What causes it?

Certain foods, such as those high in fat or carbohydrate, are harder for your body to break down. During pregnancy they spend longer in your intestine than they would if you weren't pregnant and they create gas as they sit there. You expel this gas as flatulence.

» What does it mean for my pregnancy?

Flatulence poses no danger to your health or to that of your unborn baby, but it can be embarrassing and cause cramping. If you have cramping that doesn't feel like wind, contact your midwife.

» What can I do?

Try to avoid eating too many foods that are high in saturated fats and carbohydrates that are known for causing wind (Brussels sprouts, prunes, cauliflower, asparagus, cabbage, artichokes, beans, and so on). A balanced diet should keep flatulence to a minimum. Eating little and often will help your gut to keep up. Make sure you sit upright when you eat and slowly chew every mouthful of food.

Vaginal discharge

» What, when, and how often?

Known medically as leucorrhoea, vaginal discharge is part of your body's natural cleansing system – and it's perfectly normal to have more of it during pregnancy.

» What causes it?

During pregnancy the layer of muscle in the vagina thickens and cells lining the vagina increase in response to rises in the pregnancy hormone oestrogen. This helps the vagina to prepare for childbirth. The increase in cells mean a rise in volume of vaginal discharge.

» What does it mean for my pregnancy?

Healthy vaginal discharge is not an indicator of anything being wrong with your pregnancy. It's completely normal.

» What can I do?

If the discharge is so heavy that it could leak onto clothing, use sanitary towels to soak up excess. Consult your healthcare professional if the discharge is foul smelling or tinged with blood. He or she will need to take a swab to see if you have an infection. Consult him or her if the discharge is persistent, which could indicate premature rupture of the membranes. Avoid the temptation to "wash it away" as you could upset your body's natural cleansing and antibacterial balance, and cause thrush.

Thrush

» What, when, and how often?

Thrush – or vaginal candidiasis to give it its medical name – is a fungal infection that causes a proliferation of candida albicans (a natural yeast) in the vaginal tract. It causes increased vaginal discharge (which can smell of yeast), sometimes pain during sexual intercourse, and some soreness and itchiness in the vagina.

» What causes it?

An increase in pregnancy hormones causes the body's natural sugars to increase around the vagina, which "feeds" candida. Sometimes the infection is sexually transmitted,

but often it is the result of not wiping properly when you go to the loo (always wipe front to back).

» What does it mean for my pregnancy?

During pregnancy, thrush poses no risks to your baby, but the infection can pass to the baby during vaginal birth.

» What can I do?

Avoid using perfumed soaps and bubble baths, which can hamper the work of natural flora in your vagina at fighting the candida infection. See your healthcare professional, who will confirm the infection using a vaginal swab and may then prescribe you a topical cream or a pessary to kill the candida (don't use over-the-counter medicines and do not take oral medication for thrush). Usually one prescribed pessary will clear the problem. If you are at the start of your pregnancy, you'll probably have to wait until you are in your second trimester to have any treatment at all. Your partner will need to be treated too, as thrush can be passed back and forth between you.

Did you know...

An alternative way to relieve the symptoms of thrush is to smear the area with live yogurt or wear a sanitary towel with live yogurt on the surface (for a short period of time). You can also try a warm bath with a few drops of vinegar added to the water. You should always wear cotton underwear as it allows your vagina to breathe. Do not wear tight jeans or trousers that decrease the flow of air to this area and rub against it (if you already have thrush), making you more uncomfortable.

80% of women will experience nausea or vomiting in early pregnancy.

Constipation

» What, when, and how often?

Feeling that you need to pass a stool and either being unable to do so, or finding doing so painful or uncomfortable means that you are constipated. Stools, when they do pass, tend to be hard and dry, and may tear the delicate mucous lining of your bowel as they make their way out. This can cause some bleeding. Constipation can occur at any time during pregnancy, but is common in the first trimester.

» What causes it?

During pregnancy your intestines and bowel have slowed down because of the increase in progesterone in your system. This means that your stool spends longer in your colon, and water gets reabsorbed from it into your body, thus making the stool hard. The effects are compounded later in pregnancy because your bowel, like everything else in your abdomen, is squashed and has less room to do its job. Iron supplements (if you're taking them) can exacerbate constipation, so talk to your midwife about whether it's safe for you to stop.

» What does it mean for my pregnancy?

Constipation is uncomfortable for you and can cause embarrassing gas, but it doesn't pose any harm to your unborn baby.

» What can I do?

Keep yourself hydrated – drink at least eight glasses of water a day, as this will help to keep your stool soft. Make sure your diet contains plenty of fibre (see p.50), including dried fruits

DRINK LOTS OF WATER

such as dried apricots and prunes, which can have a laxative effect on your bowel. Eat little and often so that your bowel doesn't have too much to cope with at any one time. Keep moving: regular, gentle exercise appropriate for your pregnancy will also give your bowel a helping hand.

APRICOTS

PRUNES

DATES

FIGS

Urine infection

» What, when, and how often?

A stinging sensation when you urinate is usually the first sign of a bacterial infection in your bladder, also known as cystitis. You may experience lower back pain (in your kidney region), and pain in your abdomen.

» What causes it?

Increased oestrogen levels in your system can lead to increased levels of the E coli bacteria in your gut, which makes you more prone to urine infection. This is compounded by the slower transit of urine through your system as a result of pregnancy hormones, and the increased pressure of your uterus on your ureters – the tubes that carry urine from your kidneys.

» What does it mean for my pregnancy?

Urine infections require treatment with antibiotics. If left untreated, urine infections can lead to a more complicated kidney infection, which can increase the

Cranberries Research has been done into cranberry juice helping to prevent and alleviate the symptoms of urine infections. The results are inconclusive, but it's worth a try.

amount of fluid in your circulation, putting pressure on your heart. About 2 per cent of pregnant women in the UK develop kidney infection. This is also treated with antibiotics. You are at a small increased risk of preterm labour, and your baby may catch the infection during birth.

» What can I do?

Drink plenty of fluids throughout your pregnancy to keep flushing out your system. See your GP straight away if you suspect that you have a urine infection.

abdominal pressure – it's just a side-effect of pregnancy. If, though, the pain is unbearable it could be a sign that something else is wrong. PPGP can continue for three to six months after the birth.

» What can I do?

For both conditions relax in warm bath water. For PPGP keep your legs together when getting out of bed and into bed or in and out of a car. Sleep on your left side with a pillow between your legs (see p.114). Ask your doctor for an elasticated tubular bandage or a support belt.

Abdominal pains

» What, when, and how often?

Early on in your pregnancy, it's common to experience some cramping in your abdomen as your uterus prepares itself to provide a safe-house for your developing fetus. By the second trimester, abdominal pain may move to the sides of your abdomen. Pain later in your pregnancy is more likely to be the result of indigestion than anything more sinister.

» What causes them?

Implantation and expansion in your uterus are the most common causes of cramping during early pregnancy. Then, when your body starts to loosen up as a result of increased progesterone and relaxin levels, you may feel as though you're getting pains at the sides of your abdomen – these are just signs that your ligaments are softening to allow room in your pelvis for your growing baby. Occasionally, you may have a small internal bleed in your uterus and this can give you abdominal pain.

» What does it mean for my pregnancy?

Early stage abdominal pains are normal, but do mention them to your healthcare professional so that you can be checked to ensure all is well. If you have any pain, at any time in your pregnancy, that is accompanied by bleeding,

Inability to urinate

» What, when, and how often?

This sounds like the opposite problem to the one most pregnant women complain about, but it is exactly as it sounds – you feel the need to go to the loo, but nothing comes out.

» What causes it?

As the baby grows, your bladder is pushed up inside your abdomen, and once it's out of the way, the baby is free to lie on the urethra – the tube that allows urine to run out of your bladder. If the tube is blocked or squashed, you can't pass urine.

» What does it mean for my pregnancy?

You need to be able to drain urine from your body, otherwise toxins are reabsorbed back into your system, and you are at increased risk of kidney infection.

» What can I do?

See your doctor immediately. Usually, your baby will shift position and naturally free up your urethra, but if that doesn't happen, you may need to have a catheter inserted in order to drain urine from your bladder.

Lower abdominal pressure and "PPGP"

» What, when, and how often?

A dull ache or stabbing pain low down in your pelvic region may cause lower abdominal pressure during your

pregnancy, particularly in the later stages. "PPGP" stands for pregnancy-related pelvic girdle pain. It was formerly known as symphysis pubic dysfunction and affects one in five pregnant women. It can be incredibly painful.

» What causes it?

As your uterus grows during your pregnancy, it presses on the various bones and ligaments of your pelvis. This effect is compounded when the baby grows into the space too. PPGP is caused by hormonal changes that affect the way the pelvic joint functions.

» What does it mean for my pregnancy?

There is no danger to you or the baby from this kind of

Haemorrhoids

» What, when, and how often?

Haemorrhoids are often called "piles". They are dilated blood vessels around the inside or edge of the anus.

» What causes them?

During pregnancy a woman is more likely to get piles because the hormonal softening of the tissues around the anus. Also, the pressure from the baby's head on the blood vessels is another factor. Constipation can cause haemorrhoids to occur.

» What does it mean for my pregnancy?

Having haemorrhoids can be uncomfortable or even painful in more severe cases, but pose no risk to you or your baby.

Anal canal

Haemorrhoid

» What can I do?

Avoid getting constipated or straining when you pass a stool. Cold packs and creams can relieve the discomfort. A health-professional might be able to reduce a haemorrhoid by pushing it gently back into place.

call your healthcare provider straightaway. Cramping later in pregnancy that isn't accompanied by bleeding is probably nothing to worry about, but again mention it to your midwife.

≫ What can I do?

Most cramping is perfectly benign, but because very occasionally it is a symptom of something more significant it's always important to alert your healthcare professional. Rest as much as you can. A warm bath can help to soothe aching, stretched, and displaced muscles and ligaments.

Restless legs

≫ What, when, and how often?

A tingling, creepy-crawly sensation in your legs, often when you're lying down or trying to sleep, restless legs affects up to a 25 per cent of pregnant women in the UK and is most commonly reported in the third trimester of pregnancy. It's debilitating because it makes you feel like you want to move around all the time, even when you're trying to sleep.

≫ What causes it?

No one is really sure why pregnant women are more prone to restless-leg syndrome, but it could be that there is increased circulation through the veins, pregnancy weight gain, low iron levels, or it may be a simple side effect of increased hormone levels. Studies indicate that it tends to run in families.

≫ What does it mean for my pregnancy?

As long as the condition is not related to an iron deficiency (see above), restless legs will pose no harm to you or your baby, apart from making you feel tired if it's hampering your sleep.

≫ What can I do?

Firstly, ask your midwife to check your iron levels. Do everything you can to encourage sleep – avoid eating too late at night, exercise gently (appropriately for your stage in pregnancy), and treat yourself to a soporific warm bath before bedtime. Walking around can cause temporary relief, as can giving your legs a quick rub.

Varicose veins and vulval varicosities

≫ What, when, and how often?

Varicose veins are enlarged veins that can develop in the legs and around the vulval area. They can look unsightly.

≫ What causes them?

During pregnancy the expanding uterus puts pressure on veins in the pelvis. This leads to increased pressure in the legs and vulval area, making varicose veins and vulval varicosities more likely to form (see p.120).

≫ What does it mean for my pregnancy?

Varicose veins can become uncomfortable and itchy in the later stages of pregnancy, but they aren't dangerous.

Back pain and sciatica

≫ What, when, and how often?

Most pregnant women experience some dull aching around their lower back during pregnancy. If that pain becomes sharp or shooting it may be sciatica – especially if it runs down the buttocks and backs of the legs, too (or more often down one leg). You are most likely to experience it during your third trimester, when your uterus is expanding into your abdomen and your baby is growing rapidly.

≫ What causes them?

Lower back pain is commonly caused by the shifting centre of gravity as your baby grows and your uterus expands, causing you to stand and walk awkwardly in order to correct your balance. The loosening in your ligaments during pregnancy can also put strain on your back – all thanks to hormonal changes. Sciatica is a specific condition caused when there is compression on your sciatic nerve, which runs from your lower back down your legs. The compression may be the result of your shifting centre of gravity, whereby other muscles in your lower back contract to keep you upright and in doing so squeeze the nerve. Or it may be specifically the baby's position in later pregnancy – when your baby's head descends into your pelvis it can press on the nerve. Weight gain and your expanding uterus are also common culprits.

≫ What does it mean for my pregnancy?

There is no specific danger to your baby from lower back pain or sciatica – the effects are really only on your own wellbeing and often your mood. Living in constant pain can be debilitating.

Sciatic nerve The main nerve leading to the legs and feet.

Sciatica This artwork shows the path of the nerve and the path of the pain resulting from compression of nerve at the pelvis.

≫ What can I do?

Kegel exercises (see p.67) and swimming can help to strengthen and support your lower back, relieving the pain on the nerve. Although it's good not to let your lower back stiffen up, periods of rest when you've taken the weight off your feet will relieve pressure pain. You can try a hot compress on the sore part of your back. Ask your partner to give you a gentle lower back massage. Tell your healthcare professional that you're suffering so that he or she can keep an eye on things. If you are in severe pain you might be referred to an obstetric physiotherapist. Always consult your healthcare professional before taking anything to ease your discomfort.

Varicosities in the vagina or vulval area won't rupture during birth or pose any other problems.

≫ What can I do?

Tell your healthcare professional if you notice that you have developed a varicose vein. Wear pregnancy support tights or support underwear that a physiotherapist can prescribe.

Foot problems

≫ What, when, and how often?

Many pregnant women suffer from aching arches and cramp in their feet. Swollen ankles and feet are another common pregnancy issue.

≫ What causes them?

Weight gain can put pressure on the arches of your feet, while using the muscles in your feet to correct your balance

is also a cause of aching. Your extremities, including your feet, are particularly prone to the problems associated with increased fluid in your system, which can cause oedema, the medical name for fluid retention (see p.134).

≫ What does it mean for my pregnancy?

For the health of your baby nothing at all, but foot pain and swollen ankles can make walking around fairly debilitating. If your feet and ankles swell excessively or very suddenly, let your healthcare professional know.

≫ What can I do?

Take the weight off your feet as much as you can, raising your feet above your hips to help disperse any excess fluid. Keep your feet moving, even when you are sitting. Turning your feet at the ankle, first in one direction and then in the other can help to relieve pain and swelling. Although it may seem counterintuitive, drinking plenty of fluid will help to flush excess from your system. Aim to gain weight slowly and wear comfortable footwear with good support.

Oedema

Putting your feet up
Make sure your feet are higher than your hips when you are in a resting position.

» What, when, and how often?

Oedema is otherwise known as water or fluid retention – and it causes swelling and puffiness in your cells. Oedema can be partly responsible for a more flushed, plumped-up complexion on your face, but also for swollen ankles, feet, wrists, and fingers. Around half of all pregnant women suffer from oedema at some stage in their pregnancy, particularly in the third trimester.

» What causes it

In order to carry nutrients efficiently to your baby, your blood volume increases by up to one-third during pregnancy. However, not all this increase in volume is made up of extra red blood cells – a large proportion of it is fluid. When the fluid enters the cells in your body, it causes them to swell. Sometimes – especially when you've been stationary for a long period of time, or towards the end of the day, or if the weather is especially hot – the fluid pools in your cells, and this causes the excess swelling.

» What does it mean for my pregnancy?

Most women will experience some normal swelling during the course of their pregnancy, usually in the extremities (fingers, hands, toes, feet, and ankles). If the swelling is excessive, consult your healthcare professional.

» What can I do?

Drink plenty of fluid as this helps to flush excess fluid from your body (although it may seem counterintuitive to do so). Eat a healthy diet and aim to gain weight steadily throughout your pregnancy. Exercise regularly and appropriately for your pregnancy stage. If you notice that your extremities are swelling, keep them moving – make circles with your wrists and ankles and give your toes and fingers a stretch. Avoid too being stationary for long stretches of time – get up and walk around every 30 minutes or so to prevent fluid pooling in your legs. When you rest, try to make sure your feet are higher than your hips.

Numbness in hands

» What, when, and how often?

The very odd sensation of your hand going numb, along with pain in your thumb and first two fingers, may be the result of carpal tunnel syndrome. This condition can occur usually in the second or third trimester of pregnancy and affects around 50 per cent of pregnant women. Carpal tunnel syndrome tends to run in families; and you're likely to get it again if you've had it in a previous pregnancy. It occurs most often in the dominant hand (so your right hand if you're right-handed).

» What causes it?

Your pregnancy hormones increase the amount of fluid circulating in your system. When that fluid pools in your wrists (often during the night when you're stationary), causing swelling, it can put pressure on your median nerve, which runs down your arm into your hand. This then leads to numbness and a pins-and-needles sensation in the fingers of your hand. You'll be more susceptible to the condition if you are overweight or are carrying more than one baby.

» What does it mean for my pregnancy?

If carpal tunnel syndrome is the reason for your numbness, there are no harmful effects for your baby or your pregnancy, but you may find it hard to use your hand properly – in particular you'll probably find that you have a weak grip.

» What can I do?

Apart from eating healthily and performing wrist exercises (rather like the ankle exercises you might try for swollen ankles), all you can do is wait it out. Most cases of carpal tunnel syndrome will pass within a few months of your baby's birth. If you find the numbness lingers, you may need to have surgery to relieve the pressure on your median nerve. You might be offered a wrist support from your healthcare professional to help support your hand.

Nasal problems

» What, when, and how often?

Around one-third of all pregnant women experience nasal problems during pregnancy, commonly beginning around the middle of the second trimester and lasting until birth. Typically, the problems are frequent nosebleeds, increased nasal congestion, and snoring.

» What causes them?

Nasal congestion and snoring is caused by increased oestrogen in your system, which causes a proliferation of mucus in your nasal passages (you may also find you develop blocked ears). Nosebleeds become more frequent because the walls of the tiny capillaries in your nose thin out and are more liable to breaking.

» What does it mean for my pregnancy?

Nosebleeds that don't stop need medical attention, because they could be a sign of a circulation problem; and very loud, very prolonged snoring may be a sign of gestational diabetes. Other than those circumstances, nasal problems are just a harmless side effect of pregnancy.

» What can I do?

Talk to your healthcare professional to make sure that what you're experiencing is normal. If there is cause for concern, you will be referred to an obstetrician for further checks.

Blurred vision

» What, when, and how often?

Eye problems are extremely common during pregnancy, most noticeably many women experience blurring in their vision. Dry eyes and temporary loss of peripheral vision may also occur.

» What causes it?

The cells in your skin start to swell with increased fluid during pregnancy – and the same happens in your eyeballs. This causes the lens in your eye to thicken and distort, blurring your vision. It's possible that the effect is exacerbated because progesterone levels in your body, which cause your muscles to become more lax, may have the same softening effect on your cornea.

» What does it mean for my pregnancy?

Blurred vision can be a sign of pre-eclampsia (flashes in your eyes, too), so it's very important that you let your healthcare professional know if you experience any changes to your eyesight. Most of the time, though, it's just another side effect of pregnancy.

» What can I do?

Keep up your fluid intake to try to minimize fluid retention in your cells. Your vision should return to normal after birth, but it may take several weeks. Some women experience permanent changes to their eyesight, so if you're still having sight problems six weeks after you've had your baby, visit your optician.

PUPPP/PEP skin rash

❯❯ What, when, and how often?
Pruritic urticarial papules and plaques of pregnancy (PUPPP) and polymorphic eruption of pregnancy (PEP) is an itchy skin rash that usually appears on the abdomen (other than on the belly button) and then spreads to other parts of the body. It looks a bit like eczema, characterized by small, fluid-filled blisters. It's a condition of late pregnancy – usually occurring from around 35 weeks pregnant, but it occurs in fewer than half a per cent of all pregnancies.

❯❯ What causes it?
No one is sure what causes PUPPP, but it is most common in women carrying boys (interestingly, a study found male DNA in skin biopsies of PUPPP rash) or multiples and in first pregnancies. It rarely occurs during second or subsequent pregnancies. Some people think it may be hereditary.

❯❯ What does it mean for my pregnancy?
The most significant effect is itchiness, usually worst in the first few days of the condition. It doesn't seem to have any effect on the unborn baby, though as a precaution many hospitals recommend that the baby is induced at 39 weeks.

❯❯ What can I do?
Keep cool by wearing loose-fitting cotton clothing. You can talk to your midwife about topical treatments. The rash disappears of its own accord within a week of having the baby. In rare cases it may linger for a bit longer.

Heat rash

❯❯ What, when, and how often?
Also known as prickly heat, a heat rash is a raised red, itchy rash that affects parts of the skin where heat builds up – folds in the neck and abdomen, for example.

❯❯ What causes it?
During pregnancy you will probably feel hotter and sweatier than usual, which can cause a rash to develop where the air can't easily dry away the sweat.

❯❯ What does it mean for my pregnancy?
Nothing at all other than feeling irritated by your prickly skin. The rash is completely benign and has no side effects.

❯❯ What can I do?
Keep as cool as possible and wear loose-fitting cotton clothing. Cool and soothe your skin using a flannel that has been soaked in cold water. Avoid highly scented soaps.

Clogged milk ducts

❯❯ What, when, and how often?
Many women don't realize that milk production begins during pregnancy. Part of this process means that the milk ducts in your breasts stretch and enlarge to accommodate the increase in fluid. Sometimes, in the second half of your pregnancy, the ducts can be clogged up, making your breasts feel lumpy and tender. The lumps may even look red compared with the rest of the skin on your breast.

❯❯ What causes them?
Your breasts are busy making milk, but until your baby is born, you don't have an outlet for it. The back-up of milk can cause blockages in the ducts.

❯❯ What does it mean for my pregnancy?
A blocked duct is really a good sign that your body is making milk. It's really nothing to worry about, other than that it can cause some discomfort and tenderness. Note that if the lump isn't red or painful, it would be worth mentioning it to your healthcare professional, just in case it's a breast lump that is unrelated to your milk production.

❯❯ What can I do?
A cool flannel placed over the affected area on your breast can help to ease tenderness. Gently use your thumbs and fingers to massage around the blocked duct with the aim of freeing up the blockage. You may have some discharge from your nipple as you do this – that's fine.

Leaking milk

❯❯ What, when, and how often?
This can occur at any time from your second trimester, but is most likely to occur at the end of your pregnancy as your breasts become full. Usually you will leak colostrum rather than actual milk. Colostrum is a yellowish, thick secretion. It's more digestible and richer in nutrients than breast milk.

❯❯ What causes it?
Very simply, your breasts fill with milk but until the baby is born, there's no outlet for all the liquid. The result is that some of it gets squeezed out unintentionally from your breasts.

❯❯ What does it mean for my pregnancy?
Your body is gearing up to feed your baby once he is born. There is no relationship between leaky breasts and ability (or inability) to produce enough milk to nurse a baby.

❯❯ What can I do?
Use breast pads to soak up any fluid from your nipples. Change them regularly if you need to.

Bleeding

❯❯ What, when, and how often?
One third of pregnant women will experience some form of spotting or bleeding in their first trimester. It can be brown, pink, or bright red. Sometimes large blood clots are expelled. Bleeding or spotting can happen later on in pregnancy, too.

❯❯ What causes it?
In early pregnancy the increased levels of hormones make the surface of the cervix fragile and prone to spotting or bleeding. Later your cervix is softer and has increased blood flow to it. As a result it can bleed or become bruised.

❯❯ What does it mean for my pregnancy?
While worrying, bleeding is common in the first trimester. It doesn't neccessarily mean you have miscarried, though it should always be checked. Bleeding later in pregnancy should always be checked too, as it could be a sign of a low-lying placenta, placental abruption, or preterm labour.

❯❯ What can I do?
Speak to your healthcare professional as soon as possible. You will probably be offered an ultrasound scan to put your mind at ease and check that nothing is wrong. Report any heavy bleeding immediately, especially if it is accompanied by any pain.

Protruding navel

❯❯ What, when, and how often?
During the third trimester of pregnancy, your abdomen will be heading towards full stretch and one of the results is that your belly button may appear to "pop out". This usually occurs after the 24th week of pregnancy and happens to almost all pregnant women.

❯❯ What causes it?
The simple matter of a growing abdomen (growing baby and growing uterus) is the cause of your popped-out belly button.

❯❯ What does it mean for my pregnancy?
A protruding navel is not the sign of anything sinister going on and its only effect is that it might look like a very low third nipple if you're wearing tight-fitting clothes.

❯❯ What can I do?
Absolutely nothing. Your belly button will stop protruding and sit neatly back in its original position as soon as you've had your baby.

Standing proud If you are happy with your changing body, then show off your bump.

{ Q I don't feel very well. What medications are considered safe in pregnancy?

It's normal to fall ill from time to time during pregnancy (especially as your immune system is suppressed), but the over-the-counter (OTC) medications you would naturally turn to if you weren't pregnant aren't necessarily safe. Be extra careful and always check with your healthcare professional before taking any remedies.

Many minor ailments, such as common colds and diarrhoea, resolve themselves without medication. If you think you do need treatment, seek advice from a healthcare professional – and always let him or her know you are pregnant. Before using an OTC remedy, check with the pharmacist that it's safe in pregnancy, take it at the lowest dose possible, and limit using it to the shortest amount of time possible. Many natural medicines – and particularly herbal remedies – can be unsafe for your developing baby.

If you can, it is best to avoid **over-the-counter medications** altogether – especially in the first trimester when your baby is most susceptible to risk.

Prevention is better than cure

You can be more susceptible to infections during pregnancy because your body is suppressing its immune system in order to maintain your pregnancy. You can boost your immunity and protect yourself against infection through good diet, moderate exercise, and sensible hygiene.

» Wash your hands before preparing or eating food, and practise safe toileting habits.

» Drink plenty of water and diluted juice, too, as fluids will help to flush any infection from your system.

» Boost your intake of antioxidant foods (such as fruits and vegetables), which can support your immune system.

» Get plenty of rest as you're more likely to fall ill if you feel tired and depleted.

» Always talk to a healthcare professional before taking any natural remedy, even something as seemingly innocuous as a herbal tea.

Take care of yourself Even if you don't feel like sleeping, lying down and putting your feet up will give your body a chance to rest. Propping yourself up against a pillow can help ease congestion and an aching back.

For a blocked nose or congestion Inhale steam (with nothing added). You should also drink lots of fluids if you have a cold.

For a sore throat or cough Take lemon, ginger, and honey mixed in hot water or simple linctus (a very basic cough mixture).

COMMON AILMENTS

No medication is 100 per cent safe in pregnancy. Paracetamol is the only OTC medicine deemed safe to take without consulting a doctor, midwife, or pharmacist, but even this should be used in moderation.

AILMENT	WHAT DOES IT MEAN FOR MY PREGNANCY?	WHAT CAN I DO?
Flu and common colds	The common cold virus should not affect your baby, but severe flu may increase the risk of low birthweight. Flu can also lead to the more serious bronchitis, or even pneumonia. Colds are dehydrating so keep your fluid levels up.	Keep up your fluid intake, and use steam inhalation and hot, soothing drinks to relieve symptoms (see opposite). You can take a low dose of paracetamol if you have a high temperature but do not take any medicine containing ibuprofen or codeine. If you have flu symptoms, see your doctor, who may give you medicine to help shorten the duration of it.
Fever	A high temperature can affect your blood circulation so you should try to bring the fever down. Fever usually indicates a viral or bacterial infection.	Use a sponge dipped in cold water, cold compress, or ice bath to bring down your temperature. You can take paracetamol if needed – but you must not exceed the maximum daily dosage stated on the box. Call your doctor if your temperature is more than 40°C (104°F).
Ear, throat, chest, or urine infection	Severe bacterial infection can cross the placental barrier and affect your baby so it is important to see your doctor to get any infection treated.	Take plenty of fluids, and see your doctor. Many antibiotics are safe in pregnancy, but they must be prescribed. He or she may do tests (saliva or urine for example) to check which antibiotic would be most suitable. Take paracetamol to reduce the fever.
Diarrhoea	Diarrhoea will not harm your baby, but you must avoid dehydration. If your diarrhoea is combined with vomiting or fever, speak to your doctor.	Diarrhoea will usually stop of its own accord once your body has expelled the infection. Don't take anti-diarrhoea medication unless it is prescribed by your doctor. Rehydration solutions are safe to take, but consult your pharmacist first.
Food poisoning	The bacteria that cause food poisoning can be potentially harmful to your baby. The most dangerous of these is listeria, which can cause blood poisoning, meningitis, and pneumonia.	Let your doctor know if you suspect food poisoning and you will be advised on what, if anything, you can take to ease the symptoms. It is important to keep sipping water so that you don't become dehydrated. If you suspect listeriosis, seek help straight away.
Pain	Backache can be quite common in pregnancy, especially in the third trimester. Headache, muscular pain, and back pain will not affect your baby.	Ice and warm compresses can help muscular pain and sprains and back pain respectively, but see your doctor for persistent headaches. You can take paracetamol, but don't exceed the maximum daily dosage. Do not take any medication containing ibuprofen or codeine.
Insomnia	Insomnia is quite common in pregnancy but can stem from a variety of causes. It should not affect your baby, but will be very tiring for you.	Consult your doctor to identify the causes and discuss steps you can take. Do not use any herbal remedies, aromatherapy, or medication to induce sleep without seeking advice first.
Hayfever	While hayfever does not affect your baby, treatment of it can. Always seek advice from a pharmacist or doctor before taking any form of antihistamine.	See your doctor. Some antihistamines are fine to use in pregnancy, but it is likely that you'll be advised to use them in the form of a nasal spray or eye drops rather than tablets.
Fungal infections (such as athlete's foot)	Fungal infections such as athlete's foot or thrush have no effect on your unborn baby, but treatments for them can.	Keep the affected area clean, dry, and well-aired. Not all OTC fungal treatments are safe and you will not be able to buy them from a pharmacy when you are pregnant without a prescription. Consult a pharmacist, or speak to your doctor.
Itchy skin	Dry, itchy skin complaints can occur for a number of reasons, including eczema and pregnancy-induced pruritis gravidarum, which can be severe.	You can use emollients and barrier creams, which are available over the counter, but you should not use steroidal creams. Ask a pharmacist which are the safest options, or speak to your doctor.
Rashes	Rashes can be concentrated in one area (localized), or all over (generalized). Some rashes are harmless, but you should get them checked to find out the cause.	Ask your midwife to check your rash. If any rash (whether local or generalized) persists for more than 48 hours, see your doctor. You can use calamine lotion to relieve the symptoms of localized rashes, but not generalized ones. Cold water and ice can also help.
Cuts and scrapes	A minor cut or graze will not harm your baby, but take the usual steps to keep the wound clean and free from infection.	Clean the wound using an antiseptic and keep it dry. Although antiseptics are not thought to be hazardous to pregnancy, check with your pharmacist for the safest options to use.
Head lice	Head lice are annoying for you, but luckily don't pose a threat to your unborn baby.	Tackle the problem first with a head lice comb. Use the comb on wet hair; repeat every three days to keep clearing young lice as they hatch. You can get 4 per cent dimethicone lotion over the counter, but always let the pharmacist know you are pregnant first.
Threadworms	Threadworm infection is not known to put your unborn baby at risk, but treatment for it can.	OTC treatments are not advised when you are pregnant, but strict hygiene measures can clear the threadworms (they have a life cycle of six weeks). See your doctor for advice.

Not every pregnancy is as straightforward as it could be. Complications don't happen to most women – **they are not the norm** – but if you experience a problem you will get **lots of support** from your healthcare team. With careful attention, the majority of complications have **good outcomes**.

Complications

Types of complication

A "complication" is a medical condition that could potentially compromise your health or that of your unborn baby. Many of the checks you are offered as part of your antenatal care (and in your pre-conception care when you plan a pregnancy) are designed to identify any complications that could occur as early as possible. In many situations, your healthcare team can manage problems to keep you and your baby as safe as possible.

There are a few broad types of complication. Some women have a long-term condition, such as asthma or congenital heart disease, that warrants special attention. Sometimes previous gynaecological issues may have a knock-on effect for your pregnancy. Other complications can arise as a result of pregnancy – gestational diabetes and pre-eclampsia are examples of these. More rarely, some short-term infections can pose problems.

Plan pregnancy where possible

If you are able to, it is worth checking your immunity to certain infectious diseases before trying for a baby. You can be vaccinated before conception, but not while you are pregnant because some vaccines can harm a fetus.

If you have a pre-existing illness that requires medication and you are not already pregnant, you are strongly advised to set in place a pre-conception plan. Some medications aren't suitable for pregnancy, and some conditions need to be stabilized before you become pregnant. Giving yourself three to six months to get things planned and under control before conception can often mean the difference between a straightforward pregnancy and a difficult one.

When complications arise

If you experience a complication, your level of antenatal care might gear up with more tests, scans, and treatments. Throughout this process your medical team will explain to you what is going on in your body and its potential effects on your pregnancy, labour, birth, and baby.

Take someone with you to ultrasound scans and appointments with specialists – they can listen if you are not able to take everything in. Sometimes you may need to make difficult decisions about whether or not to take medications that can help you, but potentially affect your baby. Sometimes, a complication might dictate where, when, and how you deliver your baby, forcing you to make unexpected decisions. It's natural to feel scared or nervous. There are support groups for people in the same situation as you – ask your midwife for information on these.

{Q What happens if I catch an infectious disease while I'm pregnant?

Treatment options are limited when you are pregnant, so some infections do present risks to your pregnancy. You should contact your GP if you notice symptoms of serious infections.

Chickenpox

» What is it?
Also known as varicella, this viral infection causes fever and itchy red spots on the skin that turn into blisters.

» What does it mean for my pregnancy?
Complications from catching chickenpox are rare, but potentially serious. It can damage a fetus's eyes, brain, skin, limbs, bladder, or bowel. Risks to you include pneumonia, and inflammation in the brain and liver.

» What can I do?
If you have not had chickenpox before and come into contact with it, or if you develop symptoms, consult your doctor immediately. Antiviral therapy can help prevent any complications, although it can't cure the infection.

Measles

» What is it?
Measles causes flu-like symptoms, spots in the mouth, and a red–brown rash that lasts for just over a week. Due to vaccination programmes, measles is now rare in the UK.

» What does it mean for my pregnancy?
Developing measles increases the risk of miscarriage, stillbirth, and premature birth, especially in the first trimester. The infection can also pass to your baby during birth.

» What can I do?
See your GP urgently if you come into contact with the virus (it can take up to three weeks to develop) and you are not immune or vaccinated. You can be treated with human normal immunoglobin (HNIG), which lessens the symptoms and reduces (but doesn't eliminate) the risk to your baby.

Mumps

» What is it?
This viral infection causes fever and headache, and swelling of the cheeks and the salivary glands in the neck. Due to vaccination programmes, mumps is now rare in the UK.

» What does it mean for my pregnancy?
Mumps should not cause any birth defects in your unborn baby, but it can increase the risk of miscarriage through your fever and illness, especially in your first trimester. It can also develop into meningitis.

» What can I do?
If you lack immunity, consult your doctor as soon as you come into contact with anyone with mumps (symptoms may take two to three weeks to develop). Mumps cannot be treated but there are ways to ease the symptoms.

Rubella

» What is it?
Also called German measles, the rubella virus causes symptoms of headache, fever, joint pains, sore throat, swollen glands, and a raised red-pink rash. Due to vaccination programmes, rubella is now rare in the UK.

» What does it mean for my pregnancy?
If you contract rubella before you are 18 weeks pregnant, it can cause serious birth defects and miscarriage. The later in pregnancy the disease affects you, the lower the risk. After 18 weeks, the risks to the baby are minimal.

» What can I do?
If you have not been vaccinated, try to avoid contact with rubella. If you think you could be infected, see your doctor urgently for diagnosis. There is no treatment for rubella, but your doctor will support you and advise options if the baby has congenital rubella syndrome (CRS).

Cytomegalovirus

» What is it?
A type of herpes, cytomegalovirus (CMV) is transmitted via saliva, urine, semen, or faeces. It can lie dormant (without symptoms) and many people don't realize they have it.

» What does it mean for my pregnancy?
If you have CMV and it becomes active for the first time during your pregnancy (a primary infection), it can cause congenital disabilities and neurological problems in your baby. However, only about 1 in 2000 babies in the UK develops complications due to CMV.

» What can I do?
There is no cure for CMV, but you can try to prevent primary infection. Children under six are often carriers, so avoid contact with their faeces, urine, or saliva (kiss them on the head rather than mouth or cheeks). Many adults don't know they have the virus, so use a condom if you have sex.

Lyme disease

» What is it?
This bacterial, tick-borne infection can go undetected for many years. Symptoms include fever, chills, joint or muscle pains, facial paralysis, and a red rash with an outer red ring.

» What does it mean for my pregnancy?
Lyme disease is potentially serious for you if untreated. It increases the risk of premature birth and miscarriage.

» What can I do?
Your doctor can give you a course of antibiotics – with treatment, the outcome for you and your baby is very good. You can get infected again after treatment, if bitten again, so take precautions to prevent tick bites.

Hepatitis

» What is it?
All forms of this blood-borne virus infect the liver. Symptoms can range from vomiting and stomach cramps, to mild cold-like illness. Some people have no symptoms.

» What does it mean for my pregnancy?
Hepatitis can cause liver failure in a fetus. All women are offered hepatitis B (HBV) screening as part of antenatal care. Hepatitis C (HCV) is checked if you have risk factors.

» What can I do?
If you have HBV, your baby can be vaccinated against it at birth – this immunization has a 95 per cent success rate. Passing HCV to a baby is more rare, but if your baby is infected he will be referred for specialist assessment.

If you are not sure whether you have **immunity** to chickenpox or whether you have been **vaccinated** against measles, mumps, or rubella, your doctor can do a **blood test** to check.

{ Q I've got a medical condition already. How will it affect my pregnancy?

This section is a guide to some long-term (or chronic) conditions that can impact on pregnancy. Ideally, optimize your control of these conditions pre-pregnancy. Once pregnant, your care will be with an obstetrician as well as your midwife and doctor. Most women with these conditions have healthy pregnancies and babies, though a home- or birth-centre birth may not be recommended.

Asthma

❯❯ What is it?
This respiratory condition inflames and narrows the lung's airways, causing wheezing, coughing, chest tightness, and shortness of breath.

❯❯ Risks to your pregnancy, labour, and baby
Asthma is linked with placental problems, including low-lying placenta and placenta with poor function (reduced oxygen and nutrient supply), which slightly increases your risk of having a low birthweight baby and miscarriage.

❯❯ Medicines and tests
Asthma medication has no side effects on the unborn baby, so continue to take your medicines throughout your pregnancy. If you take oral steroids, you may need regular blood tests to check your glucose levels. Your pain relief choices may be limited during labour as diamorphine and other opioid analgesics can exacerbate asthma.

❯❯ Effects of pregnancy on your condition
If you have severe asthma at the start of pregnancy, it may become worse during pregnancy. Otherwise, asthma tends to stay the same or even improve in pregnancy, as increased levels of natural steroids can reduce attacks. Baby girls are statistically more likely to worsen asthma symptoms in the pregnant mother than baby boys.

Inflammatory bowel disease (IBD)

❯❯ What is it?
IBD describes inflammatory conditions of the digestive system, such as ulcerative colitis and Crohn's disease. It can cause pain, swelling, and cramps in the stomach, recurrent or bloody diarrhoea, extreme tiredness, and weight loss. IBD does not include irritable bowel syndrome (IBS).

❯❯ Risks to your pregnancy, labour, and baby
Whether active or inactive, IBD can slightly raise the chance of a baby being "small for dates" and premature labour. If

you are at risk of needing bowel surgery in the future, your doctors may suggest a C-section to preserve the pelvic floor muscles that are crucial to bowel function. Your baby's chance of inheriting Crohn's disease is small (5 per cent) unless both you and your partner have it (36 per cent).

❯❯ Medicines and tests
If you take methotrexate, stop taking it when you know you're pregnant (or ideally as part of your pre-conception

care) because it can cause birth defects. You can continue with other medications, but see your gastroenterologist as soon as you can for a medication review, as managing your IBD is still a priority in pregnancy. Your doctor may advise increased dosage of folic acid because some IBD medicines can interfere with folate absorption. You may have a couple of extra appointments with your gastroenterologist during pregnancy to check all is well. There is no reported ill-effect if you have to have a colonoscopy or sigmoidoscopy to check the health of your bowel during your pregnancy.

❯❯ Effects of pregnancy on your condition
If your IBD is inactive at the time you fall pregnant, and you continue your medication, the chances of a flare-up are no greater than if you were not pregnant, but you may have a flare up after the birth. Active IBD might be more difficult to control while you are pregnant. If you have a stoma or pouch, it may become squashed as your abdomen grows, which may then increase your bowel frequency.

Hypertension

❯❯ What is it?
Hypertension (high blood pressure) is a higher than recommended pressure in your arteries. This condition puts you at increased risk of heart attack and stroke.

❯❯ Risks to your pregnancy, labour, and baby
You are more vulnerable to pre-eclampsia, placental abruption, stroke, and blood clots; your baby to premature birth, low birthweight, and a slight risk of stillbirth. You will usually be encouraged to have a natural birth, if this is what you wish, unless there are specific reasons for advising a Caesarean section.

❯❯ Medicines and tests
Continue to take your medication, but consult your doctor for a medication review since some blood-pressure lowering drugs may adversely affect your baby's development. If your blood pressure is raised, it will be monitored between your regular antenatal appointments. You may be advised to take a low dose of aspirin daily in order to thin your blood, if you don't already take one. You may also be invited for additional scans to check your baby's growth. Your labour may be induced early if your blood pressure remains high and needs controlling.

❯❯ Effects of pregnancy on your condition
Pregnancy hormones dilate your blood vessels, so you

Regular monitoring is essential, whether you are managing your high blood pressure with lifestyle changes or with medication.

might find that your blood pressure decreases naturally for almost all of the nine months (rising again slightly at the end). In some cases, your doctor may even feel you are able to stop taking blood-pressure lowering drugs during pregnancy.

Thyroid problems

» What are they?
The thyroid gland regulates the body's metabolism. Disorders occur if it produces more thyroid hormones than the body needs, or not enough.

» Risks to your pregnancy, labour, and baby
Untreated hyperthyroidism (overactive thyroid) or hypothyroidism (underactive thyroid) can pose serious problems in pregnancy. Thyroid hormones play a key role in developing your baby, so your doctors will try to keep your condition under control and avoid the risks of pre-eclampsia, heart failure, kidney failure, coma, premature labour, stillbirth, or miscarriage. Pre-conception planning is very important to optimize your control of the condition as some studies suggest that a very underactive thyroid in the first trimester may affect a baby's IQ and increase the risk of learning difficulties.

» Medicines and tests
Your doctor may review your medication and possibly advise increased dosage if you need it. Hypothyroidism is sometimes treated with the synthetic hormone thyroxine during pregnancy. Your thyroid function will be checked regularly throughout your pregnancy using blood tests. You will have additional scans to check the health of your baby during your third trimester.

» Effects of pregnancy on your condition
Women with an overactive thyroid that is stable may have a relapse as pregnancy hormones can increase the circulating levels of thyroid hormone in the blood. Pregnancy can cause swelling in the thyroid gland, called a goitre.

Rheumatoid arthritis

» What is it?
This long-term inflammatory disease causes pain, swelling, and stiffness or immobility in the joints.

» Risks to your pregnancy, labour, and baby
Other than a possibility of premature labour, rheumatoid arthritis (RA) doesn't usually directly affect your pregnancy or baby. If it affects your hips or pelvis, you may need to have a Caesarean section.

» Medicines and tests
Some RA medications are not safe for the baby. Others are safe, but can cause raised blood glucose or high blood pressure for you. Talk to your doctor as soon as you discover that you are pregnant (or planning a pregnancy) to discuss your medication.

» Effects of pregnancy on your condition
Pregnancy can increase symptoms of fatigue, especially in the first trimester. In the second trimester, research suggests that in up to 70 per cent of women with RA symptoms may improve, with these improvements lasting for the first few weeks after pregnancy. However, some women experience a flare-up after this period.

Diabetes

» What is it?
Diabetes is a condition in which the body is unable to control blood glucose levels, either because it produces too little insulin, or because it cannot use the insulin it produces (see box, right). Diabetes in pregnancy can be pre-existing or can develop in pregnancy (gestational diabetes, see p.145). Here we discuss pre-existing diabetes.

» Risks to your pregnancy, labour, and baby
Diabetes increases your risk of high blood pressure and pre-eclampsia (see p.144), and of having a baby with birth defects. It also increases your risk of miscarriage, stillbirth, and preterm labour. High glucose levels in your blood mean that glucose in your baby's blood also increases, and your baby may be large at birth. Babies born to diabetic mothers may also be small at birth.

» Medicines and tests
It is very important to optimize your control of diabetes pre-pregnancy to minimize the chances of birth defects. It is also essential to continue to manage glucose levels once pregnant. Talk to your doctor as soon as you know you're pregnant for a referral to an obstetrician or a diabetes specialist. He or she will give you glucose targets to maintain in pregnancy. If you are on synthetic medicines you may switch to insulin injections, or you may carry on with your tablets. You will need to follow a glucose-friendly diet; a dietician will work out a meal plan with you. Your doctor will encourage you to test your blood glucose levels at least four times a day to make sure they remain on target. As your pregnancy progresses, you'll probably have to increase the amount of insulin you inject to keep glucose levels stable. Make sure that your friends and family know how to use the testing kits, too, just in case you have a hypo or hyper episode (both of which can lead to unconsciousness) and aren't able to test for yourself. Throughout your pregnancy, you might be offered additional growth scans to make sure your baby is growing appropriately, remembering that a large baby may indicate that your blood glucose levels are too high.

» Effects of pregnancy on your condition
Pregnancy hormones increase insulin resistance; that is, they exacerbate your body's inability to use insulin to regulate blood glucose levels. As a result, you are at a greater risk of all the complications of diabetes – hypo- and hyperglycaemia, eye problems, heart disease, and kidney disease, and you'll be monitored closely for these. If you suffer from vomiting, the concentration of acids called ketones may increase in your blood. Ketones are a by-product of burning fat stores for energy, rather than glucose. Excessively high levels can lead to serious pregnancy complications, and may be life-threatening for you. This situation is extremely rare, and most women with diabetes have healthy pregnancies, but managing your glucose levels through your diet and insulin injections is of utmost importance.

DIABETES FACTS

Here are the important facts about pre-existing diabetes and the signs to look for if haven't already been diagnosed.

» **Your body derives glucose** from the food you eat, in particular from carbohydrates, fats, and proteins in your diet.

» **The symptoms of diabetes** include having a dry mouth, frequently needing to urinate, tiredness, blurred vision, and thrush – almost all of which are also perfectly healthy symptoms of pregnancy!

» **Type I diabetes** occurs when your body makes too little of the hormone insulin, which it needs to take glucose from your blood stream and turn it into energy.

» **Type II diabetes** occurs when your body makes enough insulin, but its cells become resistant to the hormone's attempts to draw glucose from them. It is often caused by obesity.

Insulin injections Your insulin requirements will change throughout your pregnancy. It's crucial that you keep your blood-sugar under control.

Mental health problems

» What are they?
Conditions as diverse as bipolar disease, depression, psychosis, neurosis, self-harming, obsessive-compulsive disorder, addictions, and eating disorders.

» Risks to your pregnancy, labour, and baby
Medications for mental health problems can affect the health of your unborn baby. You are also at increased risk of developing antenatal depression and postnatal depression. You may feel unable to care for yourself and unwilling or unable to nurture your unborn baby; if you have an eating disorder, you may restrict your baby's access to important nutrients in utero. Studies show that babies born to women suffering from mental health problems are also at greater risk of developing depression-related conditions themselves in later life.

» Medicines and tests
Do not change or stop taking your medication without first consulting your doctor. He or she will need to make a full assessment of your condition and will devise a medication maintenance programme that you can use throughout your pregnancy to minimize the risks for your baby, while maintaining your health.

» Effects of pregnancy on your condition
Scientific studies show that the anxiety associated with being pregnant, as well as the need to reduce medication can put women with a history of mental illness at greater risk of psychosis or depression during pregnancy. However, if your condition is under control before you're pregnant, there is evidence to suggest that with the right level of support and medicine, you are not at a significantly increased risk of a relapse.

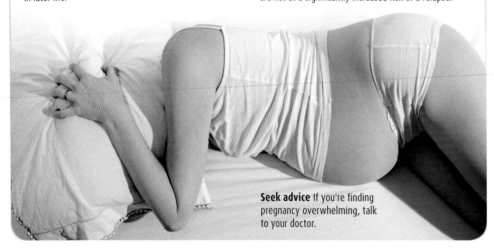

Seek advice If you're finding pregnancy overwhelming, talk to your doctor.

Epilepsy

» What is it?
A disorder of the electrical signals in the brain, epilepsy causes repeated seizures.

» Risks to your pregnancy, labour, and baby
You might experience nausea and sickness, anaemia, pregnancy-induced hypertension, or pre-eclampsia. Seizures don't harm your baby unless they're tonic clonic, clustered, or last for more than 30 minutes – all of which can starve a fetus of oxygen. Injuring yourself during a seizure could also harm the baby. Don't shower or bathe in pregnancy, or bathe your newborn, with the door locked or when there is no one in the house. There is a higher risk of premature or prolonged labour, and needing a C-section. After birth, your baby may have withdrawal from anti-epileptic drugs (AEDs) and may need an extra dose of vitamin K to help with blood clotting.

» Medicines and tests
Take your medication unless your neurologist advises you not to. Some AEDs increase the risk of newborn congenital abnormalities, but 90 per cent of women with epilepsy have healthy babies. The risks to your baby if you have a seizure are greater. A blood test can assess the levels of drugs in your body as increased blood volume in pregnancy means your usual dosage may be too diluted. Change your dosage only under medical advice. Talk to your doctor about increasing folic acid intake as some drugs inhibit its absorption (though folic acid can inhibit the efficacy of your medication). You may need a vitamin K supplement from week 36, as epilepsy drugs can affect blood clotting. You may need to avoid opioid analgesics in labour.

» Effects of pregnancy on your condition
Most women with epilepsy find that there is no change in pregnancy. Sometimes symptoms improve; in other cases seizures increase, which may continue after birth. If seizures increase, ask your neurologist to review your medication.

Congenital/acquired heart disease

» What are they?
Congenital heart disease (CHD) is a condition you're born with. Acquired heart disease (AHD) is usually caused by rheumatic fever, Kawasaki disease, or obesity.

» Effects on your pregnancy, labour, and baby
Your baby is at a slightly increased risk of developing congenital heart defects (even if your own heart disease is acquired). There may be restricted oxygen to your baby, which can cause low birthweight, premature birth, or stillbirth. You are at increased risk of fluid on your lungs – see your doctor if you experience any chest pains or abnormally increased coughing. Third-stage labour can compromise heart function, so you may be offered assisted delivery in order to keep labour as short as possible. You'll be encouraged to give birth lying on your left-hand side, as this reduces the pressure on your major blood vessels. Your breathing during the final stage of labour will be carefully guided so that you don't hold your breath. Your baby will be attached to a fetal heart monitor throughout labour, and you will probably need your own continual ECG reading. You may need to have antibiotics during labour in order to reduce your risk of heart infection.

» Medicines and tests
Your midwife may suggest increased blood pressure checks as a non-invasive measure of your circulation function. Anti-coagulant medication can cross the placenta and cause your baby's blood to thin dangerously. Your doctor will advise you on keeping you and your baby healthy.

» Effects of pregnancy on your condition
Your weight, diet, and exercise levels will be monitored over your pregnancy to ensure good nutrition and steady weight gain; excess weight during pregnancy can put a strain on your heart. The opening of your blood vessels is a natural side effect of increased progesterone. This can help blood flow to your heart, but increased blood volume and any shortening of breath can put strain on your heart.

Systemic lupus erythematosus

» What is it?
Sometimes known simply as "lupus", or SLE, this autoimmune disorder causes the immune system to attack healthy tissue in its own body by mistake.

» Effects on your pregnancy, labour, and baby
You are at increased risk of pre-eclampsia, premature labour, miscarriage, and stillbirth. If SLE has affected your kidneys, you may be at increased risk of high blood pressure. If SLE antibodies cross the placenta, this can cause a harmless skin rash in the baby at birth, and more

seriously, your baby may have a heart arrhythmia, so if you have antibodies, your baby will be monitored in pregnancy. Babies may show signs of some liver or kidney disfunction at birth. In most cases this will right itself within six months and babies generally show no long-lasting effects.

» Medicines and tests
Throughout your pregnancy, your obstetrician and midwife, as well as your SLE care team, will arrange additional visits to assess you and your baby. You'll need to see your rheumatologist at least once every three months throughout. Take your medication, unless your doctors advise you otherwise. There is a much better outcome for your pregnancy and baby if your lupus is under control.

» Effects of pregnancy on your condition
Pregnancy shouldn't cause any extra complications for sufferers of SLE as long as it's under control at conception.

Multiple sclerosis

» What is it?
Multiple sclerosis (MS) damages nerve cells in the brain and spinal cord, affecting muscle movement, balance, and vision.

» Effects on your pregnancy, labour, and baby
MS seems to have no knock-on effects for your pregnancy or baby. If MS has affected your ability to feel contractions in the muscles of your pelvis, you may need to have an assisted birth or a C-section. There is only a very small increased risk that your baby will inherit MS. You do have an increased risk of a relapse in pregnancy and after the birth.

» Medicines and tests
Consult your doctor about your medication. Many women with MS can continue to take steroids, particularly after the first trimester. You may have additional antenatal visits.

» Effects of pregnancy on your condition
Hormone levels may help to reduce the rate of MS relapse during pregnancy, particularly during the third trimester. You may experience exacerbated symptoms of fatigue, back pain, bowel dysfunction, and bladder weakness, as well as an impaired sense of balance as your baby grows and your centre of gravity shifts forward. Your increased risk of falls may mean that you need increased support when moving.

Sickle-cell disease

» What is it?
A group of genetic blood disorders, such as sickle-cell anaemia and thalassaemia. Affected haemoglobin in the red blood cells means they are unable to carry oxygen efficiently around the body, causing lack of energy, sudden attacks of pain, or ongoing pain when the tissues are starved of oxygen, and damage to internal organs over time.

» Effects on your pregnancy, labour, and baby
You have an increased risk of premature labour and a low birthweight baby. Your baby will carry the sickle cell gene (even if the baby's father has no sickle cell gene); if the father is a carrier (without symptoms), your baby has a 50 per cent chance of being born with sickle cell disease (and a 50 per cent chance of being a carrier). Your partner can be screened to work out the risk of your baby inheriting the disease. You're at increased risk of pre-eclampsia, high blood pressure, stroke, breathing difficulties, and anaemia. Your doctor may advise you to give birth in hospital, where your baby will be attached to a fetal heart monitor throughout labour. You can't have pethidine as it can cause convulsions in women with SCD, but other opiate analgesics should be fine.

» Medicines and tests
You will have lots of antenatal appointments, as well as regular visits to your haematologist and obstetrician. You may be advised to take extra folic acid and have a course of antibiotics to help protect you against infection. You may be advised to take a small daily dosage of aspirin after your first trimester to reduce the risk of high blood pressure. You will be offered an early scan at between 7 and 9 weeks to assess the viability of your pregnancy, and then growth scans for your baby once a month in your last trimester.

» Effects of pregnancy on your condition
SCD symptoms may worsen during pregnancy. Sickness can exacerbate them – consult your doctor about the best way to minimize the effects.

Phenylketonuria

» What is it?
In this genetic condition, the body cannot break down phenylalanine, which can cause brain and nerve damage.

» Risks to your pregnancy, labour, and baby
High levels of phenylalanine can cross the placenta and cause serious defects and even fatality in your unborn baby. You will need to adhere strictly to a diet regime in order to keep levels of blood phenylalanine within the range of 100–250 umol/L throughout the course of your pregnancy. Your baby could have low birthweight. Your baby will only inherit PKU if his father is a carrier, which in the UK gives him about a 1 in 100 chance.

» Medicines and tests
You will need to have blood tests up to three times a week and you will see your PKU specialist up to once a month. You may be asked to go for additional growth scans.

» Effects of pregnancy on your condition
Your protein-controlled diet will be strict. As your baby grows he will use up protein, and later his liver may produce the enzymes you cannot. As a result, the amount of protein you eat to keep your blood phenylalanine at the correct levels will increase over the course of the pregnancy – all within the strict diet prescribed by your dietician in response to your blood tests.

Cystic fibrosis

» What is it?
Known as CF, this genetic condition causes thick mucus to build up in the lungs and digestive system, making it difficult to breathe and get nutrients from food.

» Effects on your pregnancy, labour, and baby
You will probably be advised that a lung function (FEV1) of 60 per cent is necessary before you try for a baby. Pregnancy is best planned. The likelihood of having a healthy pregnancy and baby when you have CF is improving all the time. The antenatal care team can help you get a good outcome. You will pass the CF gene to your baby, who will become a carrier. He has a 50 per cent chance of developing the disease only if his father is a carrier too. You have a higher risk of gestational diabetes, your baby may be small, and there is an increased risk of premature labour, miscarriage, and stillbirth.

» Medicines and tests
Most medicines used in CF, including antibiotics, are safe to use in pregnancy. You can continue any medication unless your CF specialist advises otherwise. You will see your midwife with your CF specialist. Both will monitor your nutrition and weight gain. In some cases you may need additional scans to check the development and growth of your baby. Check with your doctor if you can continue to take pain-relief medication. Consult your CF specialist before trying to conceive.

» Effects of pregnancy on your condition
The symptoms of CF might worsen. You might find that you have trouble with breathing as your uterus expands during your pregnancy. You may also experience malnutrition as your body struggles to absorb enough nutrients. Nasal tube feeding may be advised.

Good lung function This is a key factor in having a safe pregnancy and healthy baby. Your doctors will monitor your lung function throughout your pregnancy.

{Q What significant complications can arise during pregnancy?

Pregnancy-induced complications are health issues that didn't exist before you were pregnant – and they will usually disappear after the birth of your baby. Throughout pregnancy, your midwife checks for signs of these complications. Some women have gynaecological issues that can affect pregnancy, and sometimes problems arise with the placenta that is nourishing your baby.

 Hypertension

» What is it?
It means you develop abnormally high blood pressure in pregnancy.

» What's the difference between pregnancy-induced hypertension and gestational hypertension?
There isn't a difference – both terms mean the same thing, that your high blood pressure in pregnancy is related. Your midwife took your blood pressure during your booking in appointment and will compare all subsequent blood-pressure readings to this one. In doing so she is making sure that over the course of your pregnancy there is no unexpected change – your blood pressure is expected to dip a little during pregnancy and then rise again to normal pre-pregnancy levels as you near full term. If at any point – and specifically after 20 weeks pregnant – it goes higher than 140/90mmHg, you will be diagnosed with pregnancy-induced hypertension (PIH) or gestational hypertension (GH), depending upon the term your medical practitioner chooses to use. The condition is subdivided into mild, moderate, and severe. If you have severe hypertension, this puts you at risk of a stroke, and you may have to have your blood pressure monitored up to four times a day.

 Did you know...

» **5 per cent** of all pregnant women will develop some form of pre-eclampsia
» **2 per cent** of all pregnant women develop severe pre-eclampsia
» **85 per cent** of women with pre-eclampsia also have oedema (fluid retention)
» **0.5 per cent** of women with pre-eclampsia go on to develop eclampsia

 Pre-eclampsia

» What is it?
Pre-eclampsia is a condition brought on by pregnancy. It's characterized by hypertension plus protein in urine. You have a slightly increased risk of developing the condition if you are aged 40 or over, you are a teenage mum, you are overweight, or have a pre-existing condition such as diabetes.

» My midwife says that I have pregnancy-induced hypertension. Does this mean I will get pre-eclampsia?
No, not necessarily. Although PIH can be a symptom of pre-eclampsia, it is not in itself a sign that pre-eclampsia is on its way. If you also have gestational proteinuric hypertension (protein in your urine), guidelines from the National Institute for Health and Care Excellence (NICE) say this is enough to diagnose mild pre-eclampsia. If you also have one or more of the other symptoms, you are said to have moderate or severe pre-eclampsia. If you are diagnosed with any form of pre-eclampsia, your midwife will refer you to an obstetrician who will monitor your pregnancy very carefully over the remaining weeks.

» If I have pre-eclampsia will I have to spend the rest of my pregnancy in hospital?
That depends on how severe your pre-eclampsia is. If your pre-eclampsia is mild, you are likely to have to stay in hospital for only a day or two while your blood pressure is monitored – usually up to four times a day. Often complete rest is all you need to get your blood pressure under control and you will be allowed to go home without further treatment. If you have moderate pre-eclampsia, your stay is likely to be longer and you are more likely to be given medication to bring down your blood pressure. You will probably also have a scan to check that your baby is growing well. If your due date is still a while away, you may either be advised to stay in hospital, or you will be closely managed as an outpatient, as long as your blood pressure has returned to normal and all seems well with your baby. If, however, you have severe early-onset pre-eclampsia, you will probably have to stay in hospital for the rest of your pregnancy so that you and your baby can be closely monitored. Your obstetrician may decide to deliver your baby early, although he or she will aim to deliver your baby no earlier than 37 weeks. If you develop pre-eclampsia of any severity after 37 weeks, you will usually be advised to have an early induction of labour.

» Symptoms
› Frequent or permanent headache, usually above your eyes and over your brow.
› Blurred vision, or "lightning flashes" in front of your eyes.
› Pain in your abdomen or underneath your ribs.
› Vomiting or general feelings of being unwell.
› Reduced urination (called oliguria).
› Sudden swelling in the extremities or face.

 Eclampsia

» What is it?
This is a serious condition, characterized by seizures as well as all the symptoms of pre-eclampsia. In severe cases, eclampsia can lead to unconsciousness.

» Does having pre-eclampsia mean I will definitely develop eclampsia?
No. Only around one in every 200 women with pre-eclampsia will go on to develop full-blown eclampsia.

» How will eclampsia affect my pregnancy?
If you develop eclampsia your doctors will advise you to have your baby immediately. You are also at increased risk of placental abruption, when the placenta comes away from the wall of the uterus, and HELLP syndrome (see below).

HELLP

» What is it?
A severe form of pre-eclampsia, HELLP stands for Haemolysis (breaking down of red blood cells), Elevated Liver enzymes, and Low Platelet count.

» What does it mean for my pregnancy?
HELLP puts both you and sometimes your baby in significant danger, so you will be encouraged to give birth to your baby as soon as possible, regardless of how far along you are in your pregnancy. HELLP is more likely to affect the health of the mother than the baby, so your baby has a good chance of a positive outcome unless she is very small. Very low birthweight babies will to be taken to the special-care neonatal unit in order to give them the best possible chances of survival.

Gestational diabetes

What is gestational diabetes? Does it mean I have diabetes, or my baby does?

There are two main types of diabetes, Type I and Type II (see p.141). However, if you do not usually suffer from either of these types of diabetes but you develop insulin resistance during your pregnancy, you have gestational diabetes mellitus – GDM. It's a condition that affects the mother, and potentially the baby's growth. GDM usually develops during the third trimester of pregnancy, after 25 weeks pregnant, and it will usually disappear once the baby has been born. However, if you have had gestational diabetes, you are more likely to go on to develop Type II diabetes in later life. Gestational diabetes occurs in between 2 and 5 per cent of pregnancies worldwide.

My mother has Type I diabetes, but I don't. Will I be screened for gestational diabetes?

There is no automatic screening programme in the UK for gestational diabetes. However, if you have risk factors, for example, a close family member suffers from any form of diabetes, or if a close female member of your family had gestational diabetes, your midwife will probably offer you a blood-glucose tolerance test at between 24 and 28 weeks pregnant. Screening is also offered to women of southern Asian, Afro-Caribbean, or black descent, women who have had a previous baby who weighed more than 4.5kg (9lb), who have had gestational diabetes in an earlier pregnancy, or who are obese.

Will I have to have a C-section?

Not necessarily. Clinical guidelines state that gestational diabetes alone is not a good enough reason to recommend a C-section. However, one effect on the baby is to make her "large for dates". If this applies to your pregnancy, your obstetrician may recommend a C-section as your baby's size could make labour difficult or distressing for one or both of you (see below). You'll have scans throughout the final stages of pregnancy if you have gestational diabetes, so your baby's growth will be monitored carefully and you'll be able to make a fully informed decision about how you give birth, and to weigh up your wishes against the advice of the healthcare professionals.

Will I be allowed a home birth if I have gestational diabetes? What about an active birth?

It's unlikely. If your diabetes is severe, you will most likely need to be delivered on a labour ward because of the increased risks to you and your baby during labour and birth. You will also be attached to a drip of insulin and glucose, which will make moving around tricky. Your doctor and midwife will meet with you at around 36 weeks pregnant to discuss the safest options for your baby's birth.

How will gestational diabetes affect my baby? What about after birth?

GDM can cause a baby to become large for dates, but that is the only direct effect the condition has on the baby while she is in the uterus. This does increase the risk of labour complications, as the baby may be too large to pass through the pelvis, and has an increased risk of shoulder dystocia, when the head is delivered, but there is difficulty delivering the shoulders, so a planned C-section may be advised. There are other effects that can influence the baby's wellbeing. For example, gestational diabetes can cause too much amniotic fluid to be produced, which in turn can trigger premature labour, and there may be issues stabilizing the baby's blood sugar after birth. The condition also puts you at greater risk of pre-eclampsia, which can be dangerous for both you and your baby. Finally, studies show that babies born to mothers who had gestational diabetes are more prone to obesity in later life, with the knock-on effect of increasing their risk of developing Type II diabetes.

Blood glucose meter You'll be given a blood glucose meter. This allows you to check your glucose levels through a small pin-prick sample of blood.

If you had gestational diabetes in a previous pregnancy you have a **67 per cent** chance of developing it subsequent pregnancies.

Diabetic treatments

Food choices You will be advised to eat food that will help to keep your blood glucose as stable as possible. Wholemeal bread and brown rice are both good for releasing energy gradually.

As a first step in your treatment, you'll be referred to a dietician, who will talk to you about how you can try to control your glucose levels through diet. Injecting yourself with insulin is something of a last resort.

Food and drink

You will be given guidance on dietary changes and told specifically which foods and beverages you should consume.

Exercise

Your midwife will talk to you about forms of exercise that are safe for you.

Insulin

However, if you can't control your glucose using diet and exercise alone, you will need to lower the amount of glucose in your blood either by taking metformin tablets, or through insulin injections. If you need injections, a specialist midwife will talk you through this.

Tilted uterus

» What is it?

The uterus is normally in a straight, vertical position. A tilted uterus is one that tips backwards towards the spine. It's also known as a retroverted uterus. Symptoms of tilted uterus usually include pain during sexual intercourse and pain during menstruation.

» What does this condition mean for my pregnancy? Will my uterus stay tilted after I've given birth?

The main implication for your pregnancy is that your baby may be hard to spot during an abdominal ultrasound scan. Some women with a tilted uterus have to have a vaginal ultrasound in order for the sonographer to be able to see the baby from all angles. This is simply because the baby is further away from the front of the abdomen. Other than that, complications arising directly from your uterine anatomy are extremely rare - once you have completed 12 weeks of pregnancy, your uterus will expand out of your pelvis anyway and as it grows will fill the space in your abdomen. After birth, your uterus may or may not move back into its original position - it partly depends on the strength of the muscles and ligaments around your uterus. Whatever happens, the position of your uterus after you've had your baby is unlikely to affect your chances of conceiving again in the future, so try not to worry about it.

Endometriosis

» What is it?

In this condition, pieces of tissue that are normally part of the uterine lining (also called the endometrium) are found in the abdomen and pelvis, including on the ovaries, in the bowel, and around the bladder. The endometrium is the part of the uterus that sheds during your periods. This condition can result in heavy, painful menstruation and infertility, but the cause of it is not totally understood.

» I was diagnosed with endometriosis a couple of years ago. Could it affect my pregnancy?

Once pregnant, endometriosis is unlikely to affect your pregnancy, your baby, or increase any risk factors. (The

Fibroids

» What are fibroids?

Fibroids are non-cancerous growths in the uterus, affecting a quarter of all women at some point in their lives. The most common form grow within the muscular wall of the uterus (intramuscular fibroids), although they may also appear outside the muscle wall, growing into the pelvis (subserous fibroids); dangling from the lining of the uterus (pedunculated fibroids); embedded in the inner lining of the uterus (submucosal fibroids); or on the neck of your cervix (cervical fibroids). They may be small or large, and their exact cause is unknown, although excess oestrogen makes them bigger. (This is why women who are overweight are more likely to have fibroids, because fat cells produce oestrogen.)

» How will I know if I have fibroids and what effects will they have on my body and baby?

Fibroids may cause painful and/or heavy periods, pain during intercourse, abdominal bloating, or frequent urination (if the fibroid presses on the bladder). If fibroids are large or numerous, they can affect fertility because they make it harder for the embryo to implant in the uterine lining, and they may also make it more likely for you to miscarry if you do get pregnant. If you have had fibroid treatment pre-pregnancy, this can affect your delivery options once pregnant, so talk to your doctor about this. Many fibroids are asymptomatic - in other words, a large number of women don't even discover they have them until they have a routine pregnancy scan, until the fibroids cause spotting during pregnancy, or until their midwife presses on their uterus to feel the position of the baby. Some fibroids restrict space in your uterus so that your baby doesn't have the space to grow properly. However, this is very rare. Also, as fibroids grow under the influence of pregnancy hormones, they can start to degenerate, usually in the second trimester,

Fallopian tube

Subserous fibroid

Intramural fibroid

Ovary

Submucosal fibroid
Grows under the lining

Cervical fibroid
Grows within the cervix

Sizes Fibroids can range from as small as a bean, but can also be as large as a small melon. They can be seen on X-rays.

Where are they found?
Fibroids can grow in the inner, middle, and outer layers of the uterus. Polyps can form on the cervical or uterine lining.

and this can cause pain and, rarely, premature labour.

» My fibroids are large and my midwife has said that I may have to have a C-section. Why?

There are several reasons why fibroids might mean that C-section is the safest way to deliver your baby. In pregnancy, a large fibroid may push your baby into an awkward position for delivery (called "malpresentation"), including the breech position and very occasionally presenting with a shoulder first. Cervical fibroids may block the entrance to your cervix, making it difficult for your baby to pass into the birth canal. If fibroids cause your placenta to come away slightly from your uterine lining (called a partial abruption; see opposite), your baby will continue to be well-nourished, but a pre-term C-section, as soon as your baby is big enough to survive outside the uterus, will remove the risks to the baby if the placenta comes away completely. Finally, fibroids also put you at slightly increased risk of post-partum haemorrhage (excessive bleeding after the birth) and preterm delivery. Your midwife has a duty to ensure you are fully aware of any potential complications, but it's important to remember that fibroids only very rarely cause any problems and all the situations given here are exceptional. Fibroids can be removed after pregnancy and if you do not want more children you can have a hysterectomy which means there is no risk of them reoccuring.

main problems of this condition are to do with conceiving). During your pregnancy, you may find that your symptoms of endometriosis improve or disappear, but it is likely that they will resume when your menstruation begins again after pregnancy and breastfeeding (if you are doing so) are over.

Uterus infection

» What is it?
Chorioamnionitis is an infection in pregnancy of the membranes surrounding the fetus. This is associated with prolonged rupture of the membranes (if there is a long period of time between your membranes rupturing and birth) and can affect mum and baby, so labour needs to be induced and you'll be given antibiotics. Chorioamnionitis makes a uterus infection after birth, known as endometritis, more likely. Endometritis is also more likely if you have had a C-section or a retained placenta. The infection causes pain in the lower abdomen, and you may have a high temperature. Antibiotics usually clear the infection.

» I've had an infection in my uterus in the past and may have scarring. Will this make it harder for me to carry a baby to term?
Uterine infection can cause scar tissue to develop in the uterine lining (endometrium). This, in turn, can make it harder for a fertilized egg to implant, and if it does implant, this may be less secure, increasing the risk of miscarriage. You're also at increased risk of placenta praevia (see right) and placental abruption (see below). Inform your midwife of your medical history. You will be given regular checks to monitor the progress of your pregnancy.

Cervical insufficiency

» What is it?
Cervical insufficiency is a cervix that is not rigid enough to safely hold in the membranes surrounding your baby. The cervix could open too early, in the second trimester.

» How is this diagnosed, and what does it mean?
Cervical insufficiency may be the result of a previous pregnancy that stretched the opening of the cervix too far, or of previous cervical surgery. If undiagnosed, you are at increased risk of late miscarriage, when your baby is heavy and the membranes are forced out of the cervix and rupture. However, most cases are picked up during antenatal checks, before becoming problematic. Your midwife will refer you to a gynaecologist who may scan the cervix (unless you've had a previous cervical insufficiency, in which case a scan isn't needed) and put a temporary stitch – a cerclage – into the cervix between weeks 12 and 16 to hold things in place. The stitch is removed before labour. You may be given medicine if the cervix starts to open up and shorten.

Placenta praevia

» What is placenta praevia?
More commonly known as "low-lying placenta", placenta praevia occurs when the placenta's position partially or completely covers your cervix – and thus blocks your baby's exit to the birth canal. A diagnosis of placenta praevia is not certain until late pregnancy because the placenta can move away from the internal opening of the cervix (os) as the uterus grows and stretches. The sonographer will check the position of your placenta at your second ultrasound scan (the anomaly scan). If your baby's placenta is noted to be low-lying, you will have another scan at between 32 and 34 weeks to see whether the placenta has shifted upwards. Around 90 per cent of low-lying placentas seen before 28 weeks will move to a better position by the follow-up scan. (This happens in around 50 per cent of cases if you have had a C-section in the past.) Placenta praevia can be the result of fibroids or scar tissue preventing the placenta from attaching in a good position, or it might happen by chance.

» What impact does a diagnosis of placenta praevia have on my pregnancy?
Most cases of placenta praevia require a C-section because a vaginal delivery isn't possible if the placenta is 2cm (¾in) from the edge of the cervix or closer. Your healthcare professional will talk to you about the possibility of an elective (planned) C-section in order to safely deliver your baby. There could be some extra fetal monitoring, too.

As well as blocking the cervix, placenta praevia can cause painless, bright red bleeding. If you notice this kind of bleeding, let your midwife know straight away. Heavy bleeding can put both you and your baby at risk, but most of the time it can be treated before there is any danger. In severe cases, you might need a blood transfusion. Your obstetrician might advise that you abstain from intercourse to prevent the risk of bleeding, or even advise bed rest or a hospital stay. If there is profuse bleeding or risk of premature birth, your doctor could recommend an emergency C-section.

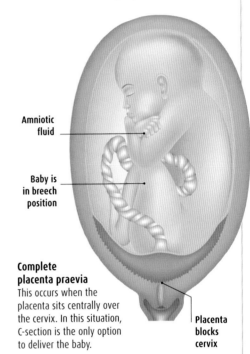

Amniotic fluid

Baby is in breech position

Complete placenta praevia
This occurs when the placenta sits centrally over the cervix. In this situation, C-section is the only option to deliver the baby.

Placenta blocks cervix

Although placenta praevia often makes a **Caesarean section necessary**, the vast majority of women deliver **healthy babies** and recover well from their operation.

Placental abruption

» What is it?
Placental abruption, when part or all of the placenta comes away from the wall of the uterus, is a serious condition that significantly impacts your baby's ability to receive nutrients and oxygen. Rarely, the entire placenta may become detached. The first signs that it might be happening are abdominal pain and bleeding. If you experience any spotting during your pregnancy, call your healthcare professional. It is a potentially life-threatening condition, so immediate attention is imperative.

» My friend's baby was stillborn following a placental abruption. What can I do to stop this happening to me?
Though you can't do anything specifically to stop a placental abruption, it's possible to carry a baby to term as long as the abruption is only mild – meaning that most of the placenta remains attached to the uterus (enough to nourish your baby). Severe or complete abruption is not treatable and is more likely to result in premature birth, or stillbirth. It is also dangerous for you, as it can result in significant blood loss. If you smoke or take drugs – stop. These habits are associated with an increased risk of placental abruption. Pre-eclampsia and a small baby also increase the risk.

» In this chapter...

Your growing baby

From feeling the first gentle movements to experiencing the fuller twists, **kicks, and hiccups**, you will marvel at the **magical changes** that are taking place inside you. As the tiny bundle of cells develops, you will become more and more aware of your baby **getting bigger and stronger** the closer you get to full term. Learn more about the placenta, your baby's developing organs, and his skeletal structure. Discover why your baby is so **unique and special**.

The biological and chemical processes that take us from a cell to a baby really are **absolutely incredible**. As soon as your pregnancy begins, your **amazing body** transforms so it can protect this **new life**, while the new life itself becomes a fully functioning human being, **one cell at a time** but at remarkable speed.

From cell to baby

The zygote of life

Your baby begins life as a single cell, created by a sperm fusing with an egg. This organism contains all the potential for new life – a full set of chromosomes (23 pairs, one in each pair from each parent). These carry your baby's unique blueprint encoded in genes. Although we often refer colloquially to this earliest stage of life as an embryo, in fact we're a few steps from an embryo yet. For the time being, your baby is a zygote. The zygote travels down the Fallopian tube and as it journeys, it is already subdividing and multiplying to make 16 cells. It's surrounded by a protective membrane called the zona pellucida, which has a very special function – it prevents the zygote from implanting in the Fallopian tube, or anywhere that isn't your uterus.

Morula to blastocyst

During its journey down the Fallopian tube to the uterus, the zygote becomes known as a morula (because the cells are grouped together and look like a mulberry, from the Latin morus). The morula is a hive of activity: its cells subdivide rapidly and eventually create a kind of bubble structure with an outer membrane (the trophoblast) containing a mass of cells (the endoderm) within a cavity. Amazingly, that bundle of cells sitting against the membrane wall will become the key to your baby's breathing and digestion among other

things. At this stage your baby becomes known as a blastocyst. The blastocyst floats around in the uterus for a while, then sends chemical messages that break down the zona pellucida. Now exposed, the "sticky" trophoblast latches onto and implants itself in the uterine wall. All this happens around seven to nine days after fertilization. Your baby has now doubled in size since fertilization and is made up of more than a hundred cells. Once implanted, the blastocyst is enveloped by the uterine lining (endometrium) and snuggles down deep within the cells of the lining. It can now receive nourishment directly from your uterus.

Embryo to fetus

At four weeks, the blastocyst can be called an embryo. The trophoblast has started to develop into the placenta (see p.154), and secretions from your uterus are nourishing the cells so that they divide and subdivide and begin to form your baby's organs, skeleton, and features. Crucially, the embryo is made up of three layers; each will develop into specific parts of your baby's body. Now that your baby is being nourished by your body, the business of becoming more "baby-like" can begin. At about 10 weeks, when his facial features are in place and most of the major organs are on their way to being formed, your baby has become a fetus – the medical name he keeps until birth.

Q How are the fertilized cells nourished before there's a placenta?

The early embryo is fed by a "yolk sac", which develops from some of the cells of the blastocyst.

Despite being called a yolk sac, there's hardly any yolk in it, but what is there provides enough energy and nutrition to see your developing baby through until the fully formed placenta takes over at around 12 weeks. The placenta doesn't begin to form until you're about four weeks pregnant (which is about two weeks after conception, since pregnancy is dated from the first day of your last menstrual period).

The early embryo is just a disc of cells; on one side there is an amniotic sac, and on the other side is the yolk sac. A basic circulatory system draws nutrients from the yolk sac and delivers them into the developing embryo cells. As the embryo grows it is enveloped by the amniotic sac, while the yolk sac remains outside, but connected to the embryo. Part of the yolk sac then triggers cells in the blastocyst to begin making the placenta. The yolk sac slowly shrinks as the placenta becomes stronger, disappearing into the umbilical cord when the placenta is fully formed. It is while the embryo is dependent on the yolk sac that it is most vulnerable – this is one of the reasons why the risk of miscarriage is highest in the first trimester and becomes lower as the placenta begins to share the job of sustaining the baby.

Amniotic sac

Embryo This is just a disc of layered cells after implanting.

Connective tissue This will eventually form the umbilical cord.

Yolk sac This feeds the embryo, but will shrink as the placenta grows.

Trophoblast The outer layer of the blastocyst

Blastocoel This is a fluid-filled cavity that the embryo can expand into.

Week 4 This illustration shows that the embryo is implanted and buried inside the uterine lining.

Q Does it matter where the cells implant in my uterus?

No and yes. The most important thing is that the bundle of cells finds a comfortable home in your uterine lining, rather than anywhere else, such as the Fallopian tubes. (If this happens, your pregnancy is termed ectopic (see p.308), which can be life-threatening for you.) Usually, your clever body draws the blastocyst towards the top (the superior wall) and back (the posterior wall) of your uterus. This is the best place for implantation because when the placenta grows, it's very unlikely to block your baby's eventual exit through your cervix. Sometimes, though, the blastocyst implants lower down in your uterus and the placenta forms too close to the cervix (this is called placenta praevia; see p.147). This can happen if, for example, you have uterine fibroids (see p.146) or a scar from a previous operation (such as a Caesarean section) that make it difficult for

the blastocyst to implant. Although your baby can develop healthily wherever in the uterus the blastocyst makes its home, the place where it implants can have consequences for your labour and your experience of birth.

Q How does my baby develop from just layers of cells?

At five weeks, the embryo is made up of three layers of cells that develop into different parts of your baby's body. These layers undergo a complex process of three-dimensional folding to form the basic bodily structures. The ectoderm is the outermost layer of the embryo and will form, among other things, your baby's nervous system, his facial features (including his eyes, nose, mouth, and ears), and his skin, nails, and hair. It also becomes your baby's anal canal. The mesoderm is the middle layer, and, will become, among other things, your baby's circulatory

system, skeletal system (including bones, cartilage, muscles, and ligaments), blood cells and bone marrow, kidneys, and reproductive organs. The endoderm is the innermost layer of the embryo and will become your baby's respiratory system, digestive system, and bladder, as well as several important glands of his endocrine (hormone) system, including the thyroid, parathyroid, and thymus glands.

100–150

cells are present in the **blastocyst** (as a result of cell division) by the time it enters the uterine cavity, ready to implant.

Q How advanced is an embryo? Which parts of my baby's body develop first?

Even in the very earliest days, your baby is already developing some primitive, functional versions of the fully fledged vital organs she'll have when she's born. As a mass of cells, the embryo is not yet akin to how we might picture a developing baby, but it is brimming with potential.

During the first 10 weeks of pregnancy, your ball of potential undergoes a process called organogenesis – the creation of your baby's vital organs. Development of the organs is far more important than your embryo's growth, which is why she grows very little in length during the first 12 weeks compared with the second and third trimesters of pregnancy. All her cellular energy is diverted into creating her organs. This requires a process of rapid cell division

and the subdivision of groups of cells into their different functions: it's called differentiation.

By just five weeks of pregnancy, your baby's thyroid, renal, adrenal, and gonadal organs (glands of her endocrine, or hormonal, system) are all present in a primitive form. The cells that will form her brain, kidneys, heart, and nerves have appeared. She has a tube that will become her gastrointestinal tract. Her lungs and stomach have divided

off from a single tube within the embryo.

Over the course of the next five weeks, all the cells that have taken on these vital roles will keep dividing, folding, turning, and forming. By the time you're 10 weeks pregnant and probably looking forward to your first scan, your baby will have a basic, functioning system of organs – a heart that beats, primitive kidneys that pass urine, and a brain that's beginning to send messages to other parts of the body.

Yolk sac This provides early sustenance for the developing embryo.

Villi Chorionic villi contain blood vessels that access the mother's blood supply in order to provide nutrients to the embryo.

Umbilical cord The cord is short to begin with. It isn't yet long enough to become coiled.

Six weeks The embryo is beginning to take on a human-looking form at this stage. Internal organs are becoming clearer and externally, the eye, ear, and limb buds are showing.

Eye

Embryo The embryo floats in the amniotic fluid.

Amniotic sac The sac will join with the outer layer of the blastocyst (the chorion) at 15 weeks.

Branchial arches These are the beginnings of the neck and lower jaw structures.

Upper limb bud This will turn into an arm as the fetus grows.

Heart This has started to beat by six weeks.

Somites These become the trunk muscles, spinal cord, vertebral column, and skin.

Q My baby's heart was beating on an early scan! Is it formed already?

At only six weeks pregnant, your baby has a simple heart that's beating, and it's doing so up to 160 times per minute.

Your baby needs a circulation system so that nutrients can pass into all her cells as they develop. At first, the yolk sac and placenta can diffuse nutrients and oxygen into her cells, but pretty soon the embryo is too large for this method and she needs a circulation system to help. That's why the heart is one of the first organs a baby develops – as early as 18 days after fertilization.

The heart begins life as two cords (the endocardial tubes) that fuse together, creating a "primitive heart tube". Once the heart tube has formed at around six weeks of pregnancy, it begins to pump blood cells. A mere three weeks later, this tiny, early heart has developed its chambers and valves.

Since your baby doesn't breathe in the uterus, she gets her oxygen from her mother through the placenta. Blood that leaves the body would normally go to the lungs to collect oxygen, but a fetus's heart has two extra connections that allow deoxygenated blood to bypass the lungs. Instead, fetal blood vessels pass out through the umbilical cord to the placenta to pick up oxygen. On the return journey, the re-routing sends oxgenated blood to the brain cells quickly. After birth, the two extra connections in the heart close.

Fusion of endocardial tubes into primitive heart tube

Ventricle

Atrium

Deoxygenated blood flow

Flow of oxygenated blood

Atrium

Ventricle

1 Primitive heart tube The two cords merge from the base upwards, forming a single primitive heart tube about 21 days after fertilization (five weeks pregnant).

2 Bending of the heart tube After forming, the heart tube begins to beat. It then elongates and loops to the right, forming a spiral and a basic circulation.

3 Final position of chambers The tube twists again to create four chambers. By nine weeks, the chambers are totally separate, and tiny valves have formed inside.

Q Is there anything I can do to encourage healthy organ development in my baby?

Yes, there are certain ways you can help.
The first 10 weeks of pregnancy are the most vulnerable time for your baby's development, as it's when her organs are most susceptible to environmental harm. If your pregnancy is planned, you may already be taking folic acid

(to encourage healthy nerve and brain development in your baby) and be avoiding toxins. But if that isn't the case for you, don't worry. As soon as you find out you're pregnant, start taking supplements of folic acid (400mcg) and vitamin D (10mcg) daily; cut out alcohol, nicotine, and any other recreational drugs if you take them (seek advice if need be); and avoid passive smoking. You can also steer clear of certain foods to lower the risk of getting harmful food poisoning (see pp.52–53).

Q What is the neural tube, and how does it relate to my baby's brain and nervous system?

The neural tube is the structure that eventually becomes your baby's brain and nervous system. It develops when you are around four weeks pregnant and at around five weeks of pregnancy, it separates to form cells that will become the outer layer of your baby's brain (the cerebellum) and other cells that will travel throughout your baby's developing body to become nerves. You may have heard of the neural tube in relation to "neural tube defects". These are conditions that can very rarely occur as a result of low maternal folic acid, among other reasons. You may be offered very accurate tests for these defects as part of your antenatal care (see p.97).

Q Why is my baby surrounded by amniotic fluid? What is it for?

Amniotic fluid protects your baby from trauma, aids lung development, helps maintain a constant temperature (slightly higher than your own), and gives your baby space to grow in. At the beginning of your pregnancy amniotic fluid is primarily made up of water and electrolytes. Around weeks 12–14 the fluid contains carbohydrates, proteins, lipids, phospholipids, and urea. As the kidneys start to function and produce urine, this passes into the amniotic fluid. By the end of your pregnancy your baby will swallow 0.5–1 litres (⁹⁄₁₀–1¾ pints) of amniotic fluid a day and replace it as urine. The volume of amniotic fluid present in the amniotic sac decreases towards the end of the pregnancy as the fetal kidneys produce smaller amounts of more concentrated urine.

Did you know...

The volume of amniotic fluid at 12 weeks is about 30ml (1fl oz), less than an egg cup full. By 32 weeks the amniotic fluid in the sac reaches its highest volume. This is usually 1 litre (1¾ pints), although this can be as much as 2 litres (3½ pints).

{Q What is the placenta and how does it work?

The placenta is your baby's life-support system. It's the means by which she receives oxygen and nutrients, it provides her with protection against disease, and it's where the waste she produces goes to be disposed of. The placenta is part of you and part of her at the same time. It's the link that enables you to nourish her while she grows inside you.

The placenta is formed

The placenta begins to form from cells in the embryo soon after the egg implants in the lining of the uterus. The embryo is surrounded by a chorionic membrane, which sends out tentacle-like projections that secure the embryo's place in the uterine wall. These projections are called "villi": they divide and branch out, and eventually fill with blood vessels from your baby's own circulatory system. Spaces around the villi fill with your blood. This whole structure – a mass of vessel-filled villi surrounded by maternal blood – is the placenta.

Villous chorion The frond-like texture of chorion creates a big surface area for gas exchange to take place

Placenta

At 12 weeks The maternal side of the placenta contains 15–20 lobes. These stop forming at this stage of gestation.

Placenta

Uterus

Endometrium

Myometrium

Perimetrium

Uterine cavity

Mucus plug

Cervix

Vagina

Your baby's lifeline In the early stages of pregnancy, your placenta grows faster than your baby. The structure of the placenta is complete by the end of the first trimester. It keeps growing in size and will end up weighing around 20 per cent of your baby's birthweight.

Umbilical cord The cord is covered in a jelly-like substance (known as Wharton's jelly after Thomas Wharton who first noted it in 1656) that prevents the cord from kinking

Uterine muscle

The uterus By 12 weeks it is too big to fit within the pelvis, so it has to flex forwards and expand into the abdomen

Fetal blood vessels These are contained in the frond-like villi and surrounded by maternal blood

...ternal blood vessels These ...g the mother's blood to intervillous spaces

Blood circulation This close up of the placenta shows how the maternal and fetal blood flow interact. The exchange of gas takes place in the intervillous spaces.

Deoxygenated blood (blue) This blood flows from the fetus to the placenta via arteries

Intervillous space The mother's blood fills the space around the villi to allow gas exchange

Gas and waste exchange This passes from the fetus's villi to the mother's bloodstream

Oxygenated blood (red) This blood flows back to the fetus through the vein after collecting oxygen and nutrients in the placenta

The umbilical cord The cord contains one vein and two arteries. The vein carries oxygenated blood and nutrients to your baby; the arteries carry deoxygenated blood and waste products away from your baby to the placenta. After birth, when the extra fetal heart ducts have closed, this will swap so that arteries carry oxygenated blood to the heart and veins carry deoxygenated blood

THE PLACENTA'S ROLE

The placenta plays a vital role in your baby's survival. It has four key functions.

» Removing your baby's waste: there are two arteries in the umbilical cord as well as arterial vessels in the villi. These carry waste and carbon dioxide-filled blood from the baby. The waste gases travel through the walls of the villi into the mother's blood and are then processed as waste by the mother's liver and kidneys.

» Protecting your baby from disease: the cells of the villi are tightly packed. This means that organisms that are made up of large cells, such as bacteria and viruses that might be in the mother's blood, can't pass into the baby's blood through the villi walls. Not all organisms are too large though, which is why it's important to avoid contracting certain diseases (such as rubella or chickenpox) by being vaccinated against them. Towards the end of your pregnancy, antibodies from your blood will pass into your baby's circulation; these provide her with a basic level of immunity that lasts several weeks after she's born.

» Protecting your baby from chemicals: many chemicals (including toxins) are also made up of cells too large to cross the placenta. This is why you can continue taking certain medications while pregnant. Certain toxins, though, such as nicotine and alcohol, can pass through the villi walls.

» Producing hormones: the placenta serves as its own endocrine system. It's an important source of progesterone to help maintain your pregnancy and prevent premature labour, and of oestrogen, to ensure your uterus expands to accommodate your growing baby and prepare your body for labour and, later, for breastfeeding. The placenta is also the source of the hormone hCG, which is the first signal your body receives that pregnancy has occurred. Growth hormones and relaxin (which softens the ligaments in your pelvis to make space for your baby and prepare your body for birth) are also produced in the placenta, along with several other hormones that optimize the transfer of nutrients and oxygen within the placenta itself.

The placenta expands in size from just a few cells to between 350g (12oz) and 700g (1½lb) in weight.

Q What's the difference between an embryo and a fetus, and what does it mean for my baby?

Your baby is called an embryo while his basic body structures and major organs form. From week 10 of your pregnancy (eight weeks after fertilization), this stage is complete and your baby becomes known as a fetus until he is born.

During the embryonic period your baby formed a face, limbs, fingers, and toes, and also rudimentary organs and body systems including the brain, heart, urinary tract, digestive tract, skin, bones, and muscles. By 10 weeks of pregnancy, the basic structures of all the major organs are present but they need further growth and development to gain the complexity of fully functioning systems that will support your baby after birth. The

graduation to fetus status marks the next stage of your baby's development. The body and organs grow rapidly; by contrast, the growth of the head slows down relative to the rest of your baby's body. The shape of the head becomes more recognizably human, and the brain and nervous system link up. By the end of your second trimester your baby will have doubled in weight and have emerging toenails and fingernails, the genitalia will be visible on

an ultrasound scan, and you'll feel him move – he may even be very active. During the third trimester, fine-tuning takes place in your baby's brain and body systems. He will be able to see and hear in utero, and taste the amniotic fluid. His body will fill out with fat deposits under the skin to keep him insulated after birth. Finally, your baby's lungs are completed, having formed millions of air sacs that will allow him to take his first breath in the outside world.

10 weeks At this stage the placenta is increasingly able to support the rapidly growing fetus and the yolk sac has almost disappeared.

Head The head takes up half the fetal length at 10 weeks. This demonstrates how much the brain needs to develop before anything else can

Umbilical cord

Chorionic villi Tertiary villi start to form and aid the transfer of nutrients

Legs and feet At 10 weeks the legs are less developed than the arms and the toes have not separated out yet

Amniotic fluid At this point in your pregnancy the fluid comes from liquids passed across the fetal skin, membranes, and placenta

Q Is it true that my baby's entire digestive system begins as a simple tube?

The whole digestive system forms its structure by 12 weeks. By the time he is born, your tiny new baby will house an incredible 2.5m (8ft) of intestines.

Your baby's digestive system begins with a "gut tube" that forms from the endoderm layer of cells (the lower layer) and connects an opening at the top of the tube (which will connect to your baby's mouth) to an opening at the bottom (eventually your baby's anus). The gut tube then develops three sections – the foregut, midgut, and hindgut – and each of these forms specific organ buds. Between six and eight weeks pregnant, the foregut develops a bulge that will become your baby's stomach. All three sections of the gut tube continually lengthen so that by the time you are nine weeks pregnant, there's so much

bowel tissue (the bowel is the collective name for the small and large intestines) that there isn't room for it to fit inside the tiny embryo. Instead, it pushes out of a hole in your baby's abdomen so that it occupies some of the space in the umbilical cord. By 10 weeks pregnant, the baby's stomach will begin to produce digestive juices – a milestone in his transition from embryo to fetus. By the time you're 12 weeks pregnant, your baby's body is large enough for his bowel to come back inside his body and his umbilical cord is empty again, apart from the vessels that belong there.

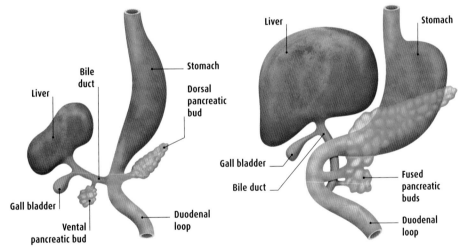

1 At nine weeks The main tube of the gut develops specialized structures that branch off from it. The early pancreas is made up of two separate buds.

2 At 10 weeks The pancreatic buds have fused. The liver and stomach are much larger, and the duodenum (part of the small intestine) is lengthening.

Q Does my baby have functioning kidneys? If so, where does the urine go?

By 13 weeks of pregnancy, your baby's urine can pass out of his newly forming kidneys, through his developing ureters, and into his tiny bladder. This urine is released into the amniotic fluid. Your baby learns to swallow at around the same time, so drinks the amniotic

fluid, swallows his urine, fills his bladder again, and so the process goes on. Although this might sound unappetizing, fetal urine is very diluted and most waste has already been filtered out of your baby's system via the placenta, which is then expelled by your waste system. The kidneys develop from 10 weeks onwards, multiplying thousands of filtration cells. The ureters that collect the urine branch into the kidneys, a process that takes until 32 weeks, when there are around two million branchings.

Q Does my baby's bowel work in the uterus?

As soon as your baby's bowel is fully formed the process of making meconium – his first poo – begins. Meconium consists of waste products such as cells from the bowel lining, amniotic fluid, mucus, and bile. It builds up and is slowly forced into the large intestine – a process helped by the peristaltic motion of your baby's bowel from 20 weeks. At roughly the same time, the muscle around his anus – the anal sphincter – tightens up, keeping the meconium in so that he doesn't poo inside the uterus.

0
Babies have no **kneecaps** when they are born. These will develop in infancy.

1
Only one organ, the **auditory ossicles** in the ear, is full size at birth.

33%
A new baby's **kidneys** are just a third of full adult size.

270
Babies have more **bones** than adults, who have 206. Many bones fuse as they grow.

30,000
The number of **tastebuds** a baby is born with reduces to 10,000 by adulthood.

{Q How does my baby's skeleton develop while she's in the uterus?

What begins as a simple framework of cartilage to protect your baby's body hardens into bone through a gradual process of ossification that continues even after your baby is born.

Body structure At 14 weeks, the fetal bones have begun to "ossify" from cartilage to bone, giving your baby enough strength to hold up and move her limbs.

Developing a supportive skeleton

Bones and muscles form early in pregnancy. At five weeks pregnant, your embryonic baby develops a sort of skeletal meshwork of connective tissue (collagen) that protects her rapidly developing organs. Over the next few weeks, this meshwork gets a blood supply, and bone cells called osteoblasts work to toughen it and form cartilage. At 10 weeks, your baby has a recognizable jaw, collarbone, shoulder blades, ribs, vertebrae, and arm and leg bones. Gradually, the osteoblast cells deposit calcium salts on the cartilage to harden, shape, and grow the bones. This process is called ossification and it continues throughout your baby's time in the uterus, and beyond until adulthood when her bones finally stop growing.

Your baby develops muscle tissue early, too: by 10 weeks she can make simple movements. By 20 to 24 weeks her nervous system is becoming connected and her musculoskeletal system has developed enough for her to bend and flex her limbs. In the third trimester of pregnancy, your baby uses 250–350mg of calcium per day to continue developing her bones. Muscle mass increases rapidly, and your baby might double in weight in the last 10 weeks of your pregnancy.

Metatarsal

Tendons and ligaments These connect bones to to muscles and cartilage

Phalanges

Ulna

Radius

Tibia

Fibula

Toes Your baby's toes separated into their individual digits at between 10 and 11 weeks of pregnancy. The small bones of her ankles have formed by the end of the first trimester

Maxilla

Mandible

Skeleton at 14 weeks There are many recognizable bones present already. They will continue to form and reform through the process of ossification for many years yet.

Ilium

Ribs At first, your baby has ribs made of cartilage at around eight weeks gestation, but these will eventually harden. The ribs protect organs in her upper body, especially her heart and lungs

ARMS AND LEGS

"Limb buds" appear on the trunk of the embryo at around five weeks of pregnancy. Her limb buds extend so that by nine weeks, her arms and legs have grown in length. These are held in shape by the long bones that have formed within them. At 14 weeks gestation, your baby's arms will probably be long enough for her to bring her hands together in front of her face, but much of her skeletal structure is still cartilage. Her limb bones will ossify from the centre outwards, leaving the tips cartilaginous (and leaving room for growth) in childhood.

SPINAL COLUMN

This is the first part of your baby's skeleton to develop. At five weeks, a rudimentary spinal cord and structures called somites form down her back (see p.49). The vertebrae form when parts of the somites (sclerotomes), split in half to allow the nerves of the spinal cord to reach through them and attach to the emerging muscles. The skeletal muscles form from another portion of the somites (the myotomes) at around seven weeks; muscle groups form first at the spine, then extend to the trunk and limbs.

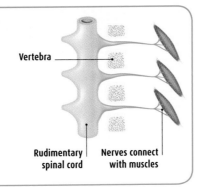

Vertebra

Rudimentary spinal cord

Nerves connect with muscles

SKULL

The flat bones that make up the sides and top of your baby's skull skip the cartilage stage and ossify directly from the membrane that surrounds her brain. By 14 weeks, your baby has a near-complete skull made up of the flat bones, the jaw, and the cartilage of the nose. The flat bones don't fuse properly, so that your baby's skull can mould to the shape of your pelvis during birth.

Parietal bone

Frontal bone

Q When are my baby's lungs fully formed? How can his respiratory system work when there's no air?

By around 36 weeks, your baby's lungs are developed enough for fully independent breathing (this is why babies born from 37 weeks onwards are considered full term), but his lungs can't inflate until there is contact with air, so "breathing" doesn't start until after birth.

Our respiratory system consists not only of our lungs, but also the nose, pharynx, larynx, and trachea. The whole respiratory tract begins life as a long tube – in fact, it's the same tube that also gives rise to most of the digestive system (see p.157). By 36 weeks, most babies' lungs are fully formed for birth, and they contain plenty of surfactant, a substance that will allow the lungs to expand and draw in air without collapsing, which makes independent breathing possible. Premature babies are supported by artificial breathing apparatus, such as a ventilator, or their oxygen levels will be controlled in an incubator.

The diagrams show how the lungs start as buds that gradually branch out and complete their development at around 36 weeks of pregnancy.

FORMATION OF THE LUNGS

First branching

Lungs at 5 weeks The lung bud branches to form left and right main bronchi. Each of the bronchial buds will develop into a lung.

Right main bronchus **Left main bronchus**

Lungs at 6 weeks The two bronchi develop differently: the left bronchus branches into two buds, and the right bronchus branches into three.

Respiratory bronchiole An early form of air sac appears at the ends of the branches

Capillary Tiny blood vessels form close to the primitive air sacs

Trachea Also known as the windpipe

Developing cartilage Sturdy rings keep the airways open

Terminal sac The old respiratory bronchiole has divided into more protrusions

Secretory cell These will produce surfactant, a substance that prevents the air sacs collapsing

Capillary These move in closer to the air sac

Right lung This has three lobes

Left lung This only has two lobes, to make room for the heart.

Right main bronchus This is at a steeper angle and is larger than the left main bronchus.

Lungs at 16 weeks There have been 20 subdivisions by this point, forming the bronchial airways. There are eight on the left and 10 on the right. The difference in number is because your baby's body is programmed to know that the left-hand lung should be smaller to leave room for his heart.

Lungs at 28 weeks There are now "terminal sacs" that will become alveoli – the air sacs where oxygen and carbon dioxide are exchanged. Until your baby takes his first breath, they're filled with amniotic fluid. The air sacs produce surfactant, a fluid that helps them to contract and expand, and prevents them collapsing.

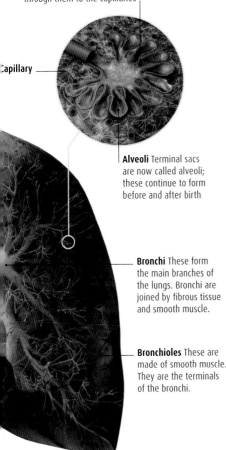

Lungs at 7 weeks The bronchial buds branch out into more buds. Secondary bronchial buds divide to form tertiary buds.

Blood-air barrier The alveoli walls are now so thin that gas can pass through them to the capillaries

Capillary

Alveoli Terminal sacs are now called alveoli; these continue to form before and after birth

Bronchi These form the main branches of the lungs. Bronchi are joined by fibrous tissue and smooth muscle.

Bronchioles These are made of smooth muscle. They are the terminals of the bronchi.

Lungs at 36 weeks Development of the lungs is usually now complete. The terminal sacs have become thin-walled alveoli that allow gas exchange with the capillaries – a process that transfers oxygen and carbon dioxide between the lungs and bloodstream.

Q At my 20-week scan it looked as though my baby was breathing, but how can that be?

Your baby can make breathing-like movements as early as 10 weeks pregnant. These are the result of the involuntary contractions in the muscles that are forming around his lungs. The contractions serve to stimulate further muscle growth and the growth of lung tissue. He begins with short practice bursts that last about 10 seconds, and by week 38 of pregnancy these practice "breaths" are in a regular rhythmic pattern of 40 "breaths" per minute, just as he will breathe after he's been born. By the time you're 24 weeks pregnant, your baby will be able to synchronize these breathing-like movements with the rhythmic pumping of his heart, just as he will when he is born.

Q Why doesn't my baby drown in his amniotic fluid?

The simple answer is that a baby doesn't drown in amniotic fluid because he doesn't actually need to breathe when in utero. The important thing for living beings is that we can access oxygen and can remove carbon dioxide from our system, but this gas exchange doesn't have to occur through breathing – in your baby it happens entirely via the placenta. Your baby's circulation, which pumps blood around his developing body, actually bypasses his lungs and goes to the placenta for oxygen until the moment of birth. When your baby is exposed to the air after birth, temperature receptors in his skin trigger the absorption of amniotic fluid from the air sacs, the circulation to the placenta "switches off", and blood starts flowing to his lungs. Then, your baby takes his first breath (which will sound a bit like a gasp), and his lungs will take over the job of breathing. Before the system of bringing oxygen into his body via the lungs is up and running, it isn't possible for your baby to drown.

Q How soon is it possible to tell whether my baby is a boy or a girl?

Although your baby's gender was determined at the moment of conception, it will be at least 14 weeks before there are outward signs. In fact, male and female fetuses look outwardly identical for some weeks (known as the "indifferent" stage) because their genitals are formed from the same structure. This is called the labioscrotal swelling, and it consists of two ridges and a rounded bud. In boys, the ridges join up to form the scrotal sac and the bud elongates to become the penis; in girls, the ridges remain separate and become the labia majora, while the bud shrinks to form the clitoris. By 14 to 17 weeks, the genitals have become obviously differentiated, and have developed enough to be clearly visible.

Internally, the sex organs begin forming at around nine weeks. Depending on whether or not your baby has a Y chromosome (which makes him male), the sex cells create either testes, seminiferous tubules, and vas deferens in your son, or ovaries, uterus, and Fallopian tubes in your daughter. The fetal ovaries contain millions of oocytes (immature egg cells) – all the eggs a female will ever have. These could become your future grandchildren. Both boys' and girls' sex organs descend from the abdomen to their correct positions after around 25 weeks. The testes have a long journey to make into the scrotal sac, which is why at birth around 1 per cent of full-term, and 10 per cent of premature male babies have an undescended testis.

At birth, your baby has in the region of **50–70 million alveoli** in his lungs, each one supplied with **hundreds** of tiny blood **capillaries** ready to exchange **oxygen** and **carbon dioxide**.

Q How many weeks does it take for my baby's face to form?

By the time you go for your scan at around 12 weeks, all your baby's facial features will be clearly recognizable – her face has been developing since the early weeks after conception.

BABY'S FACIAL FEATURE DEVELOPMENT UP TO 12 WEEKS

The following table shows some of the major milestones in the development of her facial features up to the end of the first trimester:

WEEK	FEATURES
6	» Your embryo develops dark spots on each side of her head that will become her eyes. Firstly they form "optic cups" that link to her brain via an optic stalk. The cups eventually become her retinas (the "screens" at the backs of her eyes) and irises (the coloured parts of each eye). » Minuscule indents on either side of her head are the beginnings of your baby's ears. Inner tubes that will transmit sound in your baby's ears begin to form.
7	» Her eyes start to form lenses; these are created when certain cells of the ectoderm layer fold over. Eyelids begin to form from folds of skin either side of each eye. » Skin at the sides of your baby's head begin to fold over, so that her ears begin to form. » Nostrils appear at the front of the face, and her nose starts to take shape.
8	» Changes in the ectoderm layer of your embryo mean that by eight weeks the two sides of her face have come together to shape her mouth. » Pigmentation (which gives your baby's eyes their colour) starts to collect in the iris of her eyes (see p.168). » Your baby's tongue starts to form, initially above the plate that will become the roof of her mouth.
9	» Your baby's eyes can now move around in their sockets. » Her tongue has developed taste buds.
10	» Your baby's nose starts to protrude, giving her face a more human profile. » Her eyelids start to close over her eyeballs, protecting them from light coming through your abdominal wall. This light could damage the developing retinas. » Your baby's mouth and lips are now fully formed. » Your baby's outer ears now look exactly as they will at birth, but there's still some work to be done inside before she can actually hear.
11	» The roof of your baby's mouth – her palate – is complete. » Tooth buds begin to appear inside her mouth. These will become her milk and adult teeth when the two rows eventually separate.
12	» Your baby's eyes and ears have moved upward as her head has grown, and her eyes have also moved towards the front of her face and are now more or less in their final positions. Your baby can use her mouth, jaw, and tongue to swallow and yawn.

Q I've been singing to my baby, but can she actually hear me? And can she hear my partner singing, too?

Most doctors agree that by the time a fetus is 14 weeks old, she responds to familiar sounds with a quickening of her heart rate. Certainly by 16 weeks, the three bones that transmit sound in her inner ear and the auditory pathways that take sound to her brain are developed enough to suggest that she can hear what's going on inside your body. So she'll hear the swooshing of your blood, your heartbeat, and your tummy rumbles. By 24 weeks, studies show that she'll turn her head in response to a familiar sound – in particular the sound of your voice. Sounds outside the uterus are quieter and more muffled, so it's harder for her to make them out. But hearing a voice other than yours, even if it sounds as if it's being transmitted through water, is enough to make her familiar with it, so your partner's singing definitely isn't in vain.

Q If my baby is developing taste buds, does that mean she can taste the amniotic fluid?

Absolutely! At around the same time that she learns to swallow (roughly 16 weeks pregnant), she develops receptors on her tongue that mean her taste buds can start interpreting the flavours of the amniotic fluid. Contrary to what you might think, your amniotic fluid isn't neutral-tasting: it's salty and is infused with flavours from whatever you've been eating, particularly strong flavours such as spices, onion, and garlic. Think of this as a good opportunity to get your baby used to some of your favourite foods – and to the healthy ones that you'll want her to eat when she's older!

Q When does my baby get her skin and what does it look like?

Skin begins to form from the moment a blastocyst becomes an embryo (see p.152), but until well into the second trimester, it's thin and translucent so that nutrients from the amniotic fluid can easily pass through its cells. By 15 weeks pregnant, this translucent covering is

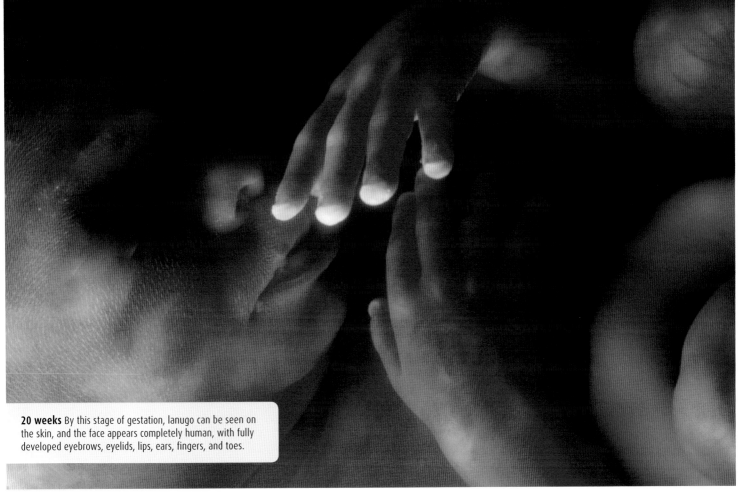

20 weeks By this stage of gestation, lanugo can be seen on the skin, and the face appears completely human, with fully developed eyebrows, eyelids, lips, ears, fingers, and toes.

made up of the three layers of skin we all have – the epidermis, which is the top layer, the dermis in the middle, and the hypodermis, the deepest layer. The skin doesn't become more "solid" looking or lose any of its permeability until you are 32 weeks pregnant. This is also when the baby's skin starts to take on the pigmentation of her complexion.

Lanugo is fine, soft, downy hair. It's the first hair to be produced by the fetal hair follicles, and it usually appears on the fetus at about 20 weeks of gestation. It is normally shed before birth, at around 28 or 32 weeks of pregnancy, but is sometimes still present at birth. It disappears within a few days or weeks of the birth. Lanugo keeps *vernix caeseosa* (a white, greasy substance) in place on your baby's skin. Vernix starts to appear at around 20 weeks and by 32 weeks it covers most of your baby's body. It's made up of skin cells, fetal skin oil, and lanugo. The Latin term *vernix caeseosa* translates as "cheesy varnish". Vernix helps to keep your baby's skin moist and protect it from exposure to amniotic fluid, which contains high levels of fetal urine (especially towards the end of your pregnancy). It is sometimes still present at birth and can act as a thick, slippery lubricator to encourage your baby's passage down the birth canal during labour.

Q Can my baby smell what's going on inside my uterus?

No one is sure. By 15 weeks pregnant, your fetus has all she needs for her sense of smell to work, but as aromas are passed through the air rather than through fluid, it's always been assumed that her sense of smell doesn't become functional until she's born and starts to breathe air. However, some research has thrown doubt over this and it's now proposed that because your baby is instantly attracted to the smell of your breast milk, she was exposed to the smell of something similar – and therefore familiar – while she was in your uterus.

Q Do my baby's eyes stay closed the whole time she's inside me?

No. Somewhere between 26 and 28 weeks pregnant, she'll screw up her eyelids in response to bright light and will start to blink. By this stage, her retinas are fully formed, so any risk of damage from bright light has passed. Not only that, but her eyebrows and eyelashes have formed, and they offer extra protection.

Q Can my baby cry tears when she is in the uterus?

Your baby has tear ducts – lacrimal glands – by the end of the first trimester. These are to ensure that her eyeballs are properly moistened throughout gestation, but whether or not they can create tears is still a mystery. Researchers believe that a fetus goes through the motions of crying (distress, frowning, and so on) in response to loud noises, but that's all we know.

Q Did you know...

>> At 7½ weeks pregnant your baby has already developed her first sense – the sense of touch.
>> At 18 weeks pregnant she has the ridges in her fingertips that will make up her unique fingerprint.
>> At 23 weeks pregnant she's covered in a soft, fine, downy hair called lanugo: this will probably almost entirely disappear by the time she's born.

Emerging senses This 22-week-old fetus is beginning to detect sounds. He can also touch and explore his facial features and even suck his thumb. His fingernails have formed, too.

We can talk in general terms about the **development of a baby** – when organs grow, when features form, when she might be ready for birth – but the only certainty is that **your baby will be unique**. From the wave of her hair to her toe-prints, she won't have a single **characteristic** that's exactly the same as any other living being.

My baby is unique

What makes babies unique?

Uniqueness comes from two main sources. Firstly, before your baby is born, the "soup" of chromosomes that she gets from each parent gives her a set of genes that might switch on or off, both in the uterus and after birth. Secondly, your baby's environment (for instance, from where you live to your morals and values) moulds her view and experience of the world. This leads to her responding to her environment in a conscious way – called learned behaviour – but it also has physical effects in her body, mutating her genetic codes so that she can adapt to life. In primitive times, this was essential to survival.

Genes are the building blocks of DNA – the hereditary blueprint that's in every cell in your baby's body. Genes give her her eye and hair colour, her fingerprints, her inherited character traits, and her inherited diseases and conditions. They're embedded in the chromosomes she receives from her parents. Present scientific thinking is that your baby (and every human being) has around 24,000 genes attached to 23 pairs of chromosomes. Apart from the chromosomes that determine gender, every chromosome has two copies of each gene. Every gene is also made up of variations of itself. Variations of the same gene are called alleles, and these can be recessive alleles or dominant ones. The dominant alleles "overpower" the recessive ones, producing a unique physical, mental, and emotional recipe for every human being.

The brain and the environment

Genes provide the raw ingredients, but other aspects of your baby's uniqueness – such as her personality, how she learns to do things, the way she responds to stimuli in her environment, how she displays her intellect, and the ways in which she forms relationships – are subject to her experience of the world around her.

From the moment of her birth, the information that your baby gets from her environment builds connections in her brain. At birth, brain imaging shows large sections of the brain waiting to form neural connections. These come with such speed that by 24 months, only small unconnected patches remain. By the age of three, your baby will have far more connections that she ever needs and a period of "synaptic pruning" begins. This eliminates and hones the connections so that brain efficiency rises.

The role of lifestyle and its influence on our genes is important when considering inherited illness. For example, we know that heart disease can also be inherited. However, while a baby might inherit a tendency towards it, her lifestyle choices can turn on or off the gene that causes the condition.

Q Which member of my family is my newborn baby going to look like most?

Your baby might have a range of features and characteristics from different members of each of your families – an aunt's hair, a cousin's sense of humour, or your mother's nose. How DNA and inheritance work can help to explain this.

Your baby shares half her DNA with you and half with your partner. In turn, you share half of your genes with each of your parents. This means that your baby shares a quarter of her genes with your parents – her grandparents.

Through each generation genes are shuffled and re-shuffled. At conception, the embryo receives 23 chromosomes from the mother's egg and 23 chromosomes from the father's sperm. These pair up to make a total of 46 chromosomes. The chromosomes contain the genes that you inherit. When the sperm fertilizes the egg, chromosomes join together and randomly exchange genes.

Likewise, even though full siblings inherit genes from the same parents, these aren't necessarily the same genes, nor the same dominant alleles. Remember, you've each passed one of two copies of every gene you have to your baby, but because the two copies of each of your genes aren't identical (every copy has variations), you won't always pass the same version of each gene to each child. Mix this up for all the genes from both of you, and it turns out that the permutations are endless.

Blue eyes, brown eyes, different shaped eyes, and noses Humans are amazingly diverse. This is due to both genetic inheritance and variation in environmental factors.

Q What determines whether I have a boy or a girl?

Your baby's gender is determined by specific chromosomes – the tube-like structures that contain her unique genetic blueprint. Healthy human beings have 23 chromosome pairs; one chromosome in each pair is inherited from each parent. The 23rd pair of chromosomes is called the sex chromosome and it determines what sex a baby will be. A woman's egg always contains the female chromosome, known as X and a man's sperm contains either an X (female) or Y (male) chromosome. An embryo that has two X chromosomes will be female, whereas one with an XY combination will be male. It is therefore the man's sperm that determines whether a baby is male or female.

Q Can environmental factors influence how my children look if they are the same sex?

Children who grow up in the same household are never in the same environment at every moment. They will have different bedrooms, different teachers, and experience different emotions. Also, how tall each child grows is partly influenced by the food they eat. One child may have weaned only on carrots and pears, but your second is more likely to wean on the foods that her big sister's now eating. What you eat plays its part, too. If your taste preferences have changed since the first pregnancy, the nutritional influence on each of your daughters will be different – and that can impact their physical characteristics.

Q Can my baby's genes determine whether or not she will be overweight later on in her life?

No, but they may predispose her to weight gain if it runs in the family. In this case, whether or not your baby turns out to be overweight will depend a lot on environmental factors. Her eating habits, stress levels, and enjoyment of sports, can all influence whether or not the genes for gaining excess weight switch on. How you eat in pregnancy can influence it as well. Your baby can taste what's in the amniotic fluid, so if she gets used to sweeter flavours, say, while she's inside you, it may be more difficult to encourage her to eat vegetables as she gets older.

Q What colour will my baby's eyes be and what determines this?

You baby's eye colour depends on how dominant and recessive alleles (variants of genes – see p.166) work.

Each person has two alleles for eye colour (and other characteristics), one inherited from each of their parents. The brown allele (B) is dominant and the blue allele (b) is recessive, so when the two come together (Bb) brown dominates over blue and the result is brown eyes. In order to have blue eyes, a person must have two blue alleles (bb). Therefore, if your baby has blue eyes but both parents have brown eyes, both you and your partner must be Bb – each of you has one brown allele and one blue allele.

A Bb mother and a Bb father have a 25-per-cent chance of having a blue-eyed baby. It becomes a 50-per-cent chance if one of you is bb and the other Bb. If one or both of you is BB, the only possible outcome is a baby with brown eyes. Of course, if you both have blue eyes (you are both bb), your baby will have blue eyes, too.

Blue eyes Many Caucasian babies' eyes look blue or grey when they are first born. It can take up to a year for the pigmentation to settle and reveal the true eye colour.

Blue and green are both recessive alleles. When blue and green are the only alleles present, they are actually co-dominant, so your baby's eye colour could take on blue, green, or a mix of the two.

EYE COLOUR

The diagram below illustrates how genes determine your baby's eye colour. This principle

PARENTS' EYE COLOUR AND GENE

Q Why is it that not all brown eyes are the same shade of brown?

No one is really sure. While the overall colour of your baby's eyes (brown, hazel, blue, or green) might be determined by one set of genes, the level of pigmentation in your baby's iris may be determined by another – perhaps many others. Pigmentation comes from melanin, which is present not only in the iris of the eye, but in hair and skin, too. So, if you have two babies and the first has dark brown eyes and the second has light brown eyes, both babies

have dominant brown alleles in the eye-colour gene. However, certain other genes caused different amounts of melanin in the eyes of the two children – resulting in different shades of brown. The more melanin that's released, the darker the pigmentation in the eye.

Q Will our baby inherit his father's height? Can we tell at birth?

Both parents' genes have a role to play in a person's final height as an adult. The mid-parental height formula estimates a child's potential growth – you simply add both parents' height in inches together, divide by two, and then add an extra $2\frac{1}{2}$ inches for a boy or subtract $2\frac{1}{2}$ inches for a girl. For instance, if mum's height is 5'4" and dad's is 5'11", a son's potential height would be 5'10" and a daughter's would be 5'5". This formula gives only a rough estimate, however, and in reality your child's health, diet, and other environmental factors play a part as well as genes. Your baby's size

at birth doesn't necessarily indicate what his adult height will be either, especially if he is premature. Mum's health, weight, and diet in pregnancy are more likely to have an affect on your baby's birthweight than genes.

Q Could my baby have curly hair if mine is straight?

In Caucasians, curly hair is determined by a dominant allele, so the answer to this depends on what pair of alleles your baby inherits from both parents. If you have straight hair, but your partner has curly hair, your baby is 50 to 75 per cent likely to have curly hair, depending upon whether your partner has two curly-hair alleles, or one curly and one straight. If you both have straight hair, then your baby's hair will probably be straight, too. If you both have curly hair, the chances are that your baby will have curly hair – although if you both are straight-hair carriers, there's still a 25-per-cent chance that your baby's hair will be straight.

Colour blindness is a condition that is passed down from parent to child and is much **more common in men** than women.

...replicated for every possible trait including hair colour, skin tone, dimples, and so on.

 BB

 bb

 Bb bb

 BB Bb

Bb bb

BB Bb

Q My baby's father is bald. Does this mean that if I have a boy, he will go bald, too?

The genetic inheritance of baldness is still not fully understood. For a long time it was thought that male pattern baldness (baldness that runs in families and begins with a receding hairline) was inherited from the mother's side. So, a baby boy was assumed to inherit baldness via his mother from his maternal grandfather rather than from his own father. However, anecdotal evidence shows that this isn't always the case, which has led researchers to look for a pattern that confirms heredity directly from father to son. Although there doesn't yet seem to be evidence that the faulty gene lies within the Y chromosome, there is some evidence that mutations in genes on chromosome 20 (which can come from a baby's mother or father) may increase the risk of a boy inheriting baldness. Environmental factors (including diet and stress levels) play a role, too. In short, while the percentages suggest that boys born to bald fathers are likely to go bald themselves, there are no certainties. As far as girls going bald is concerned, it's thought that high levels of female hormones make sure the baldness gene stays inactive.

Male pattern baldness This is the most common type of hair loss in men. It is generally thought to be caused by hormones and a genetic predisposition.

Q What causes albinism?

This is a rare genetic condition, where the genes that control melanin production are faulty.

As a result the proteins in the genes don't get the message to trigger the release of melanin in the hair, eyes, and skin, which leads to lack of pigmentation. Those affected tend to be very pale in colour, have pink or pale grey eyes, and white hair. It can cause sight problems and sensitivity to light, because eyes need melanin to make a healthy retina (the "screen" at the back of the eye). Albinism is inherited through autosomal recessive inheritance (in which both parents carry the faulty gene and the baby inherits it from both sides) and X-linked inheritance (in which the faulty gene is attached to the X chromosome in one parent).

X-LINKED INHERITANCE

An X-linked inheritance refers to conditions that occur as a result of a faulty gene within the X chromosome. The box below explains how this works.

MOTHER (XX)

A baby girl has a 50-per-cent chance of becoming a carrier of the faulty gene (and a 50-per-cent chance of not inheriting a faulty gene at all), but would not herself have the condition. This is because girls have two X chromosomes (XX) – in this case, one healthy and one carrying the faulty gene. The healthy X chromosome compensates for the carrier, and the baby girl appears healthy.

A baby boy has one X chromosome and one Y chromosome (XY), inherited from his mother and father respectively, giving him a 50-per-cent chance that he will inherit the X chromosome from his mother that carries the faulty gene. If this happens he will develop albinism, because he has no healthy X chromosome to compensate.

FATHER (XY)

A baby girl will definitely become a carrier, because in order to become a girl (XX) she must inherit the damaged X chromosome from her father.

A baby boy does not become a carrier, because to become a boy he must inherit the Y chromosome from his father.

Q Will my baby's brain be fully formed when she is born or does it carry on growing?

Your baby's brain grows faster than any other organ and, consequently, the head is still out of proportion with the rest of the body when she is born.

The brain carries on growing and developing throughout childhood and into adulthood, but is at its most sensitive during certain periods in the early years. Between conception and about the age of three a young child's brain undergoes an enormous amount of change. At birth, your baby will have around 100 billion brain cells (neurons) and that's roughly the number she has throughout her life. At this time, basic neural connections are in place, which help to control vital functions such as breathing, heart rate, digestion, and reflexes. The connections are formed at a very fast rate during the first few years and, as more links form, higher mental functions such as memory, increased attention span, language, intellect, and social skills develop. By adulthood, the neural network allows for reasoning, judgement, and original thought.

Forebrain prominence

At 5 weeks The neural tube forms the forebrain prominence.

Cranial nerves

Ear bud

Eye bud

Pharyngeal arches

At 9 weeks Swellings that will become different parts of the brain are growing and are beginning to fold into one another.

BRAIN FORMATION

During her time in the uterus, your growing baby's brain undergoes an extraordinary amount of growth and development.

WEEK	ACTIVITY
5	The neural tube divides to create separate spaces for the development of her brain cells and nerve cells – effectively beginning the formation of her brain and central nervous system.
7	The two hemispheres of your baby's brain begin to separate. The right one will go on to govern her creativity, spatial awareness, and lateral thinking; the left will influence her logic and practical thinking.
8	The synapses, which open and close the pathways to send messages between neurons, start to form. Your baby is born with relatively few synapses; most of them form within the first two to three years of life as memories and her understanding of the world are laid down.
12	Your baby's cerebellum begins to form. At the same time, the two halves of her brain begin to communicate with each other and there's a massive burst of neuron formation (called neurogenesis). Her hypothalamus and pituitary glands have formed.
14–16	Reflex responses in your baby's limbs and facial features suggest that she's now responding to stimuli in the uterus. This confirms that her brain's neurons are beginning to work, processing what she is experiencing. This coincides with maturing taste buds and the ability of the bones in her ear to transmit sound.
22–25	The formation of her brain matter is complete and her cerebral cortex starts to fold over on itself, creating her brain's typical ridged, wrinkled appearance. This increases her brain's surface area, which optimizes her chances for learning.
26–40	Your baby's nervous system is now fully developed. Her cerebral cortex begins to send out electrical impulses: researchers believe that memory has begun to develop because some of these impulses respond to the sound of familiar voices. Her cerebellum is three times bigger at 40 weeks than it was at 22 weeks, and her whole brain weighs approximately 350g (12oz).

Cerebrum The largest part of the brain and is divided into the left and right hemispheres

Cerebellum The region of the brain that is key to coordination, attention, and language

Por

Spinal cord

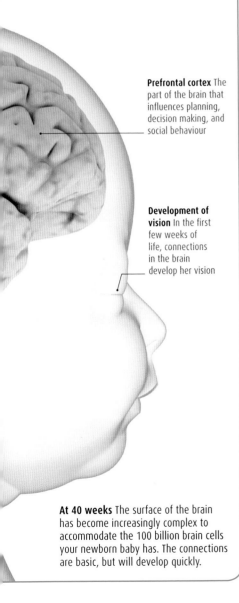

Fissures forming

Cerebellum development

Frontal lobe

Cerebrum

...ellum

...tem

13 weeks Lobes have ...ormed. The connections ...etween the cells are ...resent and the hindbrain ...ivides into two parts, the ...erebellum and brainstem.

At 25 weeks The surface of the brain is still smooth. Folds are beginning to emerge as the number of cells begins to increase.

Prefrontal cortex The part of the brain that influences planning, decision making, and social behaviour

Development of vision In the first few weeks of life, connections in the brain develop her vision

At 40 weeks The surface of the brain has become increasingly complex to accommodate the 100 billion brain cells your newborn baby has. The connections are basic, but will develop quickly.

Q I've heard that stress can affect my baby's brain development. Is this true?

Stress can affect a fetus, but it's also true that the majority of brain development happens after your baby is born. Research suggests that if you suffer from stress during pregnancy, it can have an affect on the way your baby copes with and responds to the world after she's born. However, it's not just your stress levels during pregnancy that make a difference. At birth, only a quarter of your baby's brain is "wired" with neural links; the rest are waiting to be formed by experience. So, how you teach your baby to cope with stress once she's born is very important, too, as is a consistent and loving approach to parenting.

Coping with stress in pregnancy

If you are anxious or stressed, talk to others about how you are feeling – they may be able to help you find solutions. Your partner or family members may be able to take on more at home so you can rest, or your employer may offer some flexibility if you need it. Your midwife is also there to support and advise you. Make time to rest and relax; meditation and breathing techniques, massage, and gentle exercise such as walking and yoga are all helpful for managing your stress.

Q Are baby girls' and baby boys' brains the same?

Fundamentally, yes, though after birth, when the synapses start making their connections, the genders tend to wire themselves differently. We know that girls are more likely to stare intently at faces, even when they're tiny babies, while boys tend to look around, taking in everything that's going on. Although it sounds a cliché, boys have been shown to have greater spatial awareness than girls: the parts of the brain that orient us show more connections in a little boy's brain than in a little girl's. Girls, though, tend to have better wiring for language, empathy, and communication. Of course, there's a lot of debate about whether or not "girly" behaviour and "boyish" behaviour are influenced by environmental factors. They almost certainly are, although that's not the whole story – male and female hormones play

---

a part, too. In the end, though, the incredible plasticity of brain wiring means that our brains provide us with potential, but our genes and the environment of our upbringing decide how much potential we end up fulfilling.

Q Is something wrong if my baby doesn't follow the developmental milestones, such as smiling and walking?

Usually, it is likely that your baby is just learning at her own happy pace. Very occasionally, though, being a "late" developer (measured against averages that you might read about) may be a warning of something else. All babies develop at different rates. This is due to a combination of genetics, gender, and other factors such as prematurity.

Despite the term, developmental milestones don't happen at set "miles"; they happen when your baby's ready and that's within a much broader time period than timelines generally suggest. All babies are unique and will develop in their own way. However, the order in which they acquire certain physical skills, also known as gross motor skills – strength in the head and neck, sitting up, smiling, waving, crawling, walking – is generally the same. Your baby's strength develops from the head downwards over the first 18 months. If your baby shows little or no strength in her muscles, is unresponsive to stimuli, seems unable to co-ordinate her movements, or seems to cope with the world very differently from other babies her age, talk to your doctor for guidance. More often than not, you'll be reassured that everything's fine.

Did you know...

In order to help your baby learn to walk it is crucial to play with your baby out of her pram or cot for a little while every day. This will advance her overall mobility. Encouraging activities like 'tummy time' will aid development, strengthening the neck, head, and addominal muscles that she will need to use to be able to sit, crawl, and then walk.

» In this chapter...

Practical preparations

It's important to feel **ready and prepared** for labour, birth, and life with a newborn. Gain expert, practical advice on **what you will need** for you, your baby, and your home. It's best to borrow or buy a Moses basket, car seat, feeding equipment, and pram or sling in advance of your baby arriving. Find out exactly what you need to pack in your **hospital bag** or what to have gathered ready for a home birth. This chapter also helps you think about other ways in which you can be prepared, especially if you're having a multiple birth.

As your body changes, you will want a comfortable **pregnancy wardrobe** that offers **flexibility** and **comfort aids** and props to help you to sleep and ease pregnancy niggles. You should also start buying **equipment** for **life after the birth**.

Practical tips for mum

Do I need a maternity warbrobe?

Being comfortable is key during pregnancy. In the early months when your waistband first expands, you may get away with wearing normal clothes in a larger size or borrowing your partner's tops, but for most women this isn't a solution that will work for long. Clothes designed for pregnancy use fabrics and cuts that expand in the right places as you get bigger, whereas regular clothes may simply become tighter and uncomfortable. It can seem wasteful splashing out on maternity clothes that you will wear for a brief period only, but they will see a lot of use for five or six months and will get you through any future pregnancies, too, so it is worth a little investment. Happily, it is possible to assemble a decent maternity wardrobe on a budget by borrowing them or buying them second-hand.

Keeping in season

When you start to assemble your maternity wardrobe, think about what time of year it will be towards the end of your pregnancy. If your early pregnancy is in the summer months, you may not want to splurge on maternity summer dresses or short-sleeved blouses that will see little use when you need bigger sizes. And likewise, you won't want a collection of long-sleeved, warm maternity tops if you are going to be heavily pregnant in the middle of the summer. You may be able to pick up some bargains in end-of-season sales that will be perfect in six months time.

A little support

Your growing bump can also cause pregnancy niggles such as backache, which means that getting a good night's sleep becomes increasingly difficult. Even sitting can become uncomfortable in the latter stages of pregnancy. Props such as pillows and belly support bands can be invaluable now, and some support pillows double up as feeding cushions. You may also want to consider a birthing ball, which is useful before, during, and after the birth, and inflatable cushions and pillows that can make sitting easier if you're suffering with haemorrhoids – a common pregnancy complaint – or want to avoid putting pressure on any stitches you may have after the birth.

Q I want to wear my usual clothes for as long as possible. When will I need to start wearing maternity clothes?

It is usually around the start of the second trimester that women find their waistbands start to tighten. From this point onwards, wearing your usual clothes becomes increasingly difficult and uncomfortable.

You may find early on in pregnancy that your bust size has gone up a little and your tops are fitting more snugly, but you can still wear your existing clothes. By 20 to 24 weeks, though, and perhaps earlier, your clothing choices may become restricted and you may feel that you need to start wearing purpose-made maternity wear. Invest in a few key pieces that make you feel and look good. Many women don't worry about trying to disguise their pregnancy and prefer to wear fitted clothes to flatter their new shape.

Hardworking staples Loose tunics and empire-line tops that you already own may fit comfortably until well into your second trimester.

Extending the life of your clothes

A stretchy belly band is a great pregnancy innovation. Made in soft, breathable materials, the wide band is worn over your bump and the waistband of your clothes to cover any gaps that appear between your top and bottom garments. The effect is a seamless look of clever layering. The band's snug elastic fit helps to hold your trousers up, too, so you can leave your zip or buttons undone. After the birth, it can handily cover up post-delivery flab and reduce the amount of flesh you reveal if breastfeeding.

Other options

» Expand the waistband of your trousers and jeans: thread an elastic hair band or sturdy rubber band through your trouser button hole and loop each end around the trouser button.

» Long tops will keep your emerging bump covered during your first trimester, as they won't ride up too much with your growing tummy.

» Empire-line tops, loose-fitting tops and tunics, and wrap-around tops and dresses are ideal during the transitional period when most of your clothes are too tight, but you're not big enough for maternity wear.

» Long t-shirt dresses and jersey skirts can stretch to accommodate your tummy during the transitional period.

» Borrowing your partner's clothes can come in handy from the start of your second trimester. Check if any shirts and tops will work as casual wear for weekends and evenings.

Q Which fabrics will be most comfortable in pregnancy?

You may feel hotter than usual in pregnancy due to your increased blood circulation, so opt for lighter, breathable fabrics. It is a good idea to wear light layers that you can remove or add to easily to feel just the right temperature. Natural fabrics such as jersey, wool, silk, linen, and cotton are ideal, and there are organic versions of these fabrics if you want to avoid unwanted chemical exposure and prefer their softness. Newer fabrics such as bamboo and hemp are also soft and breathable. All these fabrics are hypoallergenic and will feel very comfortable against your skin. Many women experience itchiness as their skin stretches to accommodate the baby, so avoid synthetic fabrics such as polyester, viscose, and nylon, which may irritate your skin. Look out, too, for stretchy natural-fibre clothes containing lycra, such as cotton leggings, as they will be most comfortable to wear as your bump grows.

You may find that as your bump grows, you **prefer** to wear clothes that are designed to **flatter your new, curvier figure** and show off your bump rather than hide it away.

Q What are the most useful items to buy for my pregnancy wardrobe?

Dressing a rapidly growing bump can seem tricky at first, but you can get great mileage from a small collection of key maternity items, especially if you mix and match with your existing accessories to suit the occasion.

You may like to build up your pregnancy wardrobe gradually, buying a few core pieces – perhaps one or two pairs of maternity trousers or jeans, a dress, and a couple of tops – and then add one or two new items to suit your ever-changing shape. If you buy maternity clothes in neutral colours, it will be easy to mix and match them with floaty tunics or wrap-around tops, and existing clothes such as cardigans and jackets that you can carry on wearing unbuttoned. Neutral pieces can also be styled with scarves or jewellery to give you a range of outfits.

A good pair of maternity jeans can be very versatile and work as both daytime and evening wear. They come in a variety of styles and waist options: some have a stretchy, expandable "bandeau-style" belly panel; some are designed with elastic side pieces that allow the waistband to stretch as you get bigger; and others have a low-rise waistband that sits beneath your bump. Look for stretchy cotton denim that is soft and comfortable to wear, even in the latter stages of pregnancy.

As well as a pair of maternity jeans, you may want to invest in:

» **A pair of plain trousers** to wear with a shirt or top and cardigan or jacket for work, or with a dressier top for evenings out.

» **A maternity dress or tunic.** Wrap-around styles are perfect, as you can let them out as you grow, or choose an empire-line tunic, which is flattering and works well with stretchy leggings.

» **Tops such as T-shirts, vests,** and long-sleeved tops, depending on the season.

» **Maternity tights** and leggings.

One of the most **hard-working** and **valuable** items in your pregnancy wardrobe is likely to be a pair of **maternity jeans**.

Sizing

Many maternity clothing lines advise you to stick with your pre-pregnancy size when buying maternity wear, but proportions are not necessarily the same across brands. If you can, try on some items first to check how a clothing brand regulates its sizing. Some stores have pillows in different sizes that replicate your growing bump – you can wear these when you try on clothes to see if the size is correct and works for you.

You might be tempted to buy regular clothes in bigger sizes, but beware the larger overall proportions they will have. It is likely they will fit poorly on the shoulders and arms and that hemlines will ride up at the front and won't hang properly over your bump.

Maternity trousers If you find a comfortable, well-fitting pair of maternity jeans, you should be able to wear them right up until the birth, and beyond.

Q I have a limited budget. Where can I find stylish but inexpensive maternity wear?

While your pregnancy is wonderful news, it does bring with it a financial cost, as you also need to factor in the nursery and travel equipment your baby will require. Fortunately, it's perfectly possible to be financially prudent and keep costs low when putting together your maternity wardrobe. Most high-street chains and larger supermarkets now stock good maternity ranges, which typically include many affordable basics that won't break the bank. If the timing works out and you plan ahead, you may be able to get some good deals in end-of-season sales that could be in the right season by the end of your pregnancy.

Be open, too, to any offers of maternity clothes from friends, sisters, and cousins who may be happy to pass on their entire maternity wardrobe, even if they are a slightly different size; many maternity items, particularly tops, can fit a range of sizes. You can always consider a clothes swap if that makes you feel easier about accepting the clothes.

Bargain hunting

Buying second-hand maternity clothes is well worth considering, as they are often in extremely good condition since many items will have been worn just a handful of times. Check out the local second-hand shops in your area that may sell maternity clothes, and also research or ask about any local NCT (National Childbirth Trust) "nearly new" clothes sales, which can be a great place to hunt down some maternity bargains. Car boot sales can be another great place to find clothes for a steal, and also have a look at maternity "bundles" on auction websites where new mums auction their maternity wardrobe in one lot.

Are your **shoes** feeling tight? You're not imagining things – some women find that their shoe **size increases** as **relaxin** loosens their foot ligaments. The new shoe size can be permanent.

Q Do I have to forego high heels completely?

There's no edict banning high heels in pregnancy, but most podiatrists advise against them once your bump starts to grow, so save them for special occasions.

High heels change your posture, increasing the strain on your knees and encouraging you to arch your back to compensate for the change in weight distribution. This effect is exacerbated in pregnancy due to your softened joints and ligaments (caused by the hormone relaxin) and your changing centre of gravity, so wear high heels only occasionally to prevent aches and pains.

Comfort and support

During pregnancy, you will find low-heeled, wide-fitting, supportive shoes that preserve your foot arch much more comfortable for everyday wear. It's common for feet to swell in pregnancy, caused by extra fluids in the body (known as oedema). Some women even find that their feet go up a half or whole size, again due to relaxin causing the ligaments in the feet to spread. Choose shoes with a slight, firm heel of 2.5cm (1in), to discourage you from leaning backwards. Beware of completely flat shoes as they offer little in the way of cushioning and comfort as your weight increases.

Higher heels It may not come as a surprise that the higher the heel, the more pressure you place on your forefeet. Choosing slightly lower heels, when you wear non-flat shoes, can help to reduce the strain on your feet, lower back, and knees.

7.5cm (3in) high: 76% pressure

5cm (2in) high: 57% pressure

WEARING HEELS IN PREGNANCY

When you're pregnant, wearing high heels is more of a balancing act than usual. Your growing belly throws your weight forwards, forcing you to adjust your spine, knees, and leg alignment to maintain your balance.

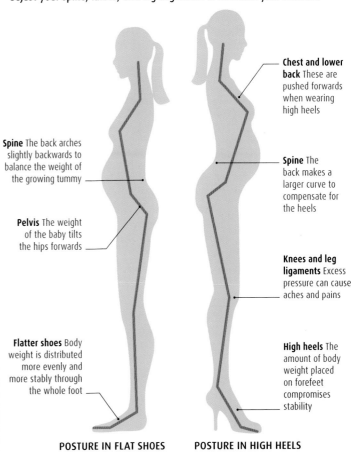

Chest and lower back These are pushed forwards when wearing high heels

Spine The back arches slightly backwards to balance the weight of the growing tummy

Spine The back makes a larger curve to compensate for the heels

Pelvis The weight of the baby tilts the hips forwards

Knees and leg ligaments Excess pressure can cause aches and pains

Flatter shoes Body weight is distributed more evenly and more stably through the whole foot

High heels The amount of body weight placed on forefeet compromises stability

POSTURE IN FLAT SHOES   POSTURE IN HIGH HEELS

Q Should I buy a special maternity swimsuit, or make do?

This depends on how much swimming you plan to do during pregnancy. If you want to swim regularly – swimming is a perfect pregnancy exercise, after all – it's worth investing in a pregnancy swimsuit specially designed to support your growing bump and bust and adapt with your changing body, while also providing comfort and ease of movement. However, if all you need a swimsuit for is a two-week holiday in the sun, then you may be able to get away with an existing stretchy swimsuit, or a bikini or tankini that fits under and over your bump.

Pregnancy swimming costumes If you are swimming regularly for exercise, a supportive maternity costume is a worthwhile investment.

Q I will be heavily pregnant in the winter. Will I need to buy a maternity coat?

If you wish to invest in a special maternity coat, by all means do so, but you may find that a winter coat will make you feel uncomfortably warm, even if the weather is cold. Before you shop for extra layers of maternity clothing, it's worth bearing in mind that your natural body temperature will be higher towards the end of your pregnancy as your blood circulation increases. A maternity coat may not be necessary, and since a coat is quite a large investment, you may prefer to keep warm by wearing knitted layers instead. You could put on a lighter waterproof mac, shawl, fleece, or scarf over these knitted items so that you can remove one or more layers if you do get hot.

Q Why are maternity bras important? Won't my usual bras be fine to wear in pregnancy?

While a few women find that their breasts don't change size significantly during pregnancy, most women do go up around two to four cup sizes during these nine months as their breasts respond to hormonal changes and prepare for milk production.

It's not just your cup size that can increase in pregnancy: your ribcage also expands, sometimes by as much as 10cm (4in). The average woman goes up two band sizes in pregnancy. Additionally, your breasts can get heavier and feel tender. All of these changes mean it is important to ensure that your breasts are comfortable and well supported.

Soft and supportive

Wearing a well-fitted, supportive bra during pregnancy can help to prevent or reduce stretch marks, ensure good posture, and relieve tension on your shoulders and back. If your breasts don't change size during pregnancy, your usual bras may suffice, but it is still likely that your breasts will feel more tender than usual, and you will want to make sure that any bra you do wear is comfortable. Good maternity and nursing bras are made from soft materials, are usually non-wired, and offer extra support at the shoulders and back. Maternity bras also have enough stretch and flexibility to allow your breasts some room to continue growing.

Maternity and nursing bras are designed to offer **the right support** and are made of soft, breathable fabrics to provide **maximum comfort**.

Go for a fitting Have a professional bra fitter check your size accurately. She will also take into account how your breasts may change through pregnancy.

Did you know...

Don't guess your new bra size! Many women end up with uncomfortable, poorly fitting bras when guessing – which is the last thing you want in pregnancy or after the birth. You can find professional bra fitters in specialist lingerie shops and the lingerie departments of many department stores – and the service is usually free. The fitter will usually measure beneath your bust line and around the bust (over your clothes or with your bra on), ask you to try on a fit bra to gauge your correct cup size, or judge by eye which bra size you need.

Q When do I need to go and get fitted for a maternity bra?

This varies from woman to woman, but as soon as your normal bra starts to feel tight, it's time to get fitted for a maternity bra. If your bra leaves red marks on your skin, it is too tight. It is quite possible that you need to change your bra size two or three times during pregnancy as your breasts continue to grow.

Usually, the end of your first trimester is a good time to check how your bra is fitting, if you haven't already done so – some women start wearing maternity bras earlier if their bust is too tender to wear their usual bras. During the second trimester, your bump and ribcage start to expand too, so it's worth getting re-measured then as well.

Q I've heard that my breasts will get even bigger after the birth. When should I get a nursing bra?

It's a good idea to buy at least one nursing bra before your baby arrives so you don't have to go shopping straight after the birth. Breasts usually stop growing by 36 weeks of pregnancy, so at this point a trained bra fitter can estimate what size your breasts will be after the birth. Your breasts will get bigger when your milk comes in (even if you don't intend to breastfeed), and you might need one or two larger nursing bras. Once your milk supply settles down, your breasts usually get a bit smaller again, so buy bras that you can tighten as your breasts change shape.

Q I'm almost 35 weeks and my maternity bra is feeling tight. Can I avoid getting a new bra now?

If your cup size still feels fine, but your bra is tight around your body, you could buy a bra extender. This cheap accessory is simply three or four extra sets of eyes that you attach to your existing bra strap so that you can let your bra out a few more centimetres as your ribcage expands. This saves you buying a new maternity bra at this late stage.

Q What's the difference between a maternity bra and a nursing bra?

Nursing bras allow easy access during breastfeeding, usually via a clasp that allows you to pull the cup material down. This enables you to feed your baby without having to remove your bra. These bras are designed to avoid placing pressure on your breast tissue, which could lead to blocked ducts and problems with feeding. Maternity bras don't have an access system, but are stretchier and designed to adapt to growing breasts during pregnancy. Women who don't plan to breastfeed sometimes prefer maternity bras after the birth as they don't need accessible cups.

Q I prefer underwired bras. Can I carry on wearing these?

It's generally recommended that you avoid wearing underwired bras during pregnancy and while nursing. As your breasts swell, the rigid underwire may dig into your skin and breast tissue, which is especially uncomfortable in pregnancy and can obstruct the blood flow to the breasts. Once you're breastfeeding, pressure from an underwired bra could lead to blocked milk ducts, obstructing the flow of milk, and even leading to mastitis (see p.274–75).

Most maternity and nursing bras are non-wired, but if you definitely prefer underwired bras (those with larger busts might find they offer more support), there are some underwired maternity bras that contain a more flexible wire made from a lightweight alloy. These mould more easily around the breast and avoid putting pressure on breast tissue.

Q My midwife suggested that I wear a bra at night, but that sounds rather uncomfortable. Is this really necessary?

If your breasts are very tender, you may find that a lightweight non-wired soft bra will help you to feel more comfortable at night. You can even buy a soft sleep bra that is designed for maximum comfort while you sleep, or you could try wearing a crop-top bra. After the birth, if you are leaking milk and using breast pads, then wearing a bra at night will make it easier to keep the pads in place (see p.275).

You may find that you start to outgrow your usual bra from as early as **8 to 10 weeks** into pregnancy. It's worth being measured **every couple of months** by a professional bra fitter to check that your current bra still **fits** you **properly**.

Q What do I look for when choosing maternity and nursing bras?

Comfort and support are key. Don't be tempted to estimate your new bra size – it's definitely worth asking a trained bra fitter to measure you and ensure that you buy styles of maternity and nursing bras that fit you perfectly.

Look for bras made of breathable cotton or cotton and lycra with some stretch in the cup. Wide adjustable shoulder straps will provide good support for your bigger breasts, but make sure the straps don't dig in. Likewise, the back strap should fit comfortably close to your body without being too tight, and should sit straight – if it rides up, the bra is too big.

A wide, curved underband at the front accommodates your growing bump. Choose maternity and nursing bras with four sets of hooks and eyes on the back panel so you can adjust the fit of your bra. Your ribcage expands in pregnancy and shrinks back after the birth, so when you're buying a bra early in pregnancy, make sure it fits on the tightest hook so you can let the strap out as your body changes; then when buying a nursing bra towards the end of pregnancy, choose one that fits on the loosest setting. Check that you can open and close the nursing bra cup easily with one hand.

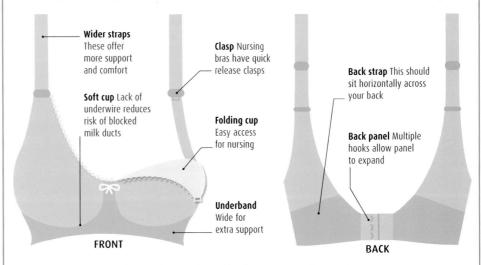

Wider straps These offer more support and comfort

Soft cup Lack of underwire reduces risk of blocked milk ducts

Clasp Nursing bras have quick release clasps

Folding cup Easy access for nursing

Underband Wide for extra support

Back strap This should sit horizontally across your back

Back panel Multiple hooks allow panel to expand

FRONT

BACK

Bra anatomy Maternity and nursing bras are designed in the same way, with supportive back and shoulder straps. Seamless bras are good if your nipples are tender. Nursing bras have fastenings on the shoulders or central panel that open and close each cup easily.

Q How much use is a birthing ball? Is it worth investing in one?

A birthing ball can be a valuable aid during labour, and it can help you perform exercises in pregnancy to prepare you for the birth. It also provides an alternative support if you find sitting uncomfortable or have poor posture.

Despite their name, birthing balls are really the same as exercise balls, made of tough anti-burst material – although some birthing balls have the advantage of a non-slip finish. It's worth buying a birthing ball early on if you do buy one, as it can be used for back support and as a base for both antenatal and postnatal exercise. If you choose to buy an exercise ball rather than a birthing ball, make sure you buy a ball that is at least 65cm (26in) in diameter, or 75cm (30in) if you are taller (1.75m/5ft 9in or more).

Comfortable exercise

Sitting on the ball while you are pregnant can help with your posture, as you need to sit straight and upright to maintain your balance without curving your back, which in turn helps to strengthen the muscles in your back and prevent backache. You can practise pelvic floor exercises (see p.67) while sitting on the ball, and perform gentle pelvis exercises (see below) during pregnancy and after the birth.

Finding your balance on the ball can be tricky as first, so ask someone to help you sit down and get up until you feel confident doing this yourself. Use the birthing ball on a carpet rather than a smooth surface for stability.

In late pregnancy, when it can be difficult to sit comfortably, a birthing ball provides a supportive base that may be more comfortable than a chair. You may find that it is easier to get into a standing position from a ball than from a chair. You also naturally lean slightly forwards when sitting on a birthing ball, which helps to move your baby into a good position before labour (see p.199).

During the first stage of labour, sitting on a birthing ball can help you to stay upright and active (see p.210) and allow you to rock your pelvis, which can help to shift your baby into a good position for the delivery. After the birth, a birthing ball may be more comfortable to sit on if you have stitches, and can provide a good route back into a gentle exercise regime.

BIRTHING BALL USES

A birthing ball can prove useful not just for labour, but throughout pregnancy and after the birth, too.

» Sitting: sit with your knees and feet apart so you feel balanced and stable. Keep your feet flat on the floor, your back straight, and your shoulders pulled back and down with your hands on your knees.

» Pelvis exercises: rotate your pelvis clockwise a few times, and then anticlockwise. Join them up by moving your pelvis in figure-of-eight movements. Then practise your pelvic floor exercises.

» Labour: gently rock your pelvis as you sit on the ball. If kneeling down feels easier during contractions, lean against the ball and wrap your arms around it for support.

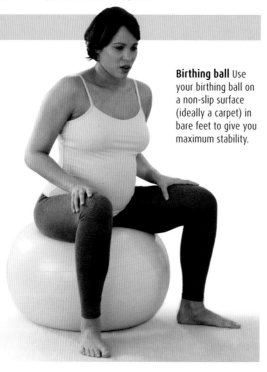

Birthing ball Use your birthing ball on a non-slip surface (ideally a carpet) in bare feet to give you maximum stability.

Tips for backache

» As well as using support aids to relieve back pain, regular gentle exercise will keep you fit and supple and help to strengthen your back and muscles. Try swimming, pregnancy yoga, or simple strengthening exercises (see p.65).

» A firm mattress will provide important support while you sleep. If your mattress sags and you're not planning on buying a new one soon, try putting a hard board under it to make it firm.

» Try a birthing ball (see left), which will help you to sit straight and ease back pain.

Q What can I use to support my back during the day? I'm getting niggling lower back pain as my bump grows.

There are a few support aids you can try, including a pregnancy belt and a lumbar support cushion. A soft, durable pregnancy belt helps to make your pelvic area more stable and support your abdomen and back. It is designed to be adjustable and fit under your bump, helping to lift and support your expanding uterus and, in turn, take the pressure off your back, relieving hip pain. Many women find these support belts helpful if they are on their feet or walking for any length of time.

Use a cushion to support your lower back when sitting in a chair or your car. Special lumbar support cushions mould to the shape of your lower back when you sit, improving your posture by stopping you sinking into the seat, and relieving stress on your back ligaments.

A soft bed mattress can exacerbate your back pain. Use a firmer mattress if you can, or place a board under your soft mattress.

Back pain is up there with the most common complaints in pregnancy, with almost three quarters of women complaining of backache at some point. See page 133 for more information on back pain while pregnant. Pregnancy-related pelvic girdle pain (PPGP) also causes pain in the lower back (see p.132 for advice). Let your healthcare provider know about your back pain, too, as he or she may be able to refer you for obstetric physiotherapy.

Q I'm planning to breastfeed. Is it worth buying a feeding cushion?

A feeding cushion is usually a V-shaped or U-shaped cushion that supports your baby while she feeds so you don't have to hold her continually, or you can use it to support your arms as you feed her so you don't get too tired or cramped.

Some women find these feeding cushions extremely useful, especially in the early weeks of breastfeeding when you and your baby are working on your technique and finding the most comfortable positions. The cushion sits around your waist and supports either your baby while she feeds, or your arms, depending on whether you want to cradle her as she feeds. Having this cushioned support under your baby or your arms stops you from craning forwards during a feeding session, so your posture is improved and your milk flow isn't hampered. However, you can try using ordinary cushions to create a similar support if you feel a feeding cushion isn't worth it. If you do invest in a feeding cushion, it can double up as a baby nest once your baby is a little older, acting as a support for her to lean against before she is able to sit up unaided.

Baby bolster Cushions have a wide section on which to lay your baby.

FEEDING CUSHION

Using a feeding cushion Sit comfortably with your back supported. Wrap the cushion around your waist and position your baby at the right angle to feed.

Q It's getting harder to get a decent night's sleep as I grow bigger. Is there anything that can help?

Strategically placed pillows can help to bolster your bump and support your legs and back. As your abdomen grows, it can be hard to find a comfortable sleeping position. After around 16 weeks of pregnancy, lying on your back puts a strain on it and becomes more difficult. You should avoid this position anyway because it puts pressure on the major blood vessels – the aorta and the major vein called the inferior vena cava – and affects the blood circulation to you and your baby, making you feel faint. Don't worry, however, if during the night you turn onto your back – if your body feels unwell it will turn naturally to a more suitable position while you are asleep. Lying on your side, specifically your left side, is thought to optimize your circulation, and is usually the most comfortable position later in pregnancy.

However, your abdomen can feel unsupported when you lie on your side, so many women find they need some support aids to be comfortable in this position (see pp.114–5).

Support pillows
You can try using one of the many pregnancy pillows available: there is a whole range of designs to choose from, and some are multi-purpose, providing support during the daytime, too, and doubling up as feeding cushions once your baby arrives. Compact wedge-shaped cushions slip under your bump when you lie on your side, and can also be used as a lower back support while sitting. For ultimate support, you can invest in a body-length pillow; these long pillows curl around your body supporting your bump, back, and legs while you sleep. After the birth, you can use them for supporting your baby's weight during feeding sessions. If you don't want to spend money on pregnancy pillows, you can use strategically placed bed pillows and cushions to create the extra support that you need.

Body-length pillows cradle your whole body while you sleep and are one of the most **popular** pregnancy accessories.

Q Which inflatable cushions are most helpful for sitting down if I've had stitches after the delivery?

If you need stitches after a tear or episiotomy (see p.217) during the birth, an inflatable cushion can help to take the pressure off your perineal area when you sit down and bring temporary relief. You are likely to feel sore and tender in the perineal area as your stitches heal, which can make sitting down uncomfortable. There are a few types to choose from:

» **C-shaped inflatable cushion** helps you avoid putting pressure on one particular area.

» **Valley-style cushion** is a uniquely designed cushion using a combination of foam and air, with two inflatable sides that you can adjust accordingly and a dip in the middle. You may be able to hire one of these cushions rather than have to buy it.

» **Doughnut-shaped inflatable cushions** with a hole in the centre are also available. These cushions will enable you to avoid putting any pressure on your perineum when you sit down, although you should avoid sitting on these types of cushion for too long, as they can compress the area, which could become uncomfortable in itself.

A CLOSER LOOK
Packing your bag

By the time you reach 36 weeks, prepare supplies for the birth itself, as you might go into labour at any point. Whether you intend to give birth in hospital, at a birthing centre, or at home, you'll need a few essential items for labour, and the equivalent of an overnight bag with extras for you and your baby after the birth. Ask about any stipulations your hospital may have about what you can and can't bring with you, and consider packing items for your birth partner, too. Lastly, don't forget your birth plan and maternity notes!

Healthy snacks Pack a stash of healthy snacks and bottled water to keep you energized and hydrated during labour. Wholegrain sandwiches or snacks provide slow-release energy. Include fresh fruit and a cereal bar in your snack bag.

You will want a few toiletries for before and after the birth. Lips can get dry in labour, so a lip balm will be welcome, and a face spray or flannel that you can wet will be refreshing and soothing during labour.

If you've had stitches, those first toilet trips can sting! Pack a small plastic jug, or an old plastic water bottle, so you can pour warm water over your perineal area as you pass urine.

Comfort aids You might want a couple of home pillows for extra comfort, and a birthing ball if the hospital doesn't supply them. And remember to pack any other aids for labour, such as essential oils, a TENS machine, or natural remedies.

Your things for after the birth You will need old underwear or disposable pants and maternity sanitary pads for postnatal bleeding. A nursing bra, breast pads, muslin squares, and nipple cream will provide all you need to start breastfeeding. Pack some nightwear, flip flops, and some loose clothing for leaving the hospital.

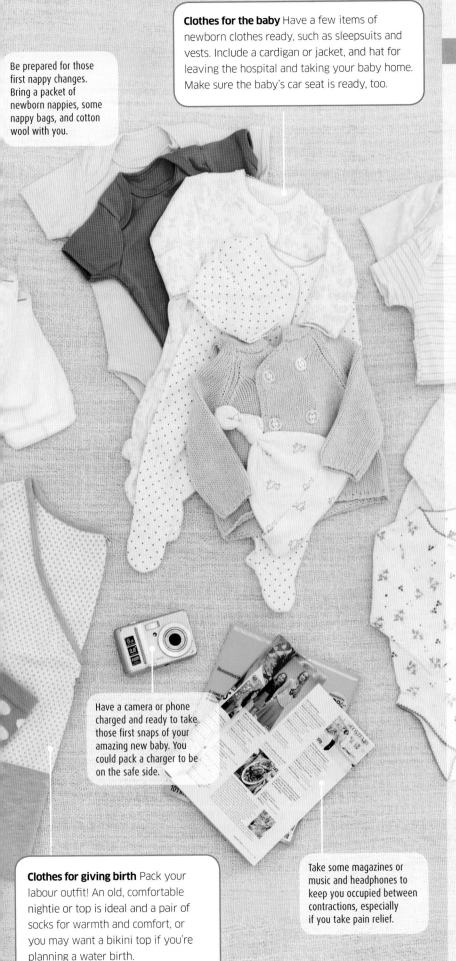

Be prepared for those first nappy changes. Bring a packet of newborn nappies, some nappy bags, and cotton wool with you.

Clothes for the baby Have a few items of newborn clothes ready, such as sleepsuits and vests. Include a cardigan or jacket, and hat for leaving the hospital and taking your baby home. Make sure the baby's car seat is ready, too.

Have a camera or phone charged and ready to take those first snaps of your amazing new baby. You could pack a charger to be on the safe side.

Clothes for giving birth Pack your labour outfit! An old, comfortable nightie or top is ideal and a pair of socks for warmth and comfort, or you may want a bikini top if you're planning a water birth.

Take some magazines or music and headphones to keep you occupied between contractions, especially if you take pain relief.

FASCINATING FACTS

It may be hard to believe some of these facts, but you'll soon find out from your own experience as a new parent.

12 nappies
This is the average number that a baby needs per day. She will wee every 1–3 hours and will poo several times a day.

40 days
In some cultures around the world, this is the time frame that mother and baby are encouraged not to leave the house in order to fully recover from the birth.

3 outfits
Most babies will need three or more outfit changes a day. Make sure you have enough clothes ready for your newborn baby's wardrobe.

16 weeks
You might look about 16 weeks pregnant straight after the birth. Your uterus still needs to go back to its pre-pregnancy size and you'll have weight from pregnancy that takes a while to lose.

5,850
This is the average number of nappies that a child will use in her lifetime.

Getting ready for your baby's arrival is truly exciting. This is an ideal time to start listing and **buying** what your **baby may need**. While you can, of course, still shop after the birth, you'll need a **core supply of basic items** ready from the outset.

Preparing for your baby

Prioritize what you need

When you begin to feel secure in your pregnancy, it's worth deciding which essentials you and your baby will need. Then buy the equipment gradually so that once your baby is born you can focus on him, rest, and recover.

There are several larger items you need to have ready for your baby, including a buggy, a Moses basket, a crib or cot, and a car seat. Purchasing these things is likely to require the most consideration. For this reason, allow yourself enough time to browse and research. You may want to test out car seats and buggies before you buy, so plan a shopping trip before you get uncomfortably big. If budget is a consideration, think about what you could accept from friends and family if they have expressed a wish to buy an item, or what you can get second-hand.

Newborn baby clothes are adorable and it's easy to be tempted to buy items now that may actually see very little wear; many first-time parents don't realize just how quickly newborns grow. Buy some essentials now and then assess your baby's needs as he grows so that baby clothes don't go to waste.

Other worthwhile purchases to buy now are nappy changing bags, a thermometer (see p.292), and simple washing equipment. Breastfeeding requires little apart from a good nursing bra, but if you are planning to bottle-feed, buy a basic set of bottles and teats. Don't panic if you think you want to breastfeed, but aren't sure how successful it will be; you can easily buy bottle-feeding equipment after the birth.

Longer-term purchases

Before you feel pressure to get a nursery ready, bear in mind that your baby will be best off in the same room as you for the first six months. And newborn babies don't need much in the way of toys for the first few weeks. Their new environment and time spent getting to know you and gazing at your face provide all the stimulation they need. If you would like to have a couple of play items to hand, look for age-appropriate toys. Babies love high-contrast patterns and looking at faces, so baby mirrors and soft books with black and white patterns or bright colours are all your little one will need at first.

Q What clothes will my baby need?

It's best to keep clothing simple for young babies. Your baby will be spending much of his first weeks feeding and napping indoors so you need only buy a limited supply of items to keep him comfortable.

Layers Try dressing your baby in layers in the beginning so that you can remove or add items easily to regulate his body temperature.

Newborn babies cannot regulate their body temperature. As they get older, this improves. As a result, it is best to dress them in a vest, adding further layers as and when required. To start with, buy no more than six to eight cotton vests with envelope-style necks and poppers around the nappy area, six all-in-one sleepsuits with poppers down the front – which are ideal for the first few months, a couple of light cardigans, a soft hat or wide-brimmed summer bonnet, a jacket or snowsuit, depending on the season, and some socks to keep his feet warm if they are uncovered. Front-fastening outfits rather than items with fiddly ties and awkward zips will be more comfortable for your baby, and make nappy changing much easier. In the winter, add vests under sleepsuits and use a lightweight cardigan when the temperature drops.

YOUR BABY'S FIRST WARDROBE

Choose baby clothes in soft, easy-care, machine-washable fabrics. Cotton is perfect for babies, as its natural fibre is gentle on your baby's sensitive skin, helps to keep him cool, is easy to wash, and is durable.

2–3 LONG SLEEVED BODY SUITS

6–8 SHORT-SLEEVED BODY SUITS – USE ON THEIR OWN IN HOT WEATHER

6–8 SLEEPSUITS, IDEALLY WITH COVERED TOES

1–2 PAIRS OF PYJAMAS; CHOOSE LIGHTER FABRICS FOR SUMMER BABIES

1–2 CARDIGANS FOR LIGHT LAYERING

2–4 EASY-ON TROUSERS OR LEGGINGS

4 PAIRS OF SOCKS

SCRATCH MITS

2 BIBS

Indoor basics All-in-one sleepsuits and body suits are ideal for day- and night-time for the first few months, then use pyjamas at night and body suits and leggings during the day. Layer with a cardigan if your baby needs extra warmth.

Outdoor essentials On hot summer days, a short-sleeved T-shirt or vest may be all your baby needs, although do use a sun hat or bonnet and sunscreen too. Otherwise layer vests or body suits with T-shirts, leggings, socks, and cardigans depending on the weather, and invest in a snowsuit or warm jacket, mittens, and a soft hat for winter.

2–3 ENVELOPE NECK T-SHIRTS

SUNHAT

JACKET OR SNOWSUIT

2 HATS

MITTENS

Q What equipment will we need for washing our baby?

In the first few weeks of your baby's life, you will probably be combining regular bathing with topping and tailing (see p.284), where you clean your baby without immersing her in a tub of water.

There's no need to bathe your newborn every day, unless she loves having a bath and finds it soothing or enjoyable; she'll only need a bath two or three times a week on average. Carefully washing your baby's face, neck, hands, and bottom – known as topping and tailing – requires very little equipment, but does need to be done thoroughly every day that your baby doesn't have a bath. Whichever you do, get everything ready beforehand and make sure that the room and the water are warm.

TOPPING AND TAILING

You will need only basic equipment:

>> **Cotton wool.** Use a fresh piece for separate areas, including around the ears and eyes.

>> **Two bowls of water,** one for each end of the body to avoid cross-infection.

WATER BOWL

BATHING

For bathing your baby you will need the following:

>> **Baby bath,** a sink, or a big bath tub. The advantage of a baby bath is that you can use it in any room. If your baby seems to dislike the water, try bathing together and soothing her as you do so.

>> **Non-slip mat** only if you are planning to use a big bath tub.

>> **Bath thermometer** can be used to check the temperature of the water is 35–38°C (95–100°F), or you can test the bath temperature with your elbow, checking it is warm, but not hot.

>> **A combined mild baby shampoo and bath product** used sparingly, although plain water is usually better for cleaning your baby at first.

>> **Soft flannels or a sponge**

>> **2–3 hooded baby towels,** to wrap your baby up in after bathing and stop her losing heat through her head.

>> **Olive oil or baby oil,** for rubbing into your baby's towel-dried skin.

Bath time This is a great opportunity to play with your baby so have everything you need prepared around you.

Q I heard that you should wash baby clothes before they are worn. Is that really necessary?

Yes, it's a good idea to wash your baby's clothes before she first wears them. This simple precaution ensures that any residues of substances from the manufacturing process that could irritate your baby's sensitive skin are removed. Use non-biological detergents to wash all your baby's clothes, bedding, and muslin squares, as these detergents don't contain enzymes, which can also prove an irritant.

Q Is it a good idea to buy a room thermometer? Where should we put it?

Making sure the room your baby sleeps in is the right temperature reduces the risk of sudden infant death syndrome (SIDS), so do buy a thermometer for the bedroom. The ideal room temperature for a baby is 16–20°C (60–68°F). If you want to ensure your baby doesn't get too hot or cold, you may like to have several thermometers around the house. Options range from affordable strip thermometers stuck to laminated board to smart digital thermometers. Remember though that if the room temperature is right, your baby won't need lots of blankets.

Q How do I choose a good changing bag and what should I stock in it?

You can choose a changing bag with a foldaway changing mat, although you don't have to buy a purpose-made changing bag; you can use a bag of your choice and buy a separate fold-up changing mat. Have the following items ready as a nappy-changing kit in the bag for when you're away from the house:
>> **A few disposable nappies** and nappy bags.
>> **Travel-sized pack** of unperfumed baby wipes (try to use baby wipes sparingly, as they can be harsh on your newborn's delicate skin).
>> **A small pot** or travel-sized pot of barrier cream to prevent or ease nappy rash.
>> **Spare clothes** for your baby and for you. When you use any of these items to change your baby while you are out, remember to restock the supplies when you get home so the bag is all ready for your next trip out.

Q How many nappies and sizes do we stock up on before the birth?

Your baby will need nappies from the outset, but it is sensible to exercise a little caution over how many you buy. While it is tempting to stock up on bargain box deals at the supermarket, you don't yet know how big your baby will be.

If you have a newborn on the larger size, she may spend very little time in newborn nappies. It may also take a while to work out which brand you prefer, and which fit your baby best.

During the first week, the number of wet nappies your baby has each day will be about six, which mounts up to 42 nappies or so. After the first week the number will gradually build up, and you can expect to change at least 10 to 12 wet nappies a day. So you may want to start off buying a couple of packs of newborn nappies to see you through the first week or so, and then assess whether you need to carry on with a newborn size or move to the next size up. Some newborn nappies have a cut-out section to accommodate the umbilical cord stump, but you don't necessarily need these – you can just turn the nappy down at the front.

Reusable cloth nappies

If you plan to use reusables, you need around 20 nappies from the outset, as well as washable wraps if you are using two-piece nappies with a cloth nappy and outer waterproof layer. There is a larger initial financial outlay involved for cloth nappies, so unless you are certain that you want your baby to wear reusables, you may prefer to wait until your daily routine has settled down and then look into the options.

12 Newborns need 12 **daily** nappy changes – **84 nappies a week.**

6–8 Older babies need **6–8 daily** nappy changes – up to **56 nappies a week.**

REUSABLE OR DISPOSABLE?

If you are undecided about which type of nappy to buy, consider these pros and cons:

» **Comfort:** disposables are more breathable, but their moisturizing, absorbing chemicals may irritate the skin. Reusables may feel softer.

» **Convenience:** disposables are more convenient when out, at daycare, or travelling. Reusables aren't as absorbent, so you may need to change a soiled nappy more frequently. Nowadays, changing a nappy, whether disposable or reusable, is quick and easy.

» **Cost:** reusable nappies are usually cheaper than disposables unless you use a laundering service.

» **Other:** disposables use resources such as trees and plastics in the manufacturing process, then collect in landfills. Washing cloth nappies uses clean water and energy, but produces only dirty water. Disposables, however, reduce the risk of infection in a group setting such as a nursery.

Disposable nappies Although these are an easy choice, consider all options before you make a decision; you may opt to use a combination of both.

Q Apart from nappies, what else will we need for nappy changing?

You will need a wipe-clean baby changing mat, cotton wool or baby wipes to clean your baby's bottom, and barrier cream. Ideally use moistened cotton wool rather than baby wipes at home to avoid skin irritations, and use a barrier cream such as zinc and castor oil to prevent or ease any nappy rash. You may also like a purpose-made nappy bin for disposable nappies. Used nappies are folded then placed in the bin shute, which seals them as the nappy moves down into the bin, locking away odours. However, this is not essential and is an extra cost to be aware of. If you are using cloth nappies, you will need a bucket to store dirty ones before washing. These are purpose-made, or you can buy a normal lidded bucket.

Q Are there any other items we need for our baby's everyday care?

There are a few more essentials that you'll need to help to make life easier with a newborn. A supply of muslin cloths is very useful for protecting your clothing during winding, and some women also like to use these to cover up a little more when breastfeeding. A soft baby brush or comb will help to gently untangle knots when your baby's hair starts to grow, and baby scissors will keep her nails trim.

If your baby is born in the summer, you will also need some sunscreen to protect her from the sun's harmful rays. The general advice used to be to avoid putting sunscreen on babies under six months because chemicals in the sunscreen could irritate their delicate skin, and to keep them out of direct sunlight instead, especially between 10am and 2pm. However, it's now recommended that as well as keeping your baby well covered and avoiding direct sunlight, you should also apply small amounts of sunscreen to exposed areas of skin. Buy at least factor 30 with a four- or five-star rating that protects against both UVA and UVB rays. Ensure that you have a wide-brimmed sunhat for her. Once your baby is a little older, if you are going to the beach, you may want to invest in a bathing suit that covers her arms and legs, offering effective protection against UV rays.

If you want peace of mind about your baby while she sleeps, a baby monitor is useful. You can buy audio devices, with a transmitter placed next to your sleeping baby and a speaker near you; audio with motion sensor pads, which sound an alarm if your baby doesn't move for a while; and video monitors that allow you to both hear and see your baby.

Q What should we buy for our baby to sleep in?

Your baby will need a Moses basket, a crib, or a cot for sleeping in. Another increasingly popular option is to opt for a co-sleeping cot which attaches to your bed, or you could try a "baby nest".

Although you can use a full-sized cot from the start, a newborn may feel cosier in a Moses basket or crib for the first few weeks, as it more closely mimics the feeling of being cocooned in the womb. A Moses basket is also easy to use as a travel cot or move around from room to room so your baby can be in the same room as you for all his sleep time, both day and night.

Some cribs are designed to be gently rocked to soothe a baby; they last longer than Moses baskets because they are bigger and so a baby can sleep in them for longer, but they are less transportable. A co-sleeping cot attached to your bed is great if you want to have your baby near you but not actually in your bed. The cot sits alongside your bed with a drop-down side so you can easily reach over to comfort your baby or gather him up for a feed without having to get out of bed. Ensure there is no gap between the cot and your bed that your baby could fall into. Another option is a baby nest, a baby mattress with sturdy sides placed in your bed, that gives your baby his own dedicated sleeping space safe from hazards such as pillows or duvets. When you do come to choose a full-size cot, make sure it conforms to all health and safety standards (right).

A Moses basket or crib **closely mimics** the feeling of being cocooned in the **womb**, so is ideal in the **first few weeks**.

SLEEPING OPTIONS

It's personal preference as to which type of crib or cot you choose, but make sure they fit these criteria.

» Moses basket: choose one with a sturdy base and handles so that it's secure when you move it around. Babies can grow out of Moses baskets quite quickly, and you may find that at around two to three months your baby is looking a little cramped. She should be able to sleep with her arms out to the side, or flung up by her head, without touching the sides or top of the basket.

» Full-size cot: ensure the cot conforms to European Safety Standards and carries the British Safety Standards number BSEN716:2008. Gaps between the vertical bars should be no more than 6.5cm (2½in) apart so your baby can't get stuck, and the space from the top of the mattress to the top of the cot must be at least 50cm (19½in). Some have an adjustable mattress that can be lowered as your baby grows.

Did you know...

Your newborn will be too young to play with toys, but he will be stimulated by his surroundings from early on. Young babies can't focus far, but they enjoy looking at black and white patterns, high-contrast colours, and baby mirrors. Your baby will also enjoy watching a colourful mobile hung above his cot. Make sure this is secure and out of his reach. Some mobiles have a wind-up music box attached, which babies can find very soothing, or you could place a music box in the room. Young babies love to touch, so find a couple of first soft books with different textures for him to explore.

Q What bedding does my baby need in his basket or cot?

You need one or two mattress protectors for if his nappy leaks in the night, three or four sheets, and two to three blankets so you have spare bedding as items are washed. Choose cotton sheets and lightweight cellular baby blankets: babies' hands and feet often feel colder than the rest of their body, so are not a reliable measure of their temperature. Feel the nape of his neck, or chest, to gauge his temperature as he sleeps, and adjust the bedclothes as necessary. You can buy fitted cot sheets or cot-sized flat sheets. It's absolutely essential to tuck the flat sheet in properly so he can't get tangled up in any loose ends. Or try a lightweight baby sleeping bag suitable for newborns instead of sheets and blankets.

Q Are there any must-have items of furniture for the baby we should invest in other than a cot?

As you will be spending a fair amount of time nursing, comforting, and perhaps reading to your baby, a chair is a worthwhile addition. Chairs marketed for feeding your baby are available, although these can be pricey. Whichever chair you choose, make sure it is comfortable for you with good back and arm support, and that you can place your feet flat on the floor. Dedicated changing tables are also handy and come in a variety of designs with shelves, drawers, and cupboard space though, again, these can be costly. Alternatively, a chest of drawers large enough to put a changing mat and some nappies on top is just as good, and good storage is essential in a nursery.

Keep the **colour scheme** of the nursery fairly neutral and use pictures, accessories, and wall-hangings to **add colour and fun**, since they are easiest to change as your baby grows.

Q We're starting to plan the nursery now. What do we need to think about first?

If you are planning to refurbish a room to turn it into a nursery, take the time now to research and buy appropriate lighting and chemical-free paints, as there is no immediate rush. The best and safest place for your baby to sleep for the first six months is in a Moses basket or cot in the same room as you, to help reduce the risk of sudden infant death syndrome (SIDS) (see p.287). So you won't need a fully functioning nursery the moment your baby arrives home. Having said that, it's best to paint the room at least two to three months before your baby moves into it so you can air the room. Avoid using any paints that give off potentially harmful paint fumes and choose a brand that is free from harmful chemicals and toxins. Look for information that stipulates the paint has low, or zero, VOC levels. Volatile organic compounds, or VOCs, are gases found in products such as household paints that emit harmful chemicals.

Think, too, about the nursery lighting. A night-light and/or dimmer switch will stop you and your partner stumbling around in the dark during night-time feeds, nappy changes, and midnight comforting sessions. And for many parents, black-out blinds are a must, ensuring that a baby isn't nudged out of sleep by early morning sunlight, especially in the summer.

Q We have been offered a second-hand cot. Should we buy a new mattress?

A new mattress is best. This is because there is evidence that a mattress that isn't in the best condition can increase the potential risk of SIDS, or cot death, which usually occurs during sleep.

Q How do we make sure the nursery is a safe space?

You should think first about the layout of your baby's room and the most appropriate place to position the cot, and then arrange the rest of the furniture and equipment accordingly.

Avoid placing your baby's cot near a window or any area where it will get hit by direct sunlight, and ensure that it isn't next to any curtain cords or pulls that your baby could get tangled up in. And once your baby starts to pull himself up to standing, you will need to make sure that there are no pieces of furniture near his cot that he could climb on to, or shelves that he could pull things off. Make sure that all the furniture is sturdy, or well anchored to the wall, so your baby won't be able to pull anything on top of himself. A plain wooden floor is ideal, as it is easy to keep clean and dust-free.

NURSERY SAFETY ESSENTIALS

Run through these safety essentials to check that everything is in order before you move your baby into the room.

» Temperature: keep the room at an even temperature and ensure that it doesn't get too hot. Use a room thermometer to keep the temperature at around 16-20°C (60-68°F).

» Smoke alarm: install a new smoke detector either in the nursery or just outside it. Choose an optical (or photoelectric) light sensor alarm, which has an infa-red LED that pulses a beam of light every few seconds to check for smoke particles.

» Baby monitor: situate a baby monitor, if you use one, well out of your baby's reach, but near enough to his cot so that you can hear him immediately if he cries or seems to be distressed.

» Hazards: ensure that there are no cords, pulls, toys, or decorations such as a hanging mobile so near to the cot that your baby could get tangled up in them. If you have a rug, secure it to the floor with double-sided tape so that no one can slip on them.

You can make it easier to control your baby's **temperature** as he sleeps by choosing **cotton sheets** and **lightweight cellular baby blankets** for his bedding so you can **add or remove layers** if he is too hot or cold.

When choosing a new mattress, look for firmness and breathable covers that can be removed and washed. The least expensive are foam mattresses, which may come with a waterproof covering, but have the least longevity and lose their shape most quickly. Coiled spring interior mattresses are better as they have inner springs sandwiched between layers of felt or foam to offer sturdy support.

Coir (coconut fibre) or other natural fibre mattresses are the firmest, most durable, and more expensive. Hypoallergenic mattresses have a removable quilted top layer that can be washed at a high temperature to remove any dust mites. Whichever mattress you choose, check that the label states it meets British Standard BS 1877-10:1997 and fits the cot properly.

Q I'm planning to breastfeed my baby. Is there anything I can do now to prepare?

One of the best things you can do to prepare for breastfeeding is to attend a breastfeeding course during pregnancy. These are usually short sessions of a couple of hours long, and may be available free in some hospitals, or you can pay for a private one. It's best to attend a course in your last trimester so that all the information is fresh in your mind when your baby arrives. You will either be shown a DVD of breastfeeding, or an experienced mum may come along to demonstrate how it's done. Experts will talk about how to latch your baby on, which positions you can try, and how to get a good milk supply established. The course leader may also discuss potential pitfalls and issues such as how to avoid nipple confusion by not introducing a bottle or dummy too early, and how to prevent and treat sore nipples. Look for courses run by an accredited lactation counsellor or consultant. You may also like to read up on the subject before you give birth so you feel fully prepared. See pages 266-77 for more information on breastfeeding.

Q I've heard of breastfeeding pillows. Is it worth buying one?

Breastfeeding can be a wonderful experience for mother and baby and it is vital that you are comfortable so that you can enjoy your time together. However it is not always easy. When feeding, it is important that you bring your baby up to nipple height rather than lean towards him. In the early weeks when your baby is very small, a good, supportive pillow will allow you to do this without having to take his weight in your arms. There are specially designed breastfeeding pillows and these can be more supportive than a normal pillow.

Similarly, most normal chairs are too high for breastfeeding so many recommend a feeding chair. These should be low and supportive in the right places for you to maintain good feeding positions. You may need to place pillows behind your back for extra support. Your lap should be flat or slightly raised so that your baby tips towards and not away from you. A feeding chair and pillow may reduce the chances of breastfeeding problems.

Q Is there anything I need to buy for breastfeeding?

One of the many benefits of breastfeeding is that it is very economical, but there are a few items you can buy that will support your breastfeeding experience and add to your comfort.

A nursing bra is essential, so it's worth buying two or three comfortable nursing bras. Make sure that the bras you buy have a clasp that you can release with one hand (see p.179), as your arms will be full with a newborn once you start to breastfeed. The bra cups should also open down completely so that nothing presses on your breast tissue and leads to blocked ducts or mastitis. Even if you want to decide about whether or not to breastfeed once your baby arrives, you should buy at least one bra before the birth, as it's not so easy to go shopping once your newborn has arrived. Breast pads, nipple cream, and muslin cloths are all additional, but affordable, items.

Breast pumps

You may want to wait to see if you need a breast pump once you have got into a routine with breastfeeding, but a manual or electric pump can prove invaluable if you have to bottle feed your baby at some point.

> Buy at least one **nursing bra** before the birth, as it will be more difficult to go shopping after.

WHAT YOU NEED TO BUY

With the exception of a breast pump, buy everything before the birth and pack them in your bag for the birth so you can start using them straight away.

» A professionally fitted, supportive nursing bra will be your main purchase. You can get fitted for a bra from about 36 weeks of pregnancy, when a bra fitter will be able to predict what size you will need after the birth (see p.178). You may also want to buy a soft night-time bra to hold your breast pads in place too.

» Disposable or washable breast pads help to collect milk that leaks when you're not feeding. Slim and discreet pads are available that are extremely absorbent; those without a plastic lining are less likely to irritate your skin and nipples.

» Nipple cream helps to protect and treat sore nipples. Look for pure, hypoallergenic, lanolin-based creams that are paraben-free.

» Muslin cloths are useful for draping over your shoulder after feeding to mop up any milk your baby possets. They can also provide some cover if you wish when you're breastfeeding in public, or you can use a shawl or scarf.

» Breast pumps enable you to express your milk (see p.272). Manual pumps have a suction cup or shield attached to a bottle, and a pump handle that you operate manually, while electric pumps operate essentially in the same way, but there is an electric motor that operates the pump action to make it a much faster process.

» Front-opening nightie or pyjamas to enable you to feed easily at night. There are breastfeeding tops that are designed to make breastfeeding easier too.

Q There are a lot of bottles and teats to choose from for bottle-feeding. What should we look out for?

All bottles and teats can be used with both formula milk and with breast milk you have expressed using a pump. There is no right or wrong choice. All of the items will be easy to buy once your baby arrives, so you shouldn't need to stockpile too many supplies before the birth.

Standard baby bottles are popular. These are usually available in a small or large size (around 125ml/4oz and 260ml/9oz), and with these you can tailor feeds depending on your baby's age and stage. Standard bottles usually come with teats and lids, are easy to clean, and are compatible with most sterilizing systems (see p.279) and bottle coolers. Some bottles are designed to help ease colic by limiting the amount of air your baby swallows with her milk, so these are worth trying for babies who often seem to be unsettled after a feed and have uncomfortable wind. Anti-colic bottles tend to be more expensive, and those that have a valve or tube to adapt the milk flow can be trickier to keep clean. If you have a microwave, consider a self-sterilizing bottle, which can be sterilized in a microwave. Again, these are a bit pricier, but can be convenient. Ready-sterilized disposable bottles are also available; you just add the formula and discard the bottle after use. While useful for travelling, these are expensive and

wasteful if used regularly. Glass bottles, made of toughened glass, are favoured by parents who worry about chemicals used in the manufacture of plastic bottles. These are more expensive, and breakable, but more environmentally friendly.

Bottle teats

Teats can be silicone or latex and have different flow speeds. Latex teats tend to be more flexible and softer, but are less durable then silicone teats. Slow-flow teats are designed to release the milk more slowly, and these are usually best for newborns and young babies. Traditionally, teats are bell-shaped; wider teats are available that are thought to resemble the shape of a human nipple more closely, so manufacturers recommend these if you are combining breast and bottle, or trying to move a breastfed baby over to bottle-feeding. However, it's unlikely a bottle teat can truly mimic the human nipple and the unique sucking action required, and there's no evidence that these are easier to use.

WHAT YOU NEED

Keep an eye on the condition of your equipment, especially the teats, and replace them when they become damaged or worn.

›› 6–8 bottles in a combination of large and small sizes.

›› 6–8 teats suitable for newborns.

›› Formula powder.

›› A sterilizing system – either a cold-water sterilizing system or a steam sterilizer. You can also boil bottle-feeding equipment. See p.279 for how different sterilizing systems work.

›› Bottle- and teat-cleaning brushes.

Feeding bottles These are available in a variety of sizes, while teats have different flow speeds; keep an eye on which ones help your baby to feed most easily and comfortably.

Large bottle

Bottle cap Keeps both bottle and water sterile until used.

Wider latex teat

Valve-flow bottle

Traditional bell-shaped silicone teat

Q The range of buggies, pushchairs, and prams is incredible. How on earth do we choose?

When thinking about what to buy, the best starting point is to focus on your specific needs: what will suit your lifestyle, your budget, and work well for both your baby and you and your partner.

If you use public transport often or travel up and down steps regularly, you may find that a lightweight, easily foldable pushchair or buggy, or a more compact pram, meets your needs well. If you drive regularly, consider a travel system where you can alternate a chair or car seat on a chassis base, making it easy to move your baby from home to car to pushchair without disturbing him too much. Sturdy models with swivel wheels are easy to manoeuvre and great for walking in cities and towns; if you walk on rough terrain, a fixed wheel is best, making it easier to push the pram over uneven ground.

Comfort is key

You will need a model that lies flat so that it's suitable for newborns to sleep in. Some prams have adjustable seats that start off fully reclined and can be adjusted into a more upright mode as your baby grows. Check that the pushchair is well padded and has a sturdy back support, and decide whether you want your baby to face inwards towards you, or outwards. Some models have a reversible seat so you can keep an eye on and make eye contact with your newborn, and turn the seat out when your baby is older. Double check that the handle is high enough for you so you don't have to lean over and strain your back. If you and your partner are significantly different heights, you may want to choose a model with an adjustable handle.

> Make sure you **try out** the model in the shop **before you purchase** and practise using it before the birth.

HOW TO DETERMINE WHICH TRAVEL SYSTEM IS RIGHT FOR YOUR FAMILY

The following summary looks at the range of options, explaining key features and highlighting the pros and cons of different models.

RANGE	DESCRIPTION
Pushchairs	Pushchairs that have a fully reclining seat are suitable from birth and are often comfortably padded with good support for your baby's back. They have the advantage that as your baby grows, the seat can be adjusted to enable him to sit up and look around, and can be forward-facing or backward facing. Some pushchairs work as a three-in-one travel system (see below), and wheels can come in various sizes, with bigger wheels offering more suspension.
Prams	These allow your newborn to lie flat and are more traditional looking than pushchairs and buggies. Your baby has an enclosed, cosy environment, and can see you as you push him along. Models with detachable carrycots double up as travel cots for the first few months.
Travel systems	These are pushchairs that also come with a car seat and carrycot that you can slot over the chassis. Travel systems are handy for moving your baby between home, car, and outside without lifting him into different seats.
Buggies	Buggies are lightweight and easy to use and usually fit easily into a car boot, so are great for travel and shopping. While some buggies are suitable only for older, sitting babies, many models recline fully to accommodate newborns. Buggies can't be used as part of a travel system with car seats or carrycots.
Double buggies	If you have twins or a toddler who needs to be pushed around with your newborn, you will need a double buggy. These can be side-by-side or tandem buggies, where one seat is positioned behind or under the main seat. Side-by-side buggies allow your babies to see each other and have an unobstructed view. Tandem buggies mean that one child has a restricted view and can be difficult to manage on steps, but can be easier to get through tighter spaces such as shop doors. You can also buy single buggy models that can be upgraded into a double buggy when required.

Q Do I need to buy extra pushchair accessories or are they really a waste of money?

There are a few useful extra items that are worth considering if you want to buy, especially if you intend to be out in all weathers. Transparent rain covers, which attach directly onto the pushchair, pram, or buggy, can give your baby complete protection from wind and rain. Air passes beneath and through side air vents so your baby can breathe easily even while the cover remains fixed in place. Foot muffs are cosy for chilly days. Some manufacturers include this as part of the model, or you can buy a foot muff separately. On sunny days, a parasol or shade attachment will help to keep your baby protected from the sun. Very small babies often need a head support, or head hugger, that fits around their head, stopping it lolling to the side; these can be used in car seats as well as pushchairs.

Q I like the idea of carrying my baby in a sling and being hands-free. Which ones give enough support for newborns?

Front carriers and baby slings will support a newborn baby, although you need to take more care if using a sling. Front carriers hold your baby upright against your body, have safety restraints, and are suitable for newborns weighing at least 3.5kg (7½lb). Your baby can either face inwards towards you, and then when older, can face outwards. Choose fabrics that can be easily cleaned and look for styles that provide good support for your baby, have broad, comfortable shoulder straps, and if possible a hip strap, so that your baby's weight is evenly distributed across your back.

Baby slings and baby wraps are made from soft, flexible fabric. Some can be worn over your shoulder in a cradle hold; others can be adapted to hold your baby in different positions. There have been safety concerns around baby slings, that babies can suffocate if carried incorrectly. Make sure you can see your baby's face at all times, he is held as high up on your chest as possible, he is held securely against your body, and his chin isn't touching his chest, as this could hamper his breathing; and his back and neck are well supported.

Q We don't drive much. Is a car seat essential for newborns and babies?

Even if you seldom make car journeys, the law states that your baby must be in a properly fitted car seat for all car journeys, even if this is just in the taxi on the way home from the hospital.

It's recommended that your baby's car seat is rear-facing until your baby reaches the correct weight for the type of car seat you are using – see the guideline table (right). In the event of a collision your baby's head and spine will be better protected; if he is in a forward-facing seat, any sudden forward movement could seriously damage his weak neck muscles and ligaments.

A baby shouldn't spend more than a couple of hours at a time sitting in a car seat, as the semi-upright position can compress a young baby's chest, which can lead to breathing difficulties and damage his developing spine.

Safety standards

When purchasing a new car seat, ensure it conforms to British and European Safety Standards ECE R44.03 or R44.04. Choose a seat with a five-point safety harness, which offers optimum safety, and follow the manufacturer's instructions when installing and using it.

There is also a new group of car seats, known as "i-size" car seats, being introduced across Europe, which bases the size of the car seat on a child's height rather than his weight. These car seats have been through rigorous safety tests and are designed to keep your baby facing to the rear of your car for longer; with the current weight-based system, parents can be tempted to place their child in a forward-facing car seat at around nine months old.

INFANT CAR SEAT GUIDELINES

Car seats are classified into groups based on your baby's weight. Your child will move into the next car seat group when he has reached the weight limit for his seat, or his eye line is level with the top of the seat.

WEIGHT	DESCRIPTION
Group 0	Infants up to 10kg (22lb), around 6–9 months of age. Allows newborns to lie completely flat. Useful for premature babies and long car journeys.
Group 0+	Infants up to 13kg (29lb), around 12–15 months of age. Equipped with a handle for you to carry it.
Group 0+ & Group 1 combination	Infants up to 13kg (29lb), around 12–15 months of age. Keeps your baby facing to the rear until 15 months old, when it can changed to be forward-facing.

Car seat This is an essential piece of equipment, and because of strict safety regulations it should be bought new.

There are plenty of practical ways in which you can prepare for the arrival of your baby (see below). By getting things in order now, you'll feel more at ease and ready for the first few weeks.

Get ahead of the game

With all eyes on the main event, it can be easy to overlook the more practical considerations of how you will cope once your baby has made his appearance. However, it's most definitely worth putting some preparation and thought in now so you can make life as easy as possible after the birth, when you will find that caring for your new baby takes up a surprising amount of your time with little opportunity to attend to other matters.

ORGANIZE YOUR HOME LIFE

If you find yourself having sudden urges to clean the house, for example, go with it – it's all part of your nesting instinct. But don't forget to take some time for yourself now, too, and consider practical and emotional support from family and friends once your baby arrives.

Line up support

Many new parents find support and help from family and friends invaluable in the early weeks after the birth. You will probably be exhausted and interrupted nights can come as a bit of a shock. Anything that can lighten the load will be appreciated. If you are expecting twins, or you are having a planned C-section, you will need additional help such as having a close relative to stay, using a maternity nurse or a doula. Discuss how your partner will use his paternity leave.

Meet friends

Another important source of support after the birth will be other new parents – and a crucial mental boost at a time when you are adjusting to an entirely different routine. If you belong to an antenatal group, make sure you have contact details for the other mothers. Once your babies arrive, you will be very busy and it can be easier to stick to pre-arranged dates. Meeting up can help you feel connected and supported.

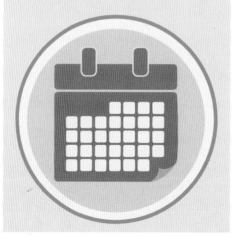

Rest & relax

It may not feel like getting organized for your baby's arrival, but taking a little time for a treat now can help you relax, increase your sense of wellbeing, and generally put you in a good place mentally and physically for your new baby. Whether it's lunch with friends, a relaxing pedicure or massage, or a cinema date with your partner, make the most of your free time now. Schedule a little treat for yourself, especially if it's something that will require much more organizing after the birth.

If you find towards the end of pregnancy that you have a sudden **burst of energy** to scrub the house thoroughly from top to bottom, put this down to a **primal nesting instinct** thought to stem from a need to **prepare for** and **protect** your new arrival.

Tidy your home

A well-documented phenomenon, the desire to clean, organize, and "nest" can take hold of many an expectant mother. It's fine to sort the house out now; having a thorough dust and clean will be one less thing to worry about when your baby arrives, and should make your environment more relaxing and enjoyable. Use eco-friendly cleaning products where you can so you don't inhale hazardous fumes. You may also want to store away clothes you won't wear until the next season to create more room in your wardrobe, or file paperwork, for example. However, be sensible and don't overdo it. And if you don't get everything organized just so, try not to fret.

Get cooking

Spend some time rustling up a few nutritious home-cooked meals for the freezer to enjoy in the weeks after the birth. First-time parents are often surprised by just how much time a new baby takes up; you may be too exhausted to spend time cooking. This will reduce the temptation to resort to unhealthy, convenience foods, and help to ensure you eat a nutritious diet while breastfeeding. Label and date items so you can keep track of what needs eating when. Have a look through your freezer and storecupboards too, and stock up on supplies. Consider setting up an online food shopping account if you don't have one already.

A QUICK CHECKLIST

Make your own checklist to refer to and tick off the tasks as they are done. You might like to include some of the following:

CLOTHES AND EQUIPMENT
» Look through everything you have bought and check that it is all there.
» Wash new clothes, muslins, and bed linen using non-biological powder.
» Pack some baby clothes in your hospital bag along with your own supplies.
» Make sure you know how the sterilizing unit works.
» Test out the pushchair.
» Fit the car seat.

GOING TO HOSPITAL
» Make sure you are familiar with the route.
» Check you have the right change for parking, if needed.
» Ask if you need a pass when you arrive.
» Check that your hospital bag is packed and ready to go.
» Make sure you have contact details of friends and family.

HOME LIFE
» Make a list of chores that will need to be done.
» Discuss with your partner how to split tasks when your baby has arrived.
» If you have other children, make a plan for what will happen to them when you go into hospital.
» Stock the freezer and store cupboard with nutritious food.
» Buy files in which to store bills and post that require a response.
» Get up to date on bills.

>> In this chapter...

Labour and birth

As labour and birth draw nearer, so does the day that you will finally meet your baby. It's natural to feel nervous, but the information in this chapter will help give you the **confidence to feel empowered** for what lies ahead. Find out about the early signs of labour, the different **stages of labour**, the best positions for each stage, and the role of a birth partner. Learn about **pain relief** and how to have a natural birth, or what to expect if you have a C-section or assisted delivery.

By the time you reach around 36 weeks of pregnancy, the prospect of **meeting your baby is tantalizingly close**. Your midwife will begin to note how she is positioned in your uterus, whether or not her **head is engaged**, and find out your wishes for your labour. Your body could also start to give you signs that your baby will soon be here.

Before labour begins

Time and space

During the last four weeks of your pregnancy, your baby grows rapidly – at a rate of about 225g (8oz) per week. The space within your uterus becomes restricted and you may feel that your baby is now squirming around rather than kicking. Keep note of the movements, and if your baby "sleeps" for longer than you would expect, or her movements are weaker or less frequent than is normal for her, call the hospital immediately. Your midwife will pay special attention to the size of your tummy over these last few weeks, to check whether your baby has plenty of amniotic fluid surrounding her and to make final predictions on the baby's size at birth.

The midwife will also work out, by palpating your abdomen, what position your baby is in. The presses may seem firm and even cause you discomfort at this stage, but don't worry as they don't harm your baby. Your midwife may be trying to nudge her into a better position, or to establish whether or not her head has engaged (see p.202), and if it has, how deeply engaged it is.

Talking about labour

During these last few weeks, you'll find that conversations with your midwife will turn to labour. You'll have the opportunity to go over your birth plan (see pp.88–89), and to raise any remaining queries. If your baby is in a breech position, or positioned across your abdomen, your midwife will talk through the implications for your labour and you'll be encouraged to discuss these with your birth partner. Remember that labour is a constantly evolving situation, so the more information you can gather now, the more confident you'll be about any decision you might have to make while you're in the delivery room.

Watching and waiting

Many women spend the last few weeks of their pregnancy eagerly watching for signs that labour might be imminent and even trying myriad old wives' tales to get the process started. Your remarkable, pregnant body is responsive to all sorts of chemical changes right now – and these can have quite surprising effects on your behaviour, mood, and wellbeing. Try to keep yourself distracted – engage in non-strenuous activities that require your concentration. Read the book that you've been meaning to try; teach yourself to knit, sew, or crochet; plant some herb pots; spend an afternoon watching movies. Don't over-exert yourself, but do try to keep busy and keep your mind off the looming question of "When?" And ignore all comments in the vein of "Still no sign, then?" Just smile and change the subject.

Q My antenatal notes tell me what position my baby is in, but what does this mean and why is it important?

The skeleton of your pelvic region is remarkably flexible, but your baby's position can influence how easy it is for her to get through the pelvic bones and under the pubic arch when the time comes. In an ideal world, your baby's position will allow the smallest point of her head to come out first, and with enough space to bend her neck, and fold in her shoulders.

PRESENTATION POSITIONS

Your baby could be lying in the uterus vertically (known as longitudinal), horizontally (transverse), or diagonally (oblique). If lying vertically, the part the baby "presents" towards your cervix can vary.

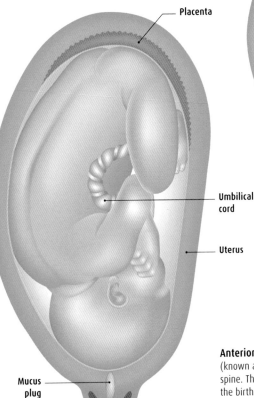

Placenta

Umbilical cord

Uterus

Mucus plug

Posterior presentation Also head downward, but your baby's spine is against your spine. From here, the baby needs to make a bigger turn as she descends through the birth canal, so labour can take longer.

Breech presentation A baby who is breech presents feet or bottom first. There are three possible breech positions – complete, frank, and footling (see p.200).

Anterior presentation Your baby is lying head down (known as cephalic) and her spine is facing away from your spine. The smallest part of your baby's head will push down the birth canal first (this is known as a vertex position). A lateral presentation (spine facing to the side) is also good.

Oblique lie If a baby is lying diagonally across the uterus, the position is called oblique. It's highly unusual for a baby to remain in this position right up until labour. Only one per cent of babies will be transverse or oblique.

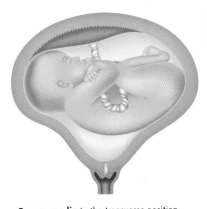

Transverse lie In the transverse position, your baby is lying straight across your uterus horizontally. The angle means the baby's body doesn't present towards the cervix.

Q How does the position of the baby affect my experience of labour?

Your baby must both descend and rotate through the birth canal to be born (see pp.214–15). In anterior or lateral cephalic presentation (vertex positions), the smallest part of the head leads the way and the baby can manoeuvre quite easily, helping to keep your labour relatively short and trouble-free. In the posterior position, a wider part of the head presents first and the baby needs to rotate more to make her descent, making labour progress more slowly. More rarely, it may mean that the baby gets stuck. Labour isn't necessarily more painful in these circumstances, but for your baby it can become distressing. If your midwife feels that labour is taking too long and the baby shows signs of stress, he or she will call an obstetrician for a second opinion. Depending upon the circumstances, you may be offered an assisted delivery or, if necessary, a Caesarean section. Babies in the transverse and oblique positions during labour are quite likely to need a Caesarean section.

37 weeks

Your baby is considered **full term** at 37 weeks. If you reach 41 to 42 weeks, you are likely to be offered induction to start your labour.

Q I'm 36 weeks pregnant and my baby is breech. Should I worry?

There's still time for your baby to turn – some babies change position up until days before birth – but your medical team will discuss your options with you.

Most babies have turned into a head-down, vertex position by 34 weeks pregnant, but it's also perfectly normal for a baby to move and swing round a few days before birth, and even during labour itself. It's an evolving process. If the baby hasn't turned by 36 weeks, your midwife will offer to try manually turning your baby with a technique called external cephalic version (ECV).

If successful, this can help avoid a Caesarean section. You will also be referred to an obstetrician to discuss the pros and cons of vaginal delivery versus Caesarean section so that you can make a fully informed decision in the event that your baby stays in a breech position. Not every situation will be the same, partly because there are three possible breech positions (shown below).

Complete (flexed) breech In this bottom-downward position the baby's legs are flexed and he is curled up, knees and chin to chest, and with ankles crossed.

Frank (extended) breech Both the baby's legs are extended so that his feet stick upward, and his bottom presents first. He might be hugging his knees.

Footling breech This baby presents his foot first: both knees are bent, but one foot is extended downwards, pressing against the cervix.

Q Can I turn a breech baby myself, or will a doctor have to do it?

If you are past 36 weeks pregnant, you should be offered an external cephalic version (ECV). This non-invasive technique involves a trained healthcare professional pressing hard on your abdomen to try to push the baby round into the cephalic (head-down) position. It's a perfectly safe procedure for both of you, and works in around half of all cases, but it may feel a bit uncomfortable at the time. If it works, ECV greatly lowers the risk of Caesarean section. If you want to help things along at home, some

mums report that adopting certain positions to "tip" the baby out of the pelvis can help give it more room to move. You could try either kneeling forward on the floor with one cheek resting on the floor and your bottom in the air, or lying on your back with a pillow beneath your hips to raise them, knees bent, feet flat on the floor. While there is no research evidence to suggest that these techniques will necessarily work, they won't harm your baby either. Just be careful you don't hurt your back or neck in the process. You can also try moxibustion, which advocates of traditional Chinese medicine believe can turn the baby. Acupuncture is also a popular therapy to try.

Q If my baby isn't lying head down, will I definitely have to have a Caesarean section?

Although Caesarean sections are often considered the safest option for breech babies, sometimes a vaginal birth is possible. If your baby presents bottom first, is of average size, and you have an average-sized pelvis, your midwife may be happy to allow a vaginal delivery, if that is your preference. If the baby presents with foot or knee first, Caesarean section is usually advised as the safer option.

Only around 3.5 per cent of births are breech (bottom downwards). A trained professional may try to turn your baby into a vertical position using ECV (see below, left), during the last few weeks of your pregnancy if he himself isn't showing signs of making the turn. If your baby is transverse (lying across your uterus), however, unless the baby can be turned manually, you will probably need to have a Caesarean section.

Q Will I be able to have a normal experience of labour if my baby is in a breech position?

Yes. The early stage of labour is more or less the same for both vertex and breech births, but you're likely to be monitored more frequently if your baby is breech. You can still move around, but your midwife may need you to remain attached to a fetal heart monitor, which would limit your movements a bit. Ask if there are any portable methods for monitoring the baby, and make a decision based on your midwife's advice. Keep emptying your bladder during your labour – every two hours or so – in order to give your baby as much space as possible to move into a good position for birth.

Remember to **monitor your baby's movements** in the uterus. Reporting changes in the **pattern of behaviour** to your midwife immediately could prevent a stillbirth.

Q I'm so huge I feel like I must be close now. Are there signs that can tell me if my labour could start before too long?

Even before you experience the symptoms of actually going into labour, if you know what to look for, you could notice your body signalling that labour is only weeks or days away.

This table describes some of the most reliable indications that your labour is approaching. The signs are organized from the very earliest possible indications at the top, to those symptoms that you should call your midwife or hospital about at the bottom. Remember that it's impossible to be prescriptive about the character of every woman's

labour, and even signs that seem genuine may stop and start, while others may not appear at all. Listen to your body, but reassure yourself that labour is impossible to miss – you'll know when it's happening! If you're at all worried or unsure, never hesitate to call your midwife, who can offer you reassurance and guidance as necessary.

EARLY SIGNS OF APPROACHING LABOUR

SIGN OF LABOUR	SYMPTOMS	HOW SOON WILL I MEET MY BABY?	ACTION
Nesting	An uncontrollable urge to clean, tidy, shop, make; a burst of energy; an overwhelming urge to protect your bump and other family members.	Could be days or weeks.	Try not to overdo it, and make sure that every energy burst is followed with quality rest; eat little and often, and drink plenty; keep an eye out for other labour signs.
Lightening	A feeling of being able to breathe more deeply yet increased pressure on your bladder and/or pelvic pressure.	Could be days or weeks.	Let your midwife know about this feeling at your next antenatal appointment; he or she will assess your baby's position.
Sleeplessness	Difficulty sleeping despite being tired; waking in the night; alarming dreams.	Could be days or weeks.	See pages 114–15 for advice on getting more and better quality sleep.
Practice contractions/ Braxton Hicks	Erratic tightening across the abdomen; tummy feels rigid when you touch it; discomfort but not pain.	More numerous practice contractions, or Braxton Hicks contractions, as you approach your due date can certainly indicate that your body is preparing for labour, but there's no need to assume that labour might be imminent.	If you're worried, unsure, or have any bright red bleeding or abdominal pain, or if you think your waters have broken (see p.206), call your midwife. Don't be anxious about possibly raising a false alarm.
Lower back pain	A dull, persistent ache across the lower portion of your back.	Lower back pain close to your due date can be a sign that your cervix is beginning to dilate; labour may be a few days away, or perhaps less.	Call the hospital if back pain is accompanied by abdominal pain or cramping, or a show (see p.206); take one or two paracetamol tablets for pain relief; distract yourself with a warm bath or other calming activity.
Diarrhoea or feeling sick	Loose or runny stools, and persistent urge to go to the loo; waves of nausea or even being sick.	No one is sure why – perhaps it is due to a hormone surge or your baby pressing against the bowel – but many women feel sick or have loose stools in the days before they go into active labour. Make sure you have everything ready, but your baby may still be a few days away.	Keep hydrated and eat little and often; call the hospital if you have diarrhoea or vomiting that persists for more than 24 hours.

Q My tummy keeps going hard and I get a tightening sensation. Is this a contraction?

You could be experiencing "practice" contractions, also known as Braxton Hicks (after the English doctor who first noted them). If the tightening sensations are short-lived and last no

longer than a minute, if they come and go without any clear pattern, but are perhaps particularly strong after you've done something strenuous, if they are uncomfortable, but not really painful and if you have no other signs of labour (see p.206), the chances are you're having "practice" contractions, rather than those of active labour. These are thought to be present throughout pregnancy, getting gradually more

noticeable and more frequent as you reach full term. You'll probably really start to notice them in the last three or four weeks. Although they are popularly thought to help the uterus tone up for real contractions, some researchers believe that in later pregnancy they begin the process of effacement – when your cervix begins to open and draw upward, becoming part of the smooth muscle of the wall of your uterus.

Q Are there any natural ways to bring on labour?

Anecdotally, there are various "natural" ways to induce labour. However, there is not enough scientific evidence to confirm that they are genuinely effective at starting off birth. Still, as long as your pregnancy has been complication-free, you are full term, and you have no reason to believe your baby could become distressed, they can be worth a go. Tell your midwife if you intend to try any of these methods.

>> Meditation and hypnosis: when you're stressed or anxious, your body releases adrenalin, which signals to your brain that now would not be a good time to give birth. In turn, this inhibits the release of oxytocin, the hormone that starts your labour. Meditation and hypnosis can help you relax, in turn removing the neurological barriers to oxytocin release.

>> Having sex: it's said that the contractions of the uterus during an orgasm can act as a catalyst for bringing on labour contractions, while the intimacy of sex itself, and of being close to someone you love and trust, releases the hormone oxytocin. Furthermore, some say that the prostaglandins (chemical messengers) in semen can soften the cervix to trigger the start of labour. Don't have sex if your waters have broken, though, as you are at increased risk of infection.

>> Nipple massage: gently rubbing your nipples and rolling them between your thumb and forefinger can release oxytocin. The aim is to simulate the action of a baby sucking on your breast, so you'll need to be methodical if you are to use this approach. Just as a breastfeeding baby would feed from one breast for 20 minutes or so, and then the other, and every few hours, for the best effects you need

to do the same. It can take up to 72 hours to have the necessary effect on your body to induce labour – so you will need to be dedicated to the cause to make this worthwhile!

>> Acupuncture: in this form of traditional Chinese medicine a qualified acupuncturist inserts tiny needles into your body along "meridians" – energy lines that interconnect to trigger certain effects throughout the physical body. Some women swear by acupuncture for induction of labour, but there is no rigorous scientific evidence that says it works. If you want to give it a go, aim to find a practitioner who is experienced in treating pregnant women, and talk to your midwife first.

>> Homeopathy: there is no firm evidence that homeopathy works for inducing labour. If you want to try a homeopathic remedy, though, make sure you consult a registered homeopath with experience of treating pregnant women. You should always talk to your midwife first.

>> Spicy foods: curries and chilli dishes stimulate your digestion and create "heat" in your body. Many women claim that the activity in the intestine and bowel has helped to bring on labour. There's no harm in giving it a go (apart, perhaps, from an increased risk of heartburn and indigestion!).

>> Fresh pineapple: pineapple stimulates your digestion (this time because it contains a digestive enzyme called bromelain), which some claim can help stimulate the uterus to begin contracting. However, it takes a lot of pineapple to raise the levels of bromelain in your system for any effect – several whole pineapples – so you are probably more likely to end up with an upset tummy in the next 24 hours than delivering your baby.

>> Herbal remedies: there are some herbs that are said to help bring on labour. These include black cohosh and evening primrose oil. Never use any herbal remedy without the expert advice from a herbalist trained in pregnancy and labour, and always talk to your midwife first.

>> Raspberry leaf tea: while evidence does suggest that raspberry leaf stimulates the action of the uterus, medically it is discouraged for the induction of labour because overstimulating the uterus can cause distress for the baby.

Q What does it mean for the baby's head to "engage"?

Known colloquially as "dropping", a baby engages when the widest part of her head has descended into the cavity in your pelvic bones (the pelvic inlet).

Engagement isn't something that happens in a single moment, but over time – usually starting between 34 and 36 weeks pregnant. It can take several weeks for a baby slowly and methodically to move herself into position. Other times, the baby will wait until labour has actually begun, allowing your contractions to provide the push she needs finally to make the move down into the pelvic

cavity. A large baby, multiple babies, fibroids in your uterus, or a badly placed placenta are all reasons why engagement might take longer. How soon or late the baby's head engages doesn't indicate when you'll go into labour or how quick your labour will be. A baby who engages at 32 weeks is no more likely to make a speedy entry into the world than one who waits until labour has started.

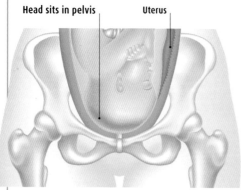

Head sits in pelvis   Uterus

Before engagement Your baby's head hovers freely above your pelvis and she is able to turn and swing around.

Cervix   Pelvic inlet

After engagement Your baby's head lies within the cavity of your pelvic bones, which can offer relief for your lungs, but you may feel your baby bearing down on your pubic bones.

Q I have reached my due date and my medical team is talking about inducing my labour. What does this mean?

Induction means artificially kick-starting labour, and it will be offered if you reach 41 weeks pregnant. After 42 weeks the placenta becomes less efficient and the risk of stillbirth increases, so induction is often recommended before that point.

Your healthcare providers will explain to you why it is appropriate to consider induction in your case, and the options available. Even if you are 41 or 42 weeks pregnant, you can request to "wait it out", but the associated risks will be discussed so that you can make an informed decision about what's best for you. If you decide you're happy for intervention to get your labour started, your midwife will begin by suggesting a cervical "sweep". Your midwife can perform the sweep at a normal antenatal appointment; she or he will insert an index finger into your vagina and make a circular, sweeping motion beyond your cervix, around the wall of your uterus, with the aim of separating the two membranes that surround the baby. This can provide the hormonal stimulation your body needs for your cervix to start softening and labour to start naturally within the next week or so. Around half of all women who have a sweep will go into labour within two days. The procedure may be repeated if you haven't gone into labour within a week. If a cervical sweep is unsuccessful, medical induction will be suggested.

MEDICAL INDUCTION METHODS

If a sweep didn't work to start your labour, your midwife will explain the medical methods available and the reasons why they are suitable for you (or not, as the case may be).

	WHAT IS IT?	WHEN AND HOW?	SUCCESS
Prostaglandin	Prostaglandin is a naturally occurring hormone that triggers the softening of the cervix. A gel or pessary containing the hormone is inserted the vagina, or you may be offered it in tablet form.	A midwife will administer the gel, pessary, or tablet in hospital. You will be asked to go home and wait. If after having gel or a tablet labour hasn't started within six hours, you'll be asked to return for a repeat dose. Two dosages is the maximum you can have. If you have had a pessary, you will be asked to return after 24 hours.	Studies show that if your cervix was already softening, a prostaglandin induction can start labour within 24 hours of treatment.
Membrane rupture	Also known as ARM (artificial rupture of membranes) and amniotomy, this technique involves a midwife deliberately breaking your waters to kick-start the labour process.	You'll be offered this if you have not had a successful prostaglandin attempt. You will usually need to be in hospital because rupturing your membranes increases the risk of infection. Your midwife will use a special hook, called an amniohook, to puncture the amniotic sac in two places, in the lower part and in the upper part.	There is no guarantee of success. However, used with oxytocin, studies show that women will generally go into labour within 24 hours of membrane rupture.
Oxytocin	This is the hormone that your body produces when it feels your baby pressing down on your cervix, and it starts labour off.	Oxytocin is the most common form of labour induction used in the UK today. It's most likely that it will be administered through an intravenous drip. Your midwife will suggest oxytocin if prostaglandin gels haven't been successful.	If this last step in the induction process hasn't worked you will be asked to consider a Caesarean section.

Q I can suddenly breathe more easily – has my baby moved position? Is that a bad sign?

If you're approaching your due date, it's more likely to be a good sign. To prepare for birth, your baby makes a descent into the lowest part of your pelvis – this is called "lightening" (or sometimes "dropping") because it "lightens" the pressure in your abdomen. The effect of your baby dropping into position is that your lungs suddenly have more space to expand, which means you can breathe more easily again.

On the flip side, you might find that the new position puts more pressure on your bladder, and you need the bathroom more often.

Q I've heard an induced labour can be more painful. Is this true?

When you go into natural labour, signals to your brain mean that your body releases endorphins, hormonal painkillers that help you to cope with labour and birth. In an induced labour, your body hasn't had the natural run-up that makes sure you have good levels of circulating endorphins from the earliest, imperceptible beginnings of labour. As a result, many women report that an induced labour is more painful than one that occurs naturally. However, try not to worry – being induced doesn't place any restrictions on the pain relief that is available to you, so ask your medical team about the options if you feel things are getting too much. Statistics show that women having an induced labour are more likely to ask for an epidural. Your baby is also slightly more likely (about 15 per cent more likely) to need an assisted birth (see p.222).

Labour is a process, a series of changes that will finally bring your baby into your arms. Although clinically there are signs, phases, and markers, **each woman's labour is different** from another's. If this is your second or subsequent baby, the experience will be unlike your previous ones – it's **unique and remarkable**.

Being in labour

Understanding the big event

Your midwife and doctors will refer to labour as having three stages. The first stage is usually the longest, beginning with the first contractions and sometimes a "show" (see p.206) that indicates your cervix has started to open, and lasting until your cervix is fully dilated. The second stage is characterized by the act of pushing your baby down the birth canal and out into the world. The third stage refers to the delivery of the placenta and membranes. It's always helpful to be aware of the terms your carers will use, but in practice labour is really just a single event that begins with a few niggling signs and ends with the emergence of your baby.

Listen to your body

Referring to labour in clinical terms – stages, centimetres, and time spans – while helpful for your medical staff, isn't really what labour is about for you. This is a magical time: the start or expanding of a family, the beginning of new life, and a time when your body performs the most natural, fundamental, and significant event. Many women worry about labour – will they "cope" with it, will they be "good" at it, will labour follow the clinical patterns they have read so much about? It's helpful to remember that clinical markers are not "rules" and there isn't one set way to give birth – try not to focus on what stage you're in, whether you are 2cm (¾in) or 9cm (3½in) dilated, or how many hours your baby has shown signs of coming. Instead, concentrate on listening to your body, responding to its signals (don't worry – they will be obvious), and focusing on the baby that you will soon be able to hold. Remain as calm as you can and stay warm. Stress inhibits the release of oxytocin, which is the hormone that triggers your contractions. Walk around if it makes you feel more at ease, or sit or stand, or lean over a birthing ball. There is no rule that says you must lie in a bed. If you need to be hooked up to a monitor for medical reasons, you can still stand or sit on a chair or ball and let gravity give you a helping hand. Make this an event that feels right for you.

Q What can I expect to happen during labour? How long is it likely to last?

As your body enters into labour and prepares to give birth to your baby, it will go through a sequence of events and stages. While no two labours are the same, this progress of labour does follow a pattern that helps the medical staff to monitor you, and encourages you that your baby is on his way.

Leaning over a birthing ball This can help you feel more at ease and comfortable during labour.

ENGAGEMENT

Towards the end of pregnancy, your baby's head drops down into the lowest part of the pelvis, or engages (see p.202), to prepare for labour and delivery. Engagement tends to happen earlier in first pregnancies, when uterine muscles that have never been stretched before can exert greater pressure to push the baby down into the pelvis.

Time it takes This sign of approaching labour can happen from several weeks before labour in first pregnancies to just as labour starts in subsequent pregnancies.

Action Your midwife will palpate your abdomen from about 36 weeks to find out whether your baby's head is engaged.

1ST STAGE – ACTIVE LABOUR AND TRANSITION

The second part of the first stage is known as "active labour". You will know it by frequent, strong contractions that are impossible to ignore. The cervix opens more quickly and at 7–9cm (3–3½ in) dilation, the active phase moves into transition, when contractions become more intense and you feel the urge to push. The first stage ends once the cervix is fully dilated, at 10cm (4in).

Time it takes In an average first labour, the cervix dilates about 1cm (½ in) an hour. Active labour can progress much quicker in subsequent labours.

Action Call the hospital when you reach active labour. You will probably be advised to time the contractions and rest at home until the contractions are closer together, about every five minutes and lasting 60 seconds.

3RD STAGE

The third stage marks the delivery of the placenta and membranes after your baby is born. This final stage can be "actively" managed, when an injection of synthetic oxytocin speeds up the delivery of the placenta, or you can deliver the placenta naturally (or "physiologically").

Time it takes An active third stage takes 5–15 minutes; and a physiological third stage takes around 20–30 minutes; these time guides are the same for first and subsequent deliveries.

Action You may need to push a little more to deliver the placenta.

Understanding **how labour works** helps you gauge when to stay at home and when to **call the midwife**.

1ST STAGE – LATENT LABOUR

The first stage of labour opens the cervix. Early labour, known as the "latent" phase, is marked by relatively mild, irregular contractions that start to thin and draw up the cervix, a process known as effacement. Then the cervix begins to dilate and will reach around 3–4cm (1¼–1½in) dilation. The pain is strong but bearable, with period-like cramping.

Time it takes This longest phase can account for as much as two-thirds of the total time of labour. It can last from several hours to a few days in a first labour; it is often much shorter in subsequent labours.

Action You'll usually be encouraged to stay at home during the latent phase. Try to get comfortable, but stay active too.

2ND STAGE

The second stage of labour begins when the cervix is fully dilated and ends with the birth of your baby. This stage is marked by a strong urge to bear down as contractions push your baby against the pelvic floor. Your midwife will support and guide you, encouraging you to push with your contractions.

Time it takes The active, pushing part of delivering your baby takes roughly 1–2 hours for a first labour, with the total second stage taking up to 3 hours. The second stage in subsequent labours often takes 2 hours or less, with 30 minutes to 1 hour needed for pushing.

Action The end is nearly in sight. Draw encouragement from your birth partner and let your midwife guide you.

Q Will I know when I'm about to go into labour? Are there signs, and what should I do if I experience them?

When you are very close to true first stage labour, there are three signs that could appear. It's not guaranteed that you will see them all – some women skip them entirely – but if you do, you should inform your midwife.

It is natural to be concerned about recognizing the signs of early labour, – unsurprisingly, it is a common worry among pregnant women – but the truth is your experience can be quite different from the next woman's. While the symptoms described below do indicate that labour is imminent, for some women active labour (see p.205) could still be a couple of days away, especially if this is their first pregnancy. Getting a

"show" or the first labour contractions indicates that your cervix has started to soften and thin (known as "effacement") in order to open and allow your baby to pass through the birth canal. The length of time this takes can vary greatly, so do listen to your body and time your contractions. If your waters break, they mostly do so once contractions have started; if it happens beforehand for you, do call your midwife.

SIGNS OF IMMINENT LABOUR

	SYMPTOMS	HOW SOON WILL I MEET MY BABY?	ACTION
A "show" (dislodging of the cervical mucus plug)	A brownish or yellowish vaginal discharge, your mucus plug has a jelly-like consistency and may look like congealed, yellowed phlegm, or be tinged dark brown with blood. It may come away in one "blob" or several. Some women never have a show; others pass the plug without noticing while going to the loo.	Even though the dislodging of the mucus plug is a sure sign that your cervix is opening out, active labour could still be a few days away, or even weeks if this is your first baby.	Call your midwife. You will probably be advised to have a relaxing bath or otherwise try to distract yourself, and to look out for first contractions. However, if you have any bright red bleeding, you are feeling unwell, or the baby has not been moving, call your midwife or hospital right away.
Labour contractions	Painful, period-like cramps that begin in the upper portion of your abdomen and spread downwards. Contractions may be irregular and spaced quite far apart at first, becoming more regularly spaced and lasting for one to two minutes each.	These "latent-phase" contractions could indicate that "active labour" is only a few hours (or less) away, but in some cases contractions will be slow and last a few days (at most).	Call your midwife or hospital. If you're going into hospital to give birth, they will probably ask you to stay at home for as long as you feel you can. If you experience any bleeding or your waters break, go to hospital or call your midwife to come to you.
Breaking waters (rupture of membranes)	This may happen as a gush or a trickle – amniotic fluid looks a lot like pale urine, so you may think you have stress incontinence.	Your baby's arrival may still be a few days away, but now that the amniotic sac has broken, your baby is at risk of infection, so will need to be delivered sooner rather than later.	Call your midwife or hospital straightaway for advice. As your baby is now at risk of infection, you will need to be carefully monitored. You should not lie in a bath, in case of infection. If the amniotic fluid is greenish in colour, go to the hospital right away (it could be meconium, a fetal bowel movement).

Q I've had a "show". Does this mean I'm in the first stage of labour?

If the show is accompanied by irregular contractions, yes, you are probably in the first "latent" stage. However, by itself, losing your mucus plug is not an indication that the first stage of labour has started, it's simply a sign that things are moving in the right direction. It's definitely time to start watching out for more certain labour signs, especially contractions that build in intensity over time.

Q I think I'm in early labour and I feel sick. Should I eat?

Giving birth to a baby is a hugely energetic event, and your body will need lots of fuel. Do try to eat if you can. The latent phase of first stage labour, when contractions are not very frequent and you are still comfortable moving around, is the best time to eat sustaining food that will keep you going through the more intense phases of labour. Foods that release energy slowly – such as wholewheat pasta,

wholemeal bread, oats, eggs, and beans – are ideal. A snack of wholemeal toast and honey, for instance, would be a good choice and is usually easy to manage. If you feel too sick to eat a meal, think back to those snacks that got you through pregnancy sickness all those months ago. Eat energy-rich, bland-tasting (and -smelling) snacks, little and often. Potatoes, rice, pasta, and couscous are all bland-tasting but full of nutrients. Unroasted, skinned almonds are an energy-rich snack. And remember to keep hydrated and drink lots of water (taking frequent tiny sips if that's all you can manage).

Q I've seen the movies – what if my waters break in the supermarket?

Labour is unpredictable, but you might be reassured to know that around 85 per cent of women experience membrane rupture only when fully dilated, at the start of the second stage of labour. So you would be very unlucky to have a sudden supermarket incident in early labour. Moreover, membrane rupture is often just a slow trickle, so you should be able to get to the loo to check with no one else being any the wiser. The further down your pelvis your baby's head is, the less fluid you will lose if your waters break. This is because the position of your baby forces most of the amniotic fluid into a sort of liquid "bubble" above his body.

That's not to say that a gush of amniotic fluid in the first stage isn't possible. If it happens in a public place, ask for help, find somewhere to sit, and call your hospital or midwife - you will need to be checked over, as your baby will no longer be protected from infection.

Q How should I time my contractions?

Time both the duration of your contractions, and the gap of time between them. Begin timing a contraction from the first moment of tightening at the top of your tummy (the "fundus"); the contraction grows in strength and becomes more painful, pushing your baby downwards. The tightening and pain should seem to move towards the lower part of the abdomen, and gradually ease - this "softer" part of the contraction helps to open out the lower part of your uterus and draw up your cervix. When the pain subsides to its weakest point, your contraction is over. Note how many seconds have passed. Also make a note of the time, as now you need to measure how long it is until your next contraction starts.

Q Do I need a stopwatch to time my contractions?

No - a simple second hand on an ordinary watch will do. If you have a smartphone, there are now some really good, free apps that will do all the work for you. Download a couple and see which you find easiest to operate; your birth partner can try them out, too.

Q What is happening when I have a contraction?

The muscles of your uterus are squeezing (or "contracting"); firstly to help open your cervix at the bottom, and then to push your baby downwards for birth.

In early labour, or the first stage's latent phase, you can feel contractions in the lower part of your uterus. They feel similar to strong period pains and start the process of opening your cervix. Later, in active labour, contractions become much stronger and begin from the top of the uterus (the fundus) and travel downwards. These contractions open the cervix much more quickly, and work to push your baby towards the cervix. The squeezing contractions briefly stop blood supply to the uterus; in the breaks between contractions, your baby is kept supplied with oxygen, but you may feel some residual pain.

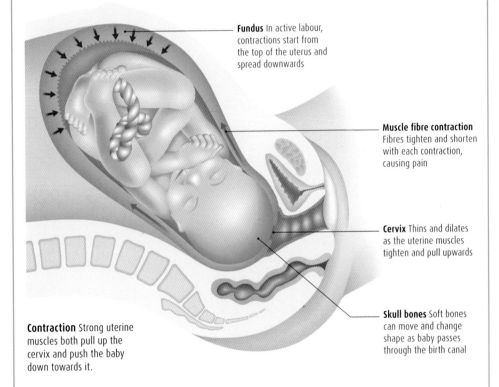

Fundus In active labour, contractions start from the top of the uterus and spread downwards

Muscle fibre contraction Fibres tighten and shorten with each contraction, causing pain

Cervix Thins and dilates as the uterine muscles tighten and pull upwards

Skull bones Soft bones can move and change shape as baby passes through the birth canal

Contraction Strong uterine muscles both pull up the cervix and push the baby down towards it.

HOW CONTRACTIONS BUILD IN FREQUENCY

At the start of labour, contractions are 15–30 seconds long, coming every 20–30 minutes. Gradually, contractions last longer, intensify, and become more frequent.

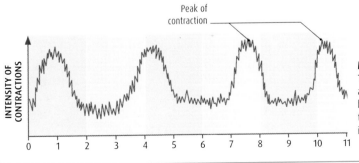

Peak of contraction

INTENSITY OF CONTRACTIONS

0 1 2 3 4 5 6 7 8 9 10 11

Maternal contractions These regular contractions are typical of a normal labour. As revealed by the trace, they gradually increase in intensity.

{Q} What is my role as the birth partner?

Studies show that women who are the least anxious during labour are most likely to have the shortest, easiest, and most positive birthing experience. Birth partners can play a key role in helping mum-to-be to remain as calm as possible, through practical help and keeping her emotionally supported during labour, and by staying calm themselves and hiding any anxiety.

How does staying calm help my partner's labour?

As your partner's contractions intensify, her brain releases endorphins, natural chemicals that boost her pain threshold and help her to cope with labour. Conversely, if your partner feels anxious, her body releases adrenaline, signalling to the brain that danger is present. The body then decides this is not a good moment to give birth and inhibits the release of endorphins and oxytocin, the hormone that controls contractions, which can in turn stall her labour.

What are the best ways to help my partner?

There are plenty of ways to keep your partner comfortable and motivated (see box, below), but two of the most important

things, from which all other practical tips stem, are to be informed about labour, and to know her preferences for labour, birth, and after the delivery. Reading up on labour (how it progresses and how your partner may feel at different points), and attending antenatal classes with your partner towards the end of pregnancy will help you to be prepared on the day. If possible beforehand, talk through your partner's birth plan with her so you can advocate for her when she is too tired or preoccupied to ask or answer questions. How she will feel once in labour is an unknown for you both, so be ready to be flexible and react to her responses on the day, whether she wants to be touched and held, or she retreats into her own space, with you close by.

THE BIRTH PARTNER'S ROLE

A continuous source of care from start to finish, a birth partner plays an active role in creating a sense of calm and helps to keep the mum-to-be motivated. Here are some practical ways you can help things go smoothly.

The build-up

» For hospital births, learn about the hospital systems in advance; for a home birth, have everything ready. Have a go at inflating the birthing pool, and know at what point you need to start filling it.
» Know how to use the birthing equipment, such as the TENS machine, a portable entonox machine, or the birthing pool.
» Provide snacks, meals, and drinks for your partner (it's important that she stays hydrated throughout labour).
» Create the atmosphere your partner would like; for example, lower the lighting if she wishes, play music, or light candles.
» Give your partner a relaxing back massage or run her a warm bath if she wishes.

On the move

» Don't go over the alcohol limit in late pregnancy so you can drive safely.
» Be informed about hospital parking (where this is and do you need change).
» Have a taxi firm number at the ready if you don't drive.
» Know where your partner's maternity notes and hospital bag are.
» Be informed about childcare arrangements for older children and implement them when the time comes.
» If a midwife or ambulance is coming to you, make sure the house number is clearly visible.
» Don't cut it fine – leave for the hospital in good time.

During labour

» Breathe with your partner during contractions.
» Support her in upright positions.
» Ask questions if she is offered an intervention so she can make an informed decision: what are pros and cons?
» Make your partner's needs and wishes heard when she is tired or emotional.
» Articulate the medical team's instructions when your partner is too distracted to hear them, and respect their professional opinion.
» Read her non-verbal signals: has she had enough talking/stroking/massaging.
» Reassure, support and encourage her.
» Sponge her face, and offer sips of water.
» Stay nourished and hydrated yourself.

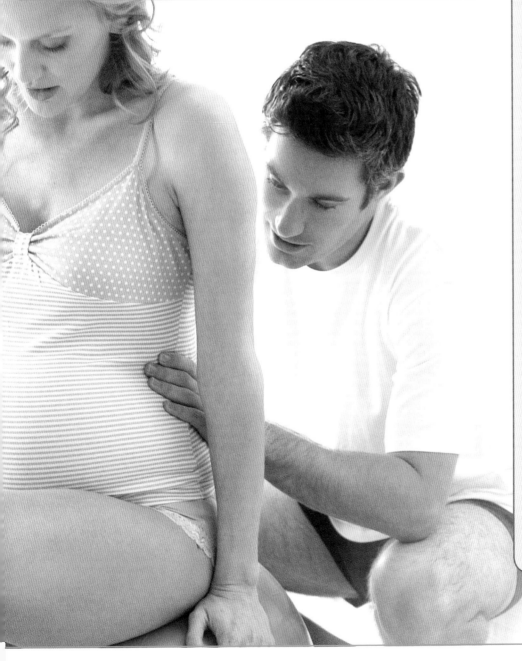

WHEN TO GO TO HOSPITAL OR STAY AT HOME

Timing contractions and helping decide when to go to hospital is a key part of your role.

Your partner may be increasingly preoccupied, which means you may need to judge when to leave for hospital. If contractions are irregular (albeit painful), and she can talk through them, it's best to stay at home. Once contractions are five minutes apart, intense, and last for around 60 seconds, head in. It may sound obvious, but factor in your distance from the hospital, and leave earlier if there's far to go.

CONTRACTION INTERVAL: 2 mins, 3 mins, 5 mins, 10 mins

CONTRACTION DURATION: 30 secs, 60 secs, 90 secs

SUDDEN BIRTH

Very occasionally, labour moves so quickly that there isn't enough time to get to hospital. If you are with your partner and she feels an overwhelming urge to push, you will need to take an active role.

» Help your partner to stay calm. Call the labour ward or 999 so that paramedics can be sent to you.

» Turn up the heating and ask your partner which room she would like to be in, then shut the door to keep the room warm. Gather about four clean towels and two or three blankets. Fold two towels and place them beneath your partner's bottom. Find a plastic bag or container that doesn't have any holes in it for the placenta to be placed in.

The birth itself

» Call 999 again and the operator will stay on the line and advise you. (Speakerphone is useful, as you'll need your hands free.) If you can see the baby's head, support it as it crowns. Check the cord, and if this is compressed around the baby before he is born, untangle it if it is loose enough to do so; if it isn't loose enough to free easily, leave it as it is and unwrap it once the baby is completely out.

» Encourage your partner to push gently with each contraction. Once the head, shoulders, and finally the body are delivered, place the baby on your partner's tummy. Leave the cord intact - it should be long enough for you to put the baby on your partner's abdomen. Dry the baby, then keep him warm with a towel and blanket. Don't pull on the cord and don't try to cut it or clamp it in any way. The cord will continue to pump blood into the baby for 10 minutes or so after the birth, then it will stop pulsating. You can leave it attached even then.

» Your partner will have one or more contractions to deliver the placenta and membranes. This should come out in one piece with the cord and the membranes of the amniotic sac attached. There'll be some bleeding, which is normal. Put the placenta in a plastic bag for the midwife to check. Keep your baby warm, listen to the paramedics, and stay calm.

Soothing touch A lower back massage can be relaxing in the early stages of labour, and may be especially welcome if contractions are causing lower back pain.

Q What are the best birthing positions to adopt during first-stage labour?

A combination of active and restful positions help you to get through first-stage labour. Active positions are thought to encourage the progression of labour and restful, supported positions allow you to have vital respite between contractions.

Follow your **instincts** and decide yourself how you want to **move, sit, or stand** during first-stage labour.

Standing upright in labour encourages your baby to move down, deep into your pelvis, and to press against your cervix. This has the effect of sending messages to your brain to release more of the hormone oxytocin, which stimulates further contractions. These become more frequent, longer, and more effective than in other birthing positions, which makes labour shorter than if you were lying down. Walking around also helps your baby to move lower into your pelvis, so labour progresses more quickly. Studies show that staying active in the first stage makes you less likely to ask for pain relief or to need a C-section, and your baby is less likely to become distressed. However, lying down and sitting positions allow you to recover from contractions, but don't stay still for too long as it will slow down your labour.

Walking up and down stairs If you have stairs near you, use them to keep active. Remember to hold on to the bannister for support.

Standing, leaning on a tall chair or stool Use a chair to support your body weight. Place a cushion under your arms for extra comfort.

Standing, leaning on bed Ease back pain by adopting this pose. This particularly helps when your baby is lying with her back against your spine.

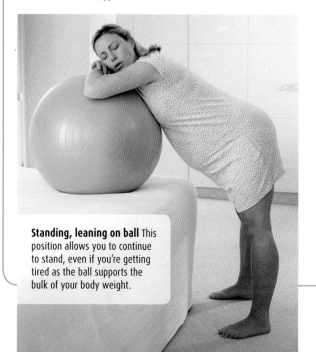

Standing, leaning on ball This position allows you to continue to stand, even if you're getting tired as the ball supports the bulk of your body weight.

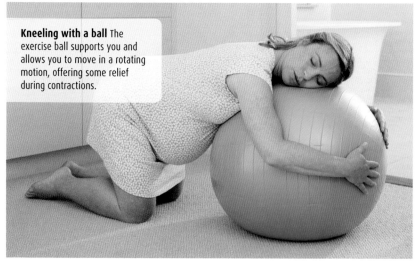

Kneeling with a ball The exercise ball supports you and allows you to move in a rotating motion, offering some relief during contractions.

Sitting, leaning on a laundry basket or stool Rest your body in this position, allowing yourself to build up your strength for the next wave of contractions.

Straddling a chair This will help open your pelvis while allowing you a rest so that you can save energy to cope with the next contraction.

Kneeling, partner support Gain comfort and physical support by kneeling on a bed and embracing your partner.

Standing, leaning forward on partner This position can make you feel close to each other and help you to relax. Your partner can support your body weight.

Side lying Lying on your right or left side can help soothe the pain and help alter your baby's position slightly if your baby is lying back to back.

Semi-prone, fetal back towards the ceiling If you know that your baby is facing right with its back against yours, you can lie on your left side for short spells. Gravity may pull the baby into a more comfortable position.

Q What are the benefits of labouring in water, and are there risks?

Women who labour in water make fewer requests for pain relief. It's thought that this is to do with the calming effect of being in water, because the measured amplitude (intensity) of contractions in fact remains the same in and out of the water. Women who labour in water also find it easier to change position as they are supported by the buoyancy of the water, and are less likely to need an episiotomy. There are no risks that specifically relate to going through your labour in water. Your midwife can monitor the baby's heart rate using a waterproof hand-held heart monitor to make sure your baby shows no signs of distress, and will take appropriate action if she does.

Q When should I get into my birthing pool?

Some experts believe that being in water during the early stages of labour can slow contractions and prolong labour. They advocate getting into the water only once you are 7cms (2¾in) dilated. Others believe that being in water eases pain and promotes relaxation, improving labour. If you are using a pool at a hospital or birthing centre, you will need to follow their protocol. At home, you can decide when to get in and out of the pool. Always make sure the water temperature is never over 37.5°C (99.5°F).

Q I want to lie on a bed, but will this make my labour more painful?

Lying down pushes the lower part of your spine against the baby's head. The added pressure when the baby tries to move past this part of your back and deeper into your pelvis can make labour more painful. Lying on your back also narrows the space that you have for your pelvic bones to separate to allow the baby through, which can increase the pain. Contractions when lying down can be more painful and less effective, lengthening your labour. If you need to lie down, don't lay flat on your back but on your left side. Lying down can be the position that is most useful for your midwife, because he or she can easily examine you. Your baby can be monitored if you are in a sitting position.

Q What does cervical dilation mean and how does it affect my labour?

In pregnancy, the cervix forms a closed, thick muscular base for the uterus. In early labour, it starts to soften, draw up, and thin (efface) and then open (dilate) so that your baby can pass into the vagina to be born.

Your midwife assesses how far and how quickly your labour is progressing by looking to see how much your cervix has thinned, or effaced, and how wide it has opened, or dilated. The width of the dilation is measured in centimetres. These changes begin in early (or latent) labour, but they can happen slowly because the contractions that act on the cervix are irregular at this point. You may feel as if your labour isn't progressing if the cervical width isn't increasing, but the cervix could still

be thinning before opening wider. Dilation can cause the mucus plug to come away from the cervix. Once the cervix has reached 3–4cm (1¼–1½) dilation, it marks your passage from the latent to the active phase of first stage labour. In active labour, contractions become stronger, longer, and more frequent and start to open up, or dilate, the cervix more rapidly. Once the cervix is 10cm (4in) dilated, you are fully dilated and at this point you will feel an urge to push, or bear down.

2cm (¾in) high

2cm (¾in) dilated

fully effaced

6cm (2¼in) dilated

10cm (4in) dilated

At around 2cm dilation The cervix is just beginning to open. This is the early (or latent) part of labour and it's likely that your contractions are still fairly irregular.

At 6cm dilation You are well established in active labour. Your contractions are now strong and regular and increasingly painful, and you may want pain relief now.

At 10cm dilation Your cervix is fully open and, once your midwife gives you the okay, you can start to push. It may feel like contractions are coming continuously now.

Q At what point should I call my midwife?

You can call your midwife as soon as strong, painful contractions begin. Your midwife will ask you questions about your contractions and how you are feeling to assess how your labour is progressing. He or she will also gauge how you are doing from the tone of your voice and how you are responding to contractions. If your contractions are painful but irregular, and you're planning to have your baby at hospital or in a birthing centre, you will probably be encouraged to labour at home for as long as you possibly can, and your carer may suggest that you take a dose of paracetamol and have a warm bath to help you cope with the pain. Studies show that labour progresses better when women are in comfortable and familiar

surroundings, where relaxation and rest support the release of oxytocin, which in turn encourages longer and more frequent contractions. Once your contractions are occurring around every five minutes and lasting at least 60 seconds, it is time to call the hospital once more to let them know you are heading in. If you're having your baby at home, your midwife will probably ask you to call again when your contractions are closer together (say, around 10 to 15 minutes apart) and lasting between 30 and 45 seconds each. Wherever you're having your baby, call your midwife (or hospital) straight away if your waters break, or if you have any bleeding. And do call at any time if you are worried, even if you've already been told to wait. Midwives are very used to reassuring and guiding women in this way the early stage of labour.

Q What happens if my early labour is very slow or it starts and stops?

Labour is never an exact science, and what can be a relatively quick experience lasting only a few hours for one mother can take days for another. It's normal for early labour to start and stop over several days, especially if this is your first baby. The timing of your contractions, and their strength and length, are the key to knowing when you've moved from the latent phase of first stage labour to a more active phase.

Q What if my baby comes quickly and I don't have time to get to hospital?

It is very unusual for this to happen with a first baby. If you do think labour is progressing too quickly for you to move to hospital, try to remain calm. First call your midwife, then either your hospital emergency number or 999 for an ambulance, then your birth partner. If you are on your own and have a friend or family member close by, get them to come over. Gather clean towels, blankets, and a plastic bag, and choose a warm, draught-free room. If you feel the urge to push, you can try to slow things down by adopting a knee-to-chest position to take pressure off the perineum: get down on all fours, rest your forearms on the floor and raise your bottom in the air. If you still feel an urge to push, go with this. Reach down to see if you can feel the baby's head, and once your baby is born, put her straight onto your tummy for warmth, dry her with a clean towel and lay another towel and blanket over her. Leave the cord intact until help arrives. When you feel another urge to push, go with this to deliver the placenta, which you can place in a plastic bag.

Q What will happen when I arrive at hospital?

Once you get to hospital, you can check in to the labour ward. Then depending on whether you appear to be in active labour, either you will be given a labour room, or you will wait on an assessment bed or in a bay so that a midwife can come and check on your progress (see opposite). If your midwife assesses that you are still in early labour, you may be sent home and given advice on when to return.

Q How will my midwife be able to tell how my labour is progressing?

Soon after your midwife arrives at your home, if you're having a home birth, or you arrive at hospital or your birthing centre, you will be checked over for several signs that indicate where you are in your labour journey and your general health. Your midwife will take your temperature and blood pressure (and will continue to check these every four hours throughout your labour), and you might be asked to give a urine sample. Between your contractions, your midwife will give you an abdominal examination to make sure your baby's head is engaged, and to assess his position, known as the "presentation" (see p.199) which indicates how your baby is likely to be born. If your midwife thinks that you are in active labour, he or she may offer you a vaginal examination to confirm this and to see how far your cervix has dilated (see box, opposite). You will be offered a vaginal examination around every four hours during your labour to see how your labour is progressing.

Q Will my baby be monitored during labour?

Your baby's heart rate will be monitored throughout labour to assess her wellbeing. Usually, your baby will be monitored intermittently. The midwife will use a hand-held Doppler device, which he or she will place against your abdomen to pick up your baby's heartbeat. If there are concerns during labour, you will be advised to have continuous monitoring, using a cardiotocograph (CTG) machine, which measures both your baby's heartbeat and the frequency of contractions. Two devices will be attached to your abdomen using straps, which means you will need to stay close to the monitoring machine. The results are printed out on a graph. If at any point your baby appears to be distressed, your medical team may suggest internal monitoring, whereby an electrode attached to a wire is passed through the cervix and placed on your baby's scalp (this doesn't hurt the baby). It is not a routine procedure and the team will always discuss with you first the reasons why it is being recommended to you.

Q Can I start pushing as soon as I feel the urge?

It is important that you wait for your midwife to give you the okay to push before you start to bear down. Towards the end of the first stage, when the cervix is around 7–9cm (3–3½in) dilated, you move into the transition phase (see box, below). You may feel a strong urge to push now, but if you do so before you are fully dilated, the cervix could swell as the baby's head bears down on it before it's ready to give way to let the baby pass through, which can make labour much more difficult. If your midwife thinks it's not yet time to push, you may be asked to take little panting breaths followed by a long, slow exhale, which can relieve your urge to bear down. Or, you may be asked to sit and draw your knees up to your chest, another way to ease the need for pushing. Pain relief, such as an epidural, can also slow things down, but your midwife will judge whether this is a good idea now, or if it is better to keep moving forwards as you are.

Q I've heard of the stages of labour, but what is "transition"?

The term "transition" describes the end of first-stage labour, as your cervix moves towards full dilation, which marks the beginning of second-stage labour.

Physiologically, during transition you may feel a strong downward, aching pressure in your lower back, and a heaviness in your perineum as your baby bears down on your cervix. This releases further hormones that cause your cervix to open that final bit – from around 7cm (3in) to 9–10cm (3½–4in) dilated.

However, rather than being a stage that is mapped by distinct physiological changes, you (and particularly your birth partner and midwife) will know that you have moved into the transition phase of labour because you will undergo some particular behavioural changes, which are listed below.

HOW YOU MIGHT ACT

» **You may start to panic** or become suddenly anxious or fearful.

» **You may appear** disorientated or confused.

» **You may start shouting** or snapping at your birth partner and his or her attempts to calm you.

» **You might demand pain relief** when previously you've been confident that you wanted to have a natural birth.

» **You may say** that you can't go on.

» **You can move "inwards"**, becoming uncommunicative and perhaps dropping in and out of sleepiness (midwives call this the "rest and be thankful" stage).

HOW YOU MIGHT BE FEELING

» **You may feel nauseous** or weak.

» **You may feel shivery**.

» **It may feel like your contractions** are coming more frequently or there is no pause between them.

» **You may feel an urge** to push or bear down.

» **There may be** bloody discharge.

Your birth partner could **learn about the behavioural changes** at this stage so that he or she understands your change in attitude!

Q I know that "second-stage labour" is when my baby is born, but what actually happens during this stage?

While intense, this is possibly the most exciting part of labour as you finally get to meet your baby. Although this stage can be tiring, many women feel encouraged that they can actively start to push their baby out now and that the end is in sight.

The second stage of labour begins when you are fully dilated at 10cm (4in), and ends with the birth of your baby. As the characteristics of transition (see p.213) pass, this signals that the second stage of labour has begun. Along with the waves of contractions, you will feel an unrelenting urge to "bear down" into your perineum (the section of muscle and skin between your anus and your vagina) as your contractions push your baby against the pelvic floor. This bearing down, known as the "Ferguson reflex", means that

your baby has reached the muscles of your pelvic floor. As the baby presses against nerve receptors there, messages flood your brain to let you know that it's time to push the baby out. Once your midwife confirms that you are fully dilated, you can do so. Your uterine muscles get some help from your diaphragm and abdominal muscles now, too: the messages to your brain lower your diaphragm and force your abdominal muscles to contract. Your whole amazing body is working to help your baby through your pelvis.

Twists and turns

Your baby's journey through the birth canal and out into the world involves a series of manoeuvres that are known as "the mechanism of labour". Rather than a straightforward descent down the birth canal and out, in fact, your baby has to make several twists and turns to be able to pass safely through your skeleton. This means that the time it takes for the second stage of your labour to progress is affected both by your baby's position in the birth canal and just how easy it is for her to turn in the

THE BIRTH

As your contractions push your baby downwards, her body rotates to enable her to emerge through the pelvic opening and out through your vagina.

1 **Your baby's body moves down** through your pelvis gradually as your uterus contracts. Your baby's head is tilted down slightly, towards her chest, and her arms and legs are folded inwards, helping her journey through the birth canal.

Intense contractions During the delivery your contractions are strong and frequent

Placenta The placenta remains attached to the wall of your uterus during the delivery

Pubic bones The hormone relaxin allows the joint that unites your left and right pubic bones to soften during delivery, making your pelvis more flexible

Umbilical cord The umbilical cord stretches out as the baby is delivered

Lowering uterus The top of your uterus lowers as your baby is delivered

Baby's body The baby's body faces your spine during delivery

2 **"Crowning"** is the term used to describe when your baby's head emerges. The rest of your baby's body will follow quite quickly as the head is the widest part of your baby and has opened the way for the body to follow.

Baby's fontanelles The fontanelles and sutures between the skull bones allow some manoeuvrability space your pelvis provides. You will feel a sense of satisfaction with every push – you are getting closer to meeting your baby.

Crowning and birth

As labour progresses and your baby's head presses against the pelvic floor, she rotates by about 45 degrees so that her face looks towards your spine. This position enables her to fit her head through your "pubic arch" – a pair of pelvic bones that form an arch. When her head makes it through these bones, your baby "crowns" – her head is out. Crowning can prompt a burning feeling, known as the "ring of fire". At this point, she turns another 45 degrees so that she can fit her shoulders through your pelvis; her head will turn, too. Once the shoulders have made the turn, they, too, emerge into the world, quickly followed by the rest of your baby's body.

Shrinking uterus Your uterus shrinks even more as your baby's body emerges

Baby's head As your baby's head emerges it needs to be supported. Her shoulders quickly follow after her head

3 The rest of your baby's body comes out soon after the head. Her shoulders will come out one after the other, followed quickly by the rest of her body.

Q Are there positions that make it easier for me to give birth?

Some positions naturally open up your pelvis so are more efficient for delivery. Ultimately, the position you choose should be the one you find most comfortable.

The more upright you are in the second stage of labour, the more you have gravity on your side to help with the descent of your baby. One of the most efficient positions to give birth is in the squatting position. This has all the benefits of standing up (see p.211), but also opens out your pelvic bones, creating space for your baby to pass through more easily. Some researchers believe that a woman who labours standing up and gives birth squatting can reduce her labour by up to an hour. If you want to squat during the final stages of your labour, you will need to have strong thighs! Ask your birthing partner to hold you under your armpits to ease the strain on your muscles. Other positions that have the same beneficial effects are resting on all-fours and the kneeling pose. For kneeling, you will need physical support as it requires good balance. If your baby is being monitored, you might have to be on a bed, but follow the guidance from your midwife.

Supported squat Your partner can support you from behind, or you can face him, putting your arms around his neck while he holds you firmly under your arms.

Kneeling on all-fours You can try doing this on top of a bed or on the floor. In this position, your birth partner can give support and gently massage your back.

Q How long will it take to push my baby out?

This partly depends upon whether or not this is your first baby. First babies may take up to three hours from the start of the second stage of labour to be born, whereas second babies can take up to two hours or less. The position of your baby within your pelvis will also affect how long she takes to be born. Your midwife will stay with you during this stage, so listen to guidance on what's happening and when to push. The midwife will monitor your progress now by looking and feeling, and will also check your baby's heart rate for about one minute every five minutes or so. Some women worry that this frequent checking means something is wrong, but it's quite normal.

Try to remember that the second stage of labour is not measured by the length of time it takes, but by forward progress – as long as your labour is progressing, even if it seems slow, you and your baby are doing fine.

Q Is there anything I can do to speed up the delivery of my baby?

An upright position can make labour quicker, but bear in mind that speed is not always best. A controlled, well-managed labour allows your perineum to stretch, minimizing damage to the pelvic floor muscles and the likelihood of tears or episiotomy (see p.217). Work with the messages your body is sending you. Breathe into a push, easing the baby down the birth canal; holding your breath makes you pull up rather than bear down. Release the push as each contraction subsides. Your baby moves back a bit, but each push makes gentle progress.

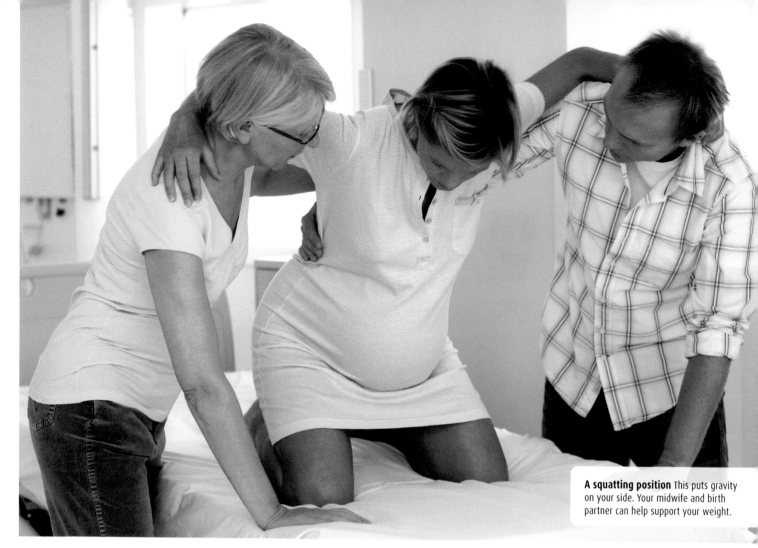

A squatting position This puts gravity on your side. Your midwife and birth partner can help support your weight.

Your birth partner's **support and encouragement** are hugely beneficial now, giving you strength to bear down and push.

Q If giving birth in a squatting position is helpful, why are women often shown lying down on their back?

There have been times in our history during which women were encouraged to lie on their backs on a bed to give birth. It is now more usual for midwives and hospitals to encourage women to do what feels right for them. It is generally acknowledged that lying "supine" is not necessarily the most comfortable or effective position to deliver a baby. There are other positions that can be more effective such as side lying, squatting, and resting on all-fours. With more upright positions, gravity can give you a helping hand to keep your labour progressing. In this way, upright positions could reduce the chances of your needing an episiotomy or an assisted birth, although they

don't improve the risk of tearing. Birthing chairs and stools (see box, above right) provide similar benefits.

Lying down can be restful, but without gravity on your side labour may be slower. You will also need to be propped up so that you don't put too much pressure on your blood vessels, which could restrict the blood flow to both you and your baby. Lying down may make it easier for a midwife to give you an internal examination and to monitor the health of your baby because you can be hooked up to a stationary heart monitor. However, the latter can be done from a sitting position, too.

An advantage of giving birth in a bed is that as soon as your baby is born, a midwife can place him on your tummy without you having to manoeuvre yourself into a comfortable and safe position, which can be especially tricky if you feel a bit unsteady after the effort of birth.

Q I'm considering a water birth. Is it safe to birth in the water or should I get out when pushing?

Yes, it is perfectly safe. Although many parents-to-be worry that a water birth poses a danger of drowning for the baby, in fact there is no known increased risk – for drowning or any other complication – compared with babies who are born out of the water. As your baby emerges into the pool, he will continue to be "fed" by the umbilical cord, giving your midwife plenty of time to lift him from the water before the breathing reflex kicks in. If you're worried, you can get out of the water to give birth.

Q I'd like to give birth lying down on my side. Is this possible?

Yes, this is completely possible. In fact, if you don't fancy the effort involved in retaining a squatting, lunging, or standing position during the second stage of labour, lying on your side is the next best thing. Studies show that giving birth in this position reduces the risk of episiotomy, assisted birth, and lowered heart rate in your baby when compared with lying on your back. Lying on your side also helps to open out your pelvis (as with squatting), which makes it easier for your baby to pass through.

Q If I am attached to a heart monitor, must I lie down or can I sit up?

As long as your position doesn't interfere with the electrodes and wires that are attached to your tummy, you can sit up if you prefer. You can even kneel on all fours, or kneel upright leaning on your birth partner's shoulders as he or she stands by the bed. Being on a bed doesn't necessarily mean you have to lie down.

Q Will having an epidural mean that I have to give birth lying down?

You will probably need to stay on your bed if you have an epidural because you will lose the sensation in your body from the waist downwards. Some hospitals will carefully monitor the administration of the epidural drug, and as you near the pushing stage they will allow it to wear off, with your consent. This will help you to be guided by your own body during the moments your baby is being born. Your midwife will advise you as to which positions you may be able to manage safely with support.

Q Does every woman tear, and will I need stitches if I do?

Around 85 per cent of women will have some perineal trauma (injury) during birth, accounting for both tears and episiotomies (see below). Tears are graded according to the amount of trauma they cause.

» A first-degree tear is a superficial wound to your vagina, damaging only a small area of the vagina's skin and fat layer and it probably won't require any stitching.

» A second-degree tear is deeper, extending into the muscle of your perineum. Your midwife will probably stitch the tear and you may need painkillers to ease the soreness for a few days.

» A third-degree tear extends into the anal sphincter, causing significant trauma. This type of tear needs to be repaired by an obstetrician in theatre, usually under epidural or spinal anaesthesia. The wound can take several weeks to heal, and you may experience some faecal incontinence while everything knits back together, but rest assured that this should only be a temporary effect.

» A fourth-degree tear is uncommon and extends into not only the anal sphincter, but also the muscular wall of your anal canal. Usually this kind of tear requires stitching in an operating theatre. Again, the wound can take weeks to heal and you may suffer some temporary faecal incontinence. Your midwife and a physiotherapist will talk to you about how you can help the damage to heal and strengthen any damaged muscles so that your recovery is as quick as possible. If at any point the soreness seems to get worse or the area around the stitches becomes inflamed, let your midwife know in case it has become infected.

Q What is an episiotomy and why might I need one?

An episiotomy is a surgical incision that opens the perineum, allowing your baby an easier passage, and you will be given one only if there is a sound clinical reason.

An episiotomy enables the midwife to control your baby's exit, but this will not be done routinely, and you will need to give your verbal consent before an incision. Your midwife will explain the reasons why the procedure is being recommended. Among those reasons are that your perineum is too rigid to stretch to allow your baby through, putting you at increased risk of a third- or fourth-degree tear (see above); to ease the delivery if you have a medical condition that makes the effort of giving birth dangerous for you, for example, if you have a heart condition or high blood pressure; if your baby is showing signs of distress (a rapid or a weak heartbeat); or if your baby is stuck and you need an assisted birth (see p.222).

The cut itself is about 3–4cm (1¼–1½) long and made with round-ended surgical scissors or with a scalpel as your baby descends into the perineum. You will have a local anaesthetic to numb the area both while the cut is being made and later when you're being stitched. The stitching will usually be done within an hour of the delivery of your baby. Once the anaesthetic has worn off, you may feel sore for about a week while the wound heals, and you may have a stinging sensation when you pass urine. Pouring warm water over the area while you pass urine can help to reduce the stinging sensation.

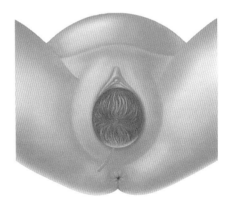

A diagonal episiotomy The cut is usually made from the back of the vagina, then out to one side. Dissolvable stitches are used to repair it.

First responses Your baby will probably respond to her new surroundings with a cry as she adjusts to life outside the womb. Hold her close to you as the sound of your voice and the rhythm of your heartbeat will soothe and reassure her.

Q What is the "third stage" of labour and what will I need to do during this stage?

Your baby has arrived, but labour is not quite over. Once you've enjoyed a first cuddle, there will be a few more contractions to deliver the placenta and membranes.

Although arguably the most exciting part of labour is over, there is still the business of giving birth to the placenta and membranes that have nourished and protected your baby during pregnancy. Your placenta, which begins to come away from your uterine lining as soon as your baby's body is out, bears down on your perineum, just as your baby had done, triggering the release of more of the hormone oxytocin, which keeps your contractions coming. Your midwife will guide you through these contractions and in most cases only a few pushes are needed to get the placenta and membranes out. You may be given an injection to help the delivery of the placenta (see below), or it may be delivered naturally. There will be some bleeding as the placenta comes away from the wall of the uterus.

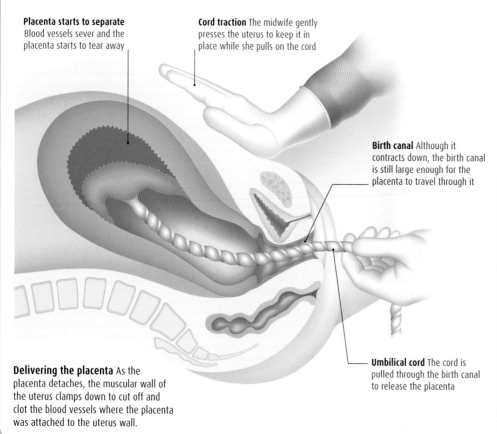

Placenta starts to separate Blood vessels sever and the placenta starts to tear away

Cord traction The midwife gently presses the uterus to keep it in place while she pulls on the cord

Birth canal Although it contracts down, the birth canal is still large enough for the placenta to travel through it

Delivering the placenta As the placenta detaches, the muscular wall of the uterus clamps down to cut off and clot the blood vessels where the placenta was attached to the uterus wall.

Umbilical cord The cord is pulled through the birth canal to release the placenta

Umbilical cord If the umbilical cord isn't cut, it will pulsate for up to ten minutes

Network of vessels In the placenta, blood vessels radiate from the umbilical cord

A healthy placenta The average full-term placenta weighs around 500g (1lb 2oz) and is 20–25cm (8–10in) in diameter. The membranes also need to come out of the uterus to avoid the risk of infection and serious bleeding.

Q I just want to get to know my new baby. How long will the third stage take?

This depends on whether you opt to deliver the placenta naturally, or to have medical assistance to deliver it. Without medical intervention, third stage labour usually takes 20–30 minutes, but it can take up to an hour. With medical intervention, this stage may take only around 15 minutes or less. For many women who decide to deliver the placenta naturally, it's just a matter of three pushes and the placenta comes out. If the process takes longer than an hour, you are at an increased risk of excessive bleeding and your midwife will talk to you about active management to deliver your placenta (see below).

Q What is an "active" third stage of labour? Should I opt for it?

An active third stage is one that is managed medically by speeding up the delivery of the placenta. There is evidence that an active third stage reduces the risk of serious bleeding after the birth, known as postpartum haemorrhage. Your midwife will offer you an injection of synthetic oxytocin hormone, which triggers contractions that help release the placenta. If you consent, you will be given the injection in your thigh around the time of your baby's birth. Following this, your midwife will pull gently on the umbilical cord, drawing the placenta away from the uterine lining and out of your vagina, with the attached membranes following behind. If you opt to deliver the placenta naturally (or physiologically), you should adopt an upright position as this can speed up the process.

Q I'd prefer not to have an injection. Are there any natural ways to help deliver the placenta?

As with the delivery of your baby, if you stand or sit, gravity will help to push out the placenta and membranes. Take care if you do stand; ensure your birth partner is there to support you, as you will probably feel wobbly after the exertion of giving birth. In addition, holding your baby "skin-to-skin" or starting to breastfeed will increase your body's release of oxytocin, which can speed up the process. Delivering your placenta naturally shouldn't affect your ability to get to know your baby – usually the cord is long enough for you to hold (and even feed) your baby while he is attached.

Q Can we keep the placenta?

If you're having your baby in a hospital or birthing centre, you'll need to check the policy on whether or not you'll be allowed to keep your placenta. Even when it's fine to do so, you'll probably have had to seek permission in advance. Hospitals won't have any containers for you to take the placenta away in, so make sure you've packed one in your hospital bag – a plastic container with a secure lid should do.

Q I always thought the umbilical cord was cut straightaway, but my midwife has said it probably won't be. Why?

When your baby is born, blood flow between him and his placenta continues through the cord for about ten minutes or so after birth. For this reason the clamping of the umbilical cord may be deferred for one to five minutes to allow the extra blood to boost your baby's iron stores. Adequate iron is important for your baby's early neurological development. Once the cord has stopped pulsating (pushing the remaining blood into your baby's body), your midwife will let you know that it's time to clamp and cut it. She will ask if your birth partner would like to cut the cord, or you may have already requested this in your birth plan. Deferred cord clamping can be carried out for both active and natural third-stage labours and C-sections.

Q I'm worried that if my partner doesn't cut the cord properly the baby will have a funny belly button. Is this the case?

The look of your baby's belly button is entirely to do with the way the umbilical cord was attached to the baby in the uterus and has nothing to do with the way it is cut after birth. If your partner wants to take an active role and cut the cord, encourage him or her to do so. Some dads feel this is a good way to play a significant role in the first moments of their new baby's life, setting the baby free in the world. If your birth partner is keen to do the honours, make a note of it in your birth plan and mention it to your midwife.

Did you know...

Some people eat the placenta. This practice is called placentophagy. While many view the placenta as a waste product of birth, others believe it can benefit the mother, delivering an iron boost and helping to ward off postnatal depression. There are references to eating it in various cultures, and while in the West the placenta has traditionally been incinerated, there is a growing trend for eating it. Evidence on the benefits is anecdotal, but there is no doubt that it is rich in nutrients and hormones.

Q What is the procedure for cutting the cord?

Cutting the umbilical cord is a significant moment when your baby makes the full transition from life in the uterus to an independent existence in the outside world.

Shortly after the birth of your baby, the midwife, doctor, or your partner will cut the umbilical cord to release your baby from the placenta. First the cord will need to be clamped to prevent bleeding from the baby or the placenta. The cord is clamped in two places. A plastic clip is placed 3–4cm (1½–2 inches) from your baby's tummy button, then a second clip is placed at the other end of the cord near the placenta. The cord is then cut between the two clamps. This procedure isn't at all painful for your baby as there are no nerves in the umbilical cord. Your baby will be left with a stump where the cord was, which will gradually blacken and fall off naturally around 10 days after the birth.

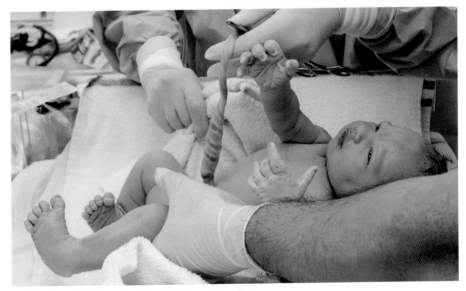

Cutting the cord This procedure is a straightforward one that can be done by your midwife or birth partner if he or she wishes.

Q What does it mean when a delivery is assisted and how is this done?

An assisted, or instrumental, delivery is when an obstetrician or midwife uses a specially designed instrument, either forceps or a ventouse suction cup, to help give birth to your baby vaginally, avoiding the need for a Caesarean section.

Forceps These are tongs, usually made of metal, that open and close like scissors and are curved to fit the shape of your baby's head. The obstetrician will carefully position the tongs either side of your baby's head, then will gently pull during a contraction to guide your baby out.

Ventouse This is a device with a plastic or metal cup at one end that is placed on your baby's head. A vacuum is created by the suction cup, making it stick to the head, then, during your contraction, the doctor or midwife will pull on the cup to help deliver your baby.

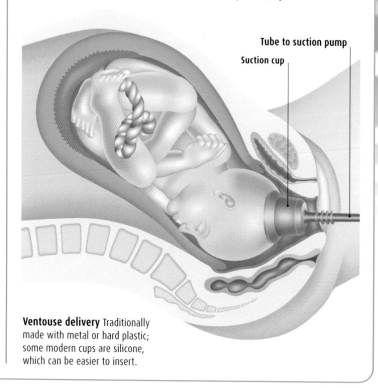

Spoon-shaped
forceps

Tube to suction pump

Suction cup

Forceps delivery Different-shaped forceps are used, depending on your baby's position and the direction in which she needs to be turned.

Ventouse delivery Traditionally made with metal or hard plastic; some modern cups are silicone, which can be easier to insert.

Q What reasons could there be for me to need an assisted delivery?

An assisted delivery is only done when there is concern for the wellbeing of either you or your baby in the second stage of labour. For example, if your baby shows signs of distress; if you have a heart condition or high blood pressure that makes the effort of natural birth dangerous for you; if your labour has been protracted and you're exhausted; or if you've had an epidural that has affected the ability of your pelvic muscles to turn your baby so that she can emerge safely. The aim is for you to have a vaginal delivery while minimizing the risks to you and your baby, and the procedure is only carried out if it is considered the safest option.

Q If I do need an assisted delivery, will they just launch in with the instruments?

Before the procedure takes place, you will be asked for your consent. This can be given verbally if the procedure is being carried out in the delivery room, or you will need to give written consent if you are moving to an operating theatre. First, you will need to be in the best position for the procedure to be carried out. The doctor or midwife will ask you to sit, leaning back slightly, with your knees drawn up, and thighs open. You could be asked to place your feet in footrests, which eases the strain on your back. You will have a catheter inserted to empty your bladder before the

procedure can begin; and you may need to have an episiotomy (see p.217) to make the opening of your vagina wide enough to allow the forceps or ventouse cup through to wrap around your baby's head. To relieve the discomfort of the procedure, you will be given either a local anaesthetic inside the vagina, known as a pudendal block, or sometimes an epidural, which may be recommended if your baby needs help rotating in your pelvis. If you do have an epidural, this makes the transition to a Caesarean section easier should the assisted delivery be unsuccessful. Your midwife will explain what is happening and why, and will encourage you to ask as many questions as you need. Your birth partner can play an important role in this situation by asking questions to help make sure you are both fully in the picture.

12.5% One in eight first-born babies in the UK are born using assisted delivery.

Q Who will perform the assisted delivery if it becomes necessary?

The procedure will be done either by an obstetrician, or by a midwife who has had specialist training in assisted deliveries. During the procedure, the delivery room may feel quite busy as you will have both a midwife (perhaps two) and an obstetrician present, and a paediatrician, who will be there just in case your baby needs attention after the birth. The presence of the paediatrician is often precautionary, but if you're concerned, ask your midwife to explain everyone's role, which he or she will be happy to do.

Q Which is better, forceps or ventouse, and will I have a choice?

Both types of delivery are considered safe and effective, but the choice of which type depends on the medical circumstances; thus it is best to be guided by your obstetrician. For example, ventouse is the preferred method if your baby needs to rotate to move down the birth canal. This method is less likely to cause injury to your vagina and/or perineum. On the other hand, forceps are gentler for the baby, but can increase the risk of trauma to you. But if your baby is in difficulty, your obstetrician's priority is to act quickly and forceps will provide the faster delivery. If your doctor begins with the ventouse and the attempt is unsuccessful, he or she may decide to try again using forceps. However, if a forceps delivery is unsuccessful, whether this is used first or after a ventouse attempt, you will usually need to have a Caesarean section.

Q How long will the assisted delivery procedure take?

Once you have been prepared for the procedure and the forceps or ventouse is attached to your baby's head, you will usually be guided through a maximum of three pushes to deliver the baby.

If your baby isn't born after three pushes, your obstetrician will decide whether to have another go, to switch to a forceps delivery (if you started with ventouse), or to send you for an emergency Caesarean section. Your midwife will be with you the whole time, explaining what is happening at each step. If you are having an assisted delivery because an epidural has made it hard for your baby to rotate, your midwife will tell you exactly when to push to help the obstetrician deliver the baby.

Q Are there risks for me if I have an assisted delivery?

You may have some vaginal or anal tearing, or need an episiotomy, which will be stitched after the birth. If there is bleeding during delivery there will be an increased risk of developing a blood clot (as with any birth where bleeding occurs). Approximately a third of women who have had an assisted delivery have some urinary incontinence afterwards, so talk to your midwife about pelvic floor exercises to help speed your recovery. Occasionally, there may be trauma to the anal sphincter (the circular muscle around your anus), which can lead to temporary faecal incontinence.

Q How can I avoid an assisted delivery in the first place?

Being well supported throughout labour, by both a midwife and a birth partner who remains with you, can help you to avoid an assisted delivery. Staying upright during labour or lying on your side can help with your baby's position and descent in the birth canal, reducing the need for an assisted delivery. Stay calm and be guided by your midwife about when to push to help prevent you becoming exhausted. Avoiding an epidural also reduces the chances that you will need help with the delivery.

Q How will my baby be affected by an assisted delivery?

An assisted delivery often leaves a mark on your baby. Swelling, bruising, and cuts are all common, but these effects soon disappear after the birth.

It's common for a baby's head to look elongated after a ventouse delivery due to the effects of the suction cup. Referred to as a "chignon", this swelling doesn't cause any damage to your baby's skull or brain, and your baby's head will return to its regular shape within 24–48 hours of the birth. Your baby may also have a small bruise, called a cephalic haematoma, where the suction was strongest, which again should disappear quickly. The stress of a ventouse birth is thought to be the reason that ventouse babies have lower than average apgar scores (see p.238) at five minutes after birth; however, these return to normal by 10 minutes. After a forceps birth, it's common for babies to have small marks on their face, and there may be cuts on the face and head, which heal and disappear quickly after the birth.

Marks and bruises These are common after an assisted delivery, but these side effects are superficial and will soon disappear.

Q I'm carrying twins and hoping to have a natural birth. How will my labour differ from having a single baby?

Many twin births have no complications, but your medical team will keep a close eye on you.

Length of labour

The dilation of the cervix (first stage) takes about the same length of time whether you are having one baby or more. Birthing the babies (second stage) may take longer, because your body has to do the job twice, but the babies are typically smaller than singletons, and can pass through the pelvis more quickly. The overall length of labour is not very different from a singleton birth.

Close monitoring

The heart rates of your babies will be more carefully monitored than if you were giving birth to only one baby. You may initially be able to walk around, especially if your babies are being monitored with handheld devices or unpluggable electrodes on your tummy. As your labour progresses closer to the second stage, and usually once your waters have broken, you may have continual monitoring that requires you to be stationary. Discuss your hospital's policy on monitoring labour for multiples well in advance of your due date so that you can manage your own expectations of the amount of freedom you're likely to have.

Birthing two babies

If both your babies are positioned head down, or one is head down and the other breech or transverse, it may be possible to deliver first one twin and then the other vaginally. The first baby opens up the birth canal as it is born, and the second baby often turns, or can be turned by palpating your abdomen, after the first is delivered. When your first twin is born you'll be encouraged to bring him to your breast and allow him to suckle (even if you don't intend to breastfeed later on) as this stimulates your body's

Amniotic sac If the babies are in separate membranes, the second baby's sac may be intact during the first baby's birth

Placenta

Emerging head The first twin is born in the usual way if he is in a vertex position

Placenta

Delivery of twins Whether or not they share a placenta, the most common presentation for twins is both head down, which makes a normal birth possible.

natural release of the hormone oxytocin and triggers your uterus to contract again, continuing your second stage labour. Your medical team will try to ensure your second twin is born within 30 minutes or so of his sibling. If your labour slows down, you may be offered an injection of oxytocin to restart the second stage for the second twin. A long delay between the two births can increase the risk of placental abruption – when your placenta comes away from the uterus lining – for the second baby, which would cut off his blood supply.

Possibility of intervention

On rare occasions – for fewer than 5 per cent of twin births – it is possible that you could need a C-section for the second baby, even if you didn't need one for the first baby. This is more likely if your second twin can't be nudged into a good position for birth, or gets into difficulty, or you become exhausted.

If you ask for pain relief, you are likely to be offered an epidural – not because labour is necessarily more painful with twins, but because pethidine can slow down the babies' heart rates and your medical team won't advise any treatment that could be high risk for multiple births. In addition to this, an epidural works as anaesthesia if you suddenly need assisted delivery or a C-section.

In almost **50 per cent of twin births** both babies present with their head downwards – sometimes the first baby is head down, and **the second turns once the first is born.**

40%

More than 40 per cent of twin births in the UK happen vaginally. But mothers expecting triplets or more are usually encouraged to opt for a Caesarean section to minimize risk.

Q Will I have to have my labour induced if I'm carrying multiples?

The majority of multiples arrive prematurely, but if yours don't, your obstetrician will recommend you are induced or scheduled for Caesarean section before 40 weeks. In all pregnancies there is a risk of stillbirth if the baby remains in utero too long, and for multiples that risk happens earlier. For twins this means early induction (see p.203) at around 37 to 38 weeks. For greater multiples, it will mean an early Caesarean section, usually at 34 weeks for triplets, and at 32 weeks for quads or more.

Q My midwife says that there might be quite a throng in my delivery room. Why?

Multiple births are more complicated than singletons, so when you go into labour there will be a team of clinicians for each baby.

A team is usually made up of a midwife or two, an obstetrician, and a paediatrician. This means that if you are having twins there will be twice as many people in the room as for a single baby; if you're having triplets there will be three times as many, and so on. The number of rescucitators (the bed-like trolleys that have oxygen equipment for newborns; see p.86) and other items of equipment in the room will also increase. This can all seem pretty overwhelming, but stay focused on your birth partner and your babies, be reassured that so many people are there to help you, and always feel free to ask what someone's role is if it's not immediately obvious.

Q Is delivering the placenta(s) and membranes different for twin births?

Usually, after a vaginal twin birth you will be encouraged to have an oxytocin injection in order to speed along the third stage of labour. A managed third-stage labour can help stem post-partum bleeding: you are at greater risk of excessive bleeding after a twin birth. The midwife will check the placenta or placentas are intact, the same as for a single birth.

If your twins are the same sex and have a placenta each and you are not sure whether they are identical or non-identical, your midwife will examine the placentas and membranes to see if it's possible to work it out. If it isn't possible, you can opt for private DNA testing if you wish to find out definitively. Of course, with many identical twins, identicality becomes fairly obvious within a few years.

Q Will my babies have to go to the neonatal unit? Will this hamper the bonding process?

If one or all of your babies are very tiny because they have been born early, they may need to spend a little time in the neonatal unit after birth to help them thrive and make sure they are continually monitored. Try not to worry. As long as it's medically safe to do so, you'll be able to hold them first. Remember that bonding with your babies began while they were in the uterus, so you already have a good start. Take photographs of each baby and of the babies together – when they aren't with you, looking at the photographs will help to trigger bonding hormones that you'd have if holding them. This can also help trigger the let-down reflex that enables you to express your own milk for your babies to drink. It will help you adjust to the idea of parenthood, too.

Full term twins in the uterus Both babies are head down – their skulls point to their mother's pelvis, and their spines are seen curving upwards. On the right, the baby's head is engaged in the pelvis, ready for birth.

It's impossible to know in advance **how you will experience** the pain of labour, and certainly levels of pain **can vary greatly** between women. Being informed about labour and what can help with the pain, though, can have a big impact on how you fare; that, in itself, will **reduce tension and fear** and will help you cope.

Pain relief in labour

Your experience of pain

The pain of labour is different from almost all other types of pain you will ever experience. Unlike pain that acts as a warning sign that something is amiss and you should stop what you're doing, labour pain is a sign that something is very right: your baby is about to be born.

The levels of pain, or perceptions of pain, women report in labour vary greatly. Some experience only moderate discomfort through much of labour, while for others the pain feels overwhelming. The nature of the pain, though, is characteristic of different stages of labour. The cramping feeling in the first stage occurs as the uterus contracts to push the baby into the pelvis. It's widespread and long-lasting: you'll feel it in your abdomen, perhaps in your lower back, and sometimes even through your buttocks and down your thighs. In the second stage, pain is more localized as the muscles and tissues of the birth canal are stretched as your baby makes her way through the vagina.

The psychology of pain

Many women worry that they won't be able to cope with the pain of labour, and that if they need medical pain relief they will somehow have "failed" in this rite of passage. Studies show that women are able to cope better if they are informed about labour pain, which helps them to feel more empowered and relaxed. Understanding where labour pain comes from, exploring the options for pain relief, and making decisions about which forms you would like to have and which, if any, you would rather avoid are all important ways to take control of your labour. And in itself, feeling in control of what's happening and the choices you're making will help you cope with labour pain. Modern methods of pain relief don't harm your baby; the fear of pain, on the other hand, can make birth traumatic not just for you but for your baby, too. Thinking about labour pain as "positive" pain that helps you achieve something incredible, can motivate you to prepare for this event, just as you would for, say, running a marathon.

Types of pain relief

Pain relief during labour is either natural or medical. Natural forms of pain relief (see p.228–29) include breathing and relaxation techniques and water births; and medical pain relief includes the use of gas and air, opioid analgesics such as pethidine and Meptid, and epidural. There is no right or wrong approach to pain relief in labour. If you start out thinking you'll be able to cope with breathing techniques alone, but then decide you need an epidural – ask for one. The most important thing is that your labour is as calm and as positive as possible.

Q What different types of pain relief are available, and when can I use them?

Some women cope with mainly natural methods of pain relief, such as breathing, for much of labour. For others, effective methods of pain relief may change as labour progresses and intensifies, and many women choose to supplement natural techniques with medical forms of pain relief.

WHAT PAIN RELIEF YOU MIGHT USE

The table below charts how different types of pain relief are commonly used during labour. The delivery of the placenta in the third stage is commonly managed without pain relief.

STAGE	HOW THE PAIN MIGHT FEEL	NATURAL PAIN RELIEF OPTIONS	MEDICAL PAIN RELIEF OPTIONS
1st stage of labour – latent phase	Contractions may stop and start, and can feel like severe menstrual pain, and there may be lower back pain. Pain is usually bearable, such that you can continue to move around and talk during contractions. Contractions gradually get closer together and stronger.	» **Breathing:** this helps you to focus during contractions. » **Meditation:** can keep you calm and focused. » **Water:** warm water is soothing and relaxing early on. » **Massage:** can ease backache and promote relaxation. » **TENS:** takes the edge off contractions and relieves backache. » **Acupuncture:** this can help you relax in early labour.	» **Analgesics:** occasionally, analgesics such as gas and air or pethidine may be used for stronger contractions now.
1st stage of labour – active phase	Contractions are regular, frequent, and intense: you're unable to talk or move through them. There may be nausea, strong pressure in the back, and pain may radiate down the legs.	» **Rhythmic breathing:** controlled breathing helps you focus and maximizes oxygen flow to the muscles. » **Meditation/massage:** these continue to be helpful. » **Water:** supportive and relieves pressure on back and pelvis.	» **Analgesics:** gas and air and opioids such as pethidine help you cope with contractions. » **Epidural:** this may be requested and set up now if pain feels unmanageable.
Transition phase	Contractions can be extremely intense now, with little rest time in between. Pressure in the lower back and rectum is strong, and you may be exhausted, overwhelmed, and nauseous. You may vomit.	» **Controlled breathing:** breathing techniques can be used if you feel panicky and out of control: use a combination of more shallow in-breaths and longer exhalations. » **Water:** you can remain in a birthing pool now if you wish to give birth in the water.	» **Analgesics:** carry on with gas and air; opioids are avoided close to delivery as they can affect the baby's breathing. » **Epidural:** can be topped up; you may be encouraged to avoid setting one up now.
2nd stage of labour	Strong, long-lasting contractions and an urge to push down. Strong pressure in the rectum and stinging or burning as the head crowns.	» **Breathing:** slow and focused exhalations can help you to bear down. Panting as the head crowns is important. Pain can feel productive as you push your baby out.	» **Analgesics:** gas and air can continue to be used during this stage.

Q Can I use more than one type of pain relief?

Yes. Most types of natural pain relief can be used alongside medical pain relief. And many women begin using gas and air, then go on to ask for opioids such as pethidine, diamorphine, or Meptid as pain gets more intense. You may want to use gas and air while you wait for an opioid to take effect, which takes 20–30 minutes. You can have opioids such as pethidine at any time up until the point at which you need to start pushing – because opioids cross into the baby's system, and can slow down his breathing, it's better that they aren't administered too close to when the baby is born. If you are given opioids, but then decide you want an epidural, that's fine, too.

Q What kinds of medical pain relief will I be able to have for a home birth?

The only medical form of pain relief definitely available for home birth is entonox (gas and air), which comes in portable cylinders. Make sure that you give the cylinder a shake before you use it, as the nitrous oxide and oxygen separate when left standing, which means you can get an undiluted gulp of nitrous oxide when you breathe in. Some midwives will also administer pethidine or Meptid (see p.230) at home births, but you will need to check the protocol in your region. These opioid analgesics come with greater risks to you and the baby, which means that some midwives prefer to use them only in a hospital environment.

Q Did you know...

Although home birth limits your access to analgesics, studies show that women who have had a home birth feel more positive about their experience of labour pain. Whether this is because they have little expectation of being able to have pain relief (so have already reached a certain level of acceptance about the pain), because they are more relaxed in their environment, or a combination of the two is unknown. At home and in hospital, the support of a midwife and a birth partner is beneficial.

Q Can breathing techniques really help me to cope in labour?

When we feel anxious or worried, we tend to hold our breath, which reduces the oxygen circulating in our blood, and we tense up, tightening muscles and restricting blood flow. In this state of hyperarousal, the perception of pain is greater, and labour becomes harder work. Conversely, calm and steady breathing lowers the heart rate, reduces anxiety, and maximizes the oxygen flow to you and your baby. If you learn breathing techniques (see p.72) before labour, you can use these to help you breathe purposefully through your contractions, focusing in particular on breathing out (releasing) as the contraction peaks, so you remain as relaxed as possible. Techniques such as Hypnobirthing (see p.73), an increasingly

popular practice that anecdotally has positive results, use breathing techniques to help you focus during contractions and breathe through the pain, rather than try to resist it.

Q My midwife asked if I was interested in using a birthing pool. How does water help labour?

Getting into a warm bath is a well-known relaxation aid. Similarly, being immersed in warm water in labour can be instantly soothing. As your muscles relax, levels of endorphins, the feel-good hormones that provide natural pain relief, increase; and it's thought that the warm water blocks pain messages from getting to your brain, reducing your perception of pain. Being in water also makes it easier to move

around as the water supports your bump, so you can rely on your own sense of balance and buoyancy to change position, rather than the strength of your birth partner or midwife. If you are using a birthing pool at home, it's up to you when you get in, but some experts believe that it's best to wait until labour is established as it's thought that warm water may slow contractions early on. The water shouldn't be above 37.5°C (99.5°F), as higher than this can raise your core temperature and distress your baby. You can stay in the pool for as long as you wish, and, if you have a midwife trained in water birth, you can give birth in it, too. If you don't have a pool, you can benefit from the soothing effects of water by lying in a warm bath.

You'll need to have someone with you while you are in water to make sure you don't become so drowsy that you fall asleep and slip under the surface, and to help you to get in and out.

Q I've heard about women using meditation in labour. How does this work?

Techniques such as meditation aim to redirect your focus away from the pain of labour to help raise your pain threshold. Meditation is simply the act of stilling the mind so that you can remain detached from the physical sensations in your body. The idea is that if you train your mind to believe that you will be able to cope with the pain of labour, you are far more likely to manipulate your experience to that end, whereas if you tell yourself labour is going to be unbearably painful, you'll almost certainly experience the full force of your pain.

Choosing a visualization or affirmation to focus on during meditation can help:
» Visualize a stream that tumbles over stones – can you see the light on the water? How fast does the water move? What sounds does it make? Does it splash or foam as it flows? The more detail you can conjure up, the more focus you have away from your pain.
» Visualize a candle flame. To keep the outbreath long and slow through a contraction, close your eyes and imagine blowing it so gently that the flame flickers, but doesn't go out.
» As a contraction starts, repeat a word or

Monitoring your baby In a birthing pool your baby's heartbeat will be monitored with a waterproof hand-held device.

phrase (in your mind or out loud), such as "love", or "calm", or your baby's name if you've chosen it. Or choose a phrase such as "I feel powerful and strong". Imagine the letters or words in front of you as you say the affirmation.

Q I'm planning to use a TENS machine for as long as possible. What do I need to know?

TENS is an acronym for Transcutaneous Electrical Nerve Stimulation. A TENS machine is a portable unit that emits low-voltage electrical impulses to your nerves via electrode pads secured either side of your spine. When you have a contraction, you push a button to send impulses to your body, which are thought to stimulate the release of endorphins and to block your pain receptors. TENS is non-invasive, has no known harmful effects on you or your baby, and allows you to move around and feel in control of your pain relief. The only place it's not possible to use your TENS machine is in water.

It can take up to an hour for endorphins to build up in your body, so as soon as you feel contractions, ask your birth partner to hook you up to the machine (it's a good idea to practice before labour starts). You'll be able to adjust the voltage of the electrical impulses to a comfortable level, increasing the frequency of the impulses as the pain gets more intense.

You may be able to borrow a TENS machine from the hospital, or you can hire one, or buy one new or second-hand. Talk to your midwife about how best to get hold of one.

Q Is acupuncture safe to use during labour, and will I be able to move?

Acupuncture is becoming increasingly common and popular as a form of pain relief during labour. This practice of inserting tiny needles at specific sites on the body is used to reduce pain sensitivity and encourage the release of endorphins. Acupuncture is safe to use during labour, but does require a trained therapist. You will need to arrange for a therapist to be present during labour, or some midwives are now trained to use acupuncture. You might want to try a few sessions in pregnancy first. In labour, the therapist is likely to work on points such as the ear, so that your movement isn't restricted.

Q I've always found massage soothing. Will it help me in labour?

Massage during labour can help you to relax between contractions, release held-in tension, and alleviate lower back pain. Touch can be also calming and increase your confidence in your ability to deal with the pain of labour.

A study published in 2013 showed that women who were given a lower back massage for 30 minutes during established first-stage labour reported significantly less pain than those who weren't. The average lengths of the labours were roughly the same in both the massage and the control groups, and the physiotherapists who performed the massage visited every woman in the control group for 30 minutes, too, but made no physical contact with them. The researchers concluded that massage has a measurably positive effect on the perception of pain.

If physical contact is something you find supportive and reassuring in everyday life, encourage your birth partner to come to the massage sessions of your antenatal classes, or find an antenatal massage class that you can both attend. Practise the techniques during your pregnancy to get a good understanding of what feels best for you (both in terms of technique and pressure levels), so your birth partner is well prepared to put the techniques into practice during your labour.

Some women find that once in labour they don't want to be touched. It's impossible to know how you'll feel on the day, but discuss this possibility with your birth partner in advance so that he doesn't take offence if you decide you don't want to be touched at all.

SOOTHING MASSAGE

Experiment with the following techniques so you can ascertain which strokes you feel comfortable with and the ones you think might be helpful during labour.

Relaxing massage Both you and your partner should be in comfortable, supported positions during a massage session so that you can both relax fully.

» **Back sweep:** sit on a birthing stool or fold yourself over a birthing ball to expose your back. Ask your partner to run his hands from the outer sides of your shoulders inwards, across your shoulder blades and down each side of your spine in one swooping, stroking motion. Repeat several times.

» **Tension release:** sit on a chair, on a stool, or on the edge of a bed and ask your partner to gently knead and squeeze the muscles of your shoulders and neck.

» **Relaxing head massage:** ask your partner to massage the top of your head, applying firm pressure with just the tips of his fingers, almost as if he is washing your hair.

» **Soothing touch:** if you don't like the idea of being stroked in labour, ask your partner to hold your palm between his two palms, gently squeezing and releasing your hand. Many women find this simple contact deeply reassuring and nurturing.

» **Foot massage:** ask your partner to use firm thumb pressure all over the soles of your feet, rubbing, pressing, and making small circles to release knots and tension.

Q Will gas and air make me feel spaced out? How can I use it so that I remain in control?

Entonox (gas and air) is effective because it gives you a short-lived "high" that has a sedative effect on your behaviour. The high hits around 20 seconds after you take a breath of entonox through a mouthpiece or mask. Inhale the entonox as soon as you feel the contraction starting, then remove the mouthpiece or mask when the contraction has gone. As long as you take a few normal breaths in between, you shouldn't feel spaced out. If you breathe in and out of the mouthpiece continually without a break, you will start to feel disorientated and you won't be able to concentrate on what your body, or midwife, is telling you to do. Birth partners can be a great help in this respect – as first stage labour reaches transition (see p.213), many women become somewhat attached to the mouthpiece and it's useful for a birth partner to be on hand to persuade you to give it up so that you can concentrate on bearing down and easing the baby out. Taking gas and air continually can also make you feel sick.

Q What is the gas in "gas and air"? Is it safe for me and my baby?

The gas is nitrous oxide – more commonly known as laughing gas – and it has been used to help women in labour since the 1930s. Today, it is mixed 50:50 with oxygen to make "entonox". When you inhale entonox the effects are almost immediate, but also cease quickly when you stop inhaling. Some women experience nausea or tingling wrists and ankles, but these side effects should not last long. The gas does cross the placenta and enters the baby's bloodstream, but it also quickly dissipates, so its effects are not considered unsafe for the baby.

35–50%
of women in the UK choose **pain relief** in the form of pethidine or Meptid during their labour.

Q What is an epidural, and how does it work?

An epidural is a procedure that injects painkilling drugs directly into the epidural space around your spinal cord through a fine tube. It works by numbing feeling below the waist, so is a very effective form of pain relief.

An anaesthetist first gives you a local anaesthetic injection to numb the section of your mid-to-low-back where the epidural goes in. He or she then inserts a long, hollow needle carrying a thin tube, or catheter, into the epidural space. (You may be asked to curl up on your side, or to sit up and bend forward for this part, as it opens the space between your vertebrae.) The anaesthetist removes the needle, leaving the catheter in place. The painkiller (a mixture of anaesthetic and narcotic) is either injected into your spine through the catheter, or pumped in via an intravenous drip or tube, to block the nerve pathways that run from your uterus to your brain. Although epidurals traditionally caused complete numbness, many now allow sensation without pain, which means you can feel to push when the time comes.

Top ups The painkilling drugs can be topped up by injecting through the small catheter placed in the spine.

Q How do I choose: pethidine, diamorphine, or Meptid?

All these forms of pain relief are opioid analgesics, meaning that they are derived from the seeds of the opium poppy, which gives us morphine. (Note that Meptid is a brand name – the generic name is meptazinol.) All of them offer limited relief from labour pain that can last for between two and four hours per dosage. They block the pain as it travels down your spinal column by "switching off" the cells in your pain receptors. Dosages are administered by your midwife, usually via an injection in your thigh, although they may also be given by intravenous drip. (The pain relief will be quicker intravenously – becoming active within two or three minutes, compared with 20–30 minutes by injection.)

Compared with Meptid, pethidine and diamorphine are likely to have more significant side effects on your baby's alertness, breathing, and feeding – it can take several days after birth for the effects of the drug to wear off in a newborn, depending upon how soon after

your last dosage she was born. Meptid is more likely to make you feel nauseous or even cause you to vomit and it is not available in every hospital (whereas pethidine and diamorphine usually are). Of the three, diamorphine is the least likely to cause nausea and vomiting. Note that none of these opioids will give you a pain-free labour, and for some women they simply don't work. Meptid tends to work fastest of all, while diamorphine often gives the most relief and is the most long-lasting. All of these drugs are useful if your first stage labour is lasting a long time and you need some sleep, as they can help you to relax.

Q Can I have pethidine, diamorphine, or Meptid if I want a water birth?

Yes, although you will need to have had the drug in your system for at least two hours before you get into the pool. This is just to make sure that you don't feel overly drowsy in the water. Of course, the water itself will help with pain relief.

INSERTING INTO THE EPIDURAL SPACE

The epidural space lies around your spinal cord, up and down its whole length. When you are given an epidural, a fine catheter is inserted directly into this space in order to administer drugs.

Epidural space

Cerebrospinal fluid

Spinal cord

Tip of catheter

Vertebra

CROSS-SECTION OF THE SPINE

LOCATION OF INSERTION POINT

A mixture of **anaesthetic** and **narcotic** injected into the spine **blocks the pain messages** from the uterus to the brain.

Q How long does an epidural take and how long does it last?

An epidural takes around 10 minutes to set up and around 15–20 minutes to become fully effective, and will last for as long as the anaesthetic is topped up. Some hospitals have pump systems that allow you to control how much anaesthetic you receive and when, leaving you to judge how much of your labour you want to be able to feel and when. Once you stop receiving the anaesthetic, the effects should wear off and you should regain the feeling in your legs within around two hours.

Q I'm worried that an epidural might damage my spine. What are the risks and side effects?

Permanent damage to your spine following an epidural is very rare – occurring in between 1 in 80,000 and 1 in 320,000 cases, depending upon the source of the statistics.

If you experience any significant discomfort or pain in your epidural site when the needle is going in or immediately after it has been withdrawn, let your anaesthetist know so that he or she can reposition the catheter if necessary. It is normal to feel a little achy in your back after an epidural, but if you have severe pain, tell your midwife or doctor.

Between 1 and 5 per cent of epidurals may lead to a "dural tap" in which the epidural needle makes a small puncture causing cerebrospinal fluid to leak from around your spinal cord. The first symptom is often a bad headache. However, just like a nick anywhere else on your body, the wound will heal and the leak will stop on its own – all you will need to do is rest. Occasionally your anaesthetist may want to plug the hole with a little of your own blood – almost like creating a scab to give the tissues beneath time to heal.

Other complications of an epidural include feelings of nausea and itchy skin, both of which are easily treated and will pass, and low blood pressure (you will probably be given an intravenous drip of medication to help prevent this side effect).

Q A pain-free labour sounds perfect! Are there any drawbacks to having an epidural?

There are several reasons why you might decide against an epidural for your labour.

» Restricted mobility: you will be limited in your ability to move around because you won't have any strength in your legs and because you will need to be attached to a fetal heart monitor. Even so-called "mobile" epidurals are still limiting – talk to your midwife about what's available in your hospital and how much freedom you'll be able to have.

» Longer labour: you may experience a slower labour because the painkilling drug can make the muscles of your pelvis weaker and so less effective at turning your baby into a good position for birth. This also slightly increases your chances of needing an assisted (instrumental) delivery (see p.222).

» Increased odds of intervention: there is a slightly increased risk of assisted delivery for women who have an epidural. Your midwife is likely to delay your pushing in second-stage labour by up to an hour to reduce the risk of your needing an assisted delivery. However, you will need to deliver your baby within four hours of the start of the second stage, otherwise your doctor will recommend a C-section.

» Limited effectiveness: even if it has been effective for the first stage of labour, an epidural doesn't always work against the pain of the second stage of labour, when there is localized sharp pain as the baby emerges.

» Risk of complications: while most doctors agree there are no risks to your baby, epidural carries certain risks for you (see left).

Did you know...

If you choose to have pethidine, diamorphine, or Meptid you will probably also be given an antiemetic – a drug that limits the side effects of nausea associated with these methods of pain relief.

You may already know that your baby will arrive **via Caesarean section** (C-section), or you may be wondering what would happen if you were told during labour that you could need an operation. Knowing what C-sections involve will **help you prepare mentally** and practically for **what lies ahead** for both you and your baby.

Caesarean section

The decision to operate

Around a quarter of all babies in the UK and around a third in the USA are born surgically. The vast majority of C-sections are done for medical reasons, of which many are known in advance, such as placenta praevia, a multiple birth, or a breech position. In these cases, you will have an "elective", or planned, C-section.

Roughly one in eight births in the UK is an "emergency", or unplanned, C-section. Some vaginal births can develop complications that mean this is the safest option for you and your baby. However, not all situations are life-threatening: a long, slow labour is the most common reason given for unplanned surgical delivery. Your medical team will always talk through the reasons why a C-section is being recommended. These discussions are open to your partner, too, but it is for you to decide and consent to. For some women, a C-section may come as a relief, whereas others may feel a sense of disappointment or failure at not having a vaginal birth. These are normal responses; asking questions about the risks and benefits will help you to make a decision you are happy with.

You can request a C-section without a medical reason if you wish, and this should be set out in your birth plan (see pp.88–89), but it is important to be fully aware of the risks and recovery implications, which are greater on balance than those for a vaginal birth. Your medical team will explain the pros and cons so that you can make a fully informed decision.

What to expect from a Caesarean section

Although having a C-section is a major operation, it can be a life-saving one. Like any operation, it can carry risks. For the mother this may mean increased blood loss (both during and after surgery), cardiac arrest, infection of the uterus or uterine lining, bladder damage, complications for future pregnancies, greater risk of future hysterectomy, and a longer hospital stay.

Your baby may experience more stress, because you won't have the benefit of the labour hormones that calm the baby. She may be born with residual fluid in the lungs and nasal passages that make independent breathing more difficult. There is a small risk (about 2 per cent) of your baby receiving a nick or cut, but this will heal within a few days. There is a possibility that your baby could be admitted to the special care unit (see p.310).

Before you are discharged, you'll be able to discuss the operation and ask any further questions about aftercare or possible complications. Your recovery will take about six weeks so it may be a good idea to get help caring for your baby at first if you can.

85%

of C-sections are carried out for **one of four reasons**: previous C-sections, lack of progress in labour, fetal distress, or breech birth.

Q What happens before surgery? Do I need to prepare myself?

For both planned and emergency C-sections, there is a set of procedures to follow.

» **Written consent:** you will need to sign a consent form to say that you agree to the operation, understand the risks, and allow the doctors to act in your best medical interests.

» **Meeting the anaesthetist:** if there's time, the consultant who will administer the drugs will explain what form of anaesthetic you will have and what its effects will be, both during and after the operation.

» **Preparing yourself:** you'll need to remove any jewellery, make-up, nail varnish, and false nails (so that the anaesthetist can monitor your skin and nail colour to check oxygen levels).

» **Being prepared by the medical team:** a midwife or nurse will shave your pubic hair around the intended incision site. For a planned C-section, you will be given a blood test for anaemia (which increases risk of blood loss) and blood type, in case a transfusion is necessary during surgery. You'll be attached to an arm cuff and chest electrodes to measure your blood pressure and heart rate throughout. You'll be given antibiotics to reduce the risk of post-operative infection, and low-blood-pressure medication if you need it. For a general anaesthetic, you will be given antacids and anti-sickness medication.

» **Immediately before surgery:** finally, you will be given your anaesthesia, and a catheter will be inserted into your ureter, to provide bladder control during surgery.

Q Why might I need a Caesarean section?

There are many reasons for a Caesarean section, but usually they are used to prevent or solve health risks to you or your baby. Nearly half are elective, planned in advance for known medical problems or by request. The remainder are advised when issues arise during labour and a quick delivery is needed.

REASONS FOR PLANNED CAESAREAN SECTION

» **Repeat C-section** could be proposed by your obstetrician if your medical history presents risk factors, such as complications with the previous procedure or a high chance of old scars tearing in a vaginal birth.

» **Breech presentation or transverse lie** (when your baby is in a bottom-down or sideways position in the uterus) might need a C-section if the baby can't be turned manually using external cephalic version.

» **Pre-eclampsia** a condition that can develop during pregnancy, could make the strain of vaginal birth dangerous for you.

» **Low-lying placenta** can block the passage of your baby or make heavy bleeding likely.

» **Twins or multiples** often require a C-section, although vaginal delivery is possible in twins if the first baby is positioned head-down.

» **Some heart conditions** make vaginal birth unsafe for the mother.

» **Maternal requests** for a C-section are sometimes made if a previous birth was difficult.

REASONS FOR UNPLANNED CAESAREAN SECTION

» **Lack of progress in labour** can happen if your cervix hasn't opened enough after a long, slow labour, or contractions are too weak. Although not life-threatening, this is the most common reason for unplanned C-sections.

» **Fetal distress** is sometimes detected during labour. Midwives monitor the baby's heart rate as standard practice for all births.

» **Unsuccessful assisted delivery** (using forceps or ventouse) can be followed by a C-section.

» **Placental abruption** is when the placenta comes away from the wall of the uterus either before or during labour. It is a rare occurrence but necessitates an emergency C-section.

» **Uterine rupture** occurs if a scar from a previous C-section tears during labour. It happens in less than 1 per cent of women with prior C-sections. Your doctor will assess the risk of rupture before planning a vaginal birth.

» **Umbilical cord prolapse** is another very rare event. If the umbilical cord slips down the cervix ahead of your baby, it can get compressed and affect the baby's oxygen supply.

Q Can I stay awake during a C-section?

In most cases, you can stay awake because you will be given either spinal anaesthesia or an epidural; both numb the lower body without making you unconscious. Spinal anaesthesia (or spinal block) is a single injection that is used only in the event of surgery. With these forms of anaesthetic, you won't feel any pain during surgery, but you might feel a bit of pushing and pulling in your abdomen. It helps to focus on music – arrange to take some music of your choice to be played in theatre. However, if a quick delivery is vital, your doctor might use general anaesthetic, which is faster to administer, but means that you will be fully asleep. General anaesthesia is only used if the benefits outweigh the risks – it can cross the placenta and make your baby drowsy, but studies show there are no long-lasting effects on the baby. The operation usually takes 40–50 minutes altogether; maybe longer if you've had a C-section before.

Q Will I be able to see my baby being born during the surgery?

In order to spare you unnecessary trauma, midwives or nurses will construct a screen between you and your tummy so that you can't see your obstetrician cut through your skin and into your uterus. However, you can usually ask for the screen to be lowered enough so that you can see your baby lifted out. The screen will be removed as soon as you've been stitched up.

Q Will a midwife be in theatre with me? Who else will be there?

Yes, your midwife will stay with you throughout your Caesarean section to offer constant reassurance to both you and your birth partner. As well as your midwife and your obstetrician, theatre staff will include an obstetric assistant, an anaesthetist and anaesthetist's nurse, two or three theatre nurses, and a paediatrician (who is on hand to check over your baby as soon as she is born). If you're having a multiple birth, there will be a paediatrician and midwife for each expected baby. All in all, the theatre can get quite busy!

Q Can my birth partner come into theatre with me?

One birth partner is usually allowed into theatre as long as you are having a spinal anaesthetic or an epidural. He or she will need to wear a surgical gown and a surgical mask, but will be allowed to sit beside you as you have your surgery. If you are having a general anaesthetic, you will usually not be permitted to have anyone in theatre with you (you'll be completely asleep). Your birth partner will be able to wait just outside the operating theatre.

Q I am HIV positive. Will I have to have a C-section?

No. The most recent guidelines from the UK's National Institute for Health and Care Excellence (NICE) recommend that women who are HIV positive and on medication that is controlling the effects of the virus are given the option of having a vaginal delivery. Overall, studies show that there is no increased risk to the baby of contracting the virus by vaginal rather than C-section. Your medical team will be able to advise you in your specific circumstances.

Q If the only reason for having a C-section is because my labour is taking a long time, can I refuse?

Yes, although your obstetrician gives his or her advice with your best interests at heart, so you should ask why he or she is suggesting the procedure, what it involves, and what would happen if you don't opt for it. Consider the risks carefully before you decide. If you choose to refuse medical intervention, your midwife and doctors will respect your wishes. They will continue to work to ensure the best outcome for you and your baby in any circumstances.

Q Who will care for my baby if I have to have a general anaesthetic?

Assuming all is well with your baby after birth, that's really a decision for you – let your midwife know your preference before you go into surgery, if possible. As a default, your birth partner will be encouraged to hold and cuddle your baby until you wake up, to have skin-to-skin contact if that is your wish, and to bottle-feed her if necessary.

Caesarean births With an epidural or spinal anaesthetic, you're awake at the moment of delivery and can see and hold your baby immediately.

Q How quickly will I be given a C-section if it is decided during labour that I need one?

That depends on the level of emergency for your C-section. The procedure will be carried out as quickly as the clinical need, and your baby could be delivered within 30 minutes or up to 75 minutes of a C-section been decided upon. Most hospitals use a two-level grading system. If either you or your baby is considered to be in danger, you'll have a Category 1 C-section, done as speedily as possible. When neither you nor your baby is in a life-threatening situation (for example, if you're too tired to keep going, or if your baby is awkwardly positioned), your C-section will be a Category 2 and there will be a little more time to prepare for theatre.

Q How is the placenta delivered when I've had a C-section? Will it have to be cut away from my uterus lining?

No, once your baby is out, you will be given an injection of synthetic oxytocin (see p.220) to actively manage the third stage of labour. This hormone will have the dual effect of helping to stem the bleeding associated with birth, and to cause your uterus to contract and separate the placenta from the lining of the uterus, just as with a vaginal birth. Your obstetrician will gently pull on the umbilical cord to separate the placenta fully and draw it out through the incision in your abdomen.

Q Will I be able to go straight to a postnatal ward with my baby after the operation?

Usually you will spend a few hours in a recovery room adjacent to the operating theatre, with your baby if possible. The medical team will check your blood pressure and heart rate regularly, and make sure you have no signs of complications relating to the operation. You will be given some painkillers and your midwife will make sure you feel able to eat and drink normally. Providing all is well and you are awake and alert, you can usually then move onto the postnatal ward.

Q What will happen during the Caesarean section?

After giving the anaesthetic, the anaesthetist will make sure you cannot feel anything. You may feel some pushing and pulling, but it should not be painful.

You will have a catheter tube inserted through your urethra to drain your bladder during the operation and once your abdomen is swabbed with antiseptic solution the operation can begin. An incision is made just below the top of your pubic hair. The obstetrican divides the layers of fat and fibrous muscle tissue before making an incision in the lower part of the uterus. If the membranes surrounding your baby have not ruptured, this will be done now. Whatever part of your baby's body is below the incision will be delivered first. Your

baby is normally delivered in the first ten minutes once surgery is underway. After the delivery, the cord is clamped and your baby can be handed to you for her first cuddle.

The low horizontal incision (known as transverse) made in your abdomen is usually 15–20cm (6–8in) long – this is the cut seen on your skin. It leaves a modest scar that fades over time. The incision made in the uterus underneath is only 5–7cm (2¼–2¾in) long, to keep scarring on your uterus to a minimum. This helps to reduce the risk of gynaecological problems later and increases your chance of having a safe vaginal birth if you go on to have another pregnancy. In unusual and very specific circumstances, a vertical (longitudinal) cut may be done. Try not to worry about scarring too much – it is just one of many changes that will take place in your body.

KEY

----- 5–7cm (2¼–2¾in) incision in uterus

----- 15–20cm (6–8in) incision in abdominal wall

Transverse incision This is the most common incision and is associated with fewer risks and a better chance of subsequent vaginal births. It leaves a discreet scar along your bikini line.

Q How soon will I be able to leave hospital? Will I have to go back to have stitches out?

You can usually leave hospital between three and four days after your C-section. Sometimes you can leave as quickly as 24 hours later (your catheter will come out around 12 hours after the operation), if your baby is well and you have made a fast initial recovery. It's very unlikely you will need to go back into hospital to have any stitches taken out. The stitches in your uterus will be dissolvable. You may also have dissolvable stitches at your abdominal incision. If you have surgical sutures or staples in your abdomen, these will be removed around five days after the operation. This may be done in hospital if you are there, or your midwife can

remove them if you have gone home. If you had a longitudinal (vertical) incision, you may need to have your stitches in for a little longer.

Q How quickly can I get out of bed and resume normal activities?

You'll be encouraged to walk around and eat and drink normally as soon as possible after your C-section, provided the anaesthetic has worn off and you aren't feeling dizzy or unwell. Movement will also decrease your chances of blood clots (an injection to prevent thrombosis is often given as well). Activities such as lifting and driving will take longer. See page 260 for some of the commonly asked questions about recovering from a Caesarean section.

Your labour is done: you have your newborn **baby in your arms**, and you are ready to get to know this tiny new person, and to start your life as a family. The medical team have a **few more checks** to make, and this **care you receive** immediately after the birth is sometimes referred to as the fourth stage of labour.

Straight after birth

Your baby's first moments

Just after your baby is born, and provided all is well, the midwife will place him on your chest to enjoy a first cuddle. Your baby will be rubbed and patted dry and have a clean towel placed over him while you hold him skin to skin. Meanwhile, the cord will be clamped and cut by the midwife, or by your partner if so planned.

Your baby will be given some initial checks (see pp.238–39), which may be done while you are holding him, then he may be weighed. Whether at home or in a hospital or birthing centre, your medical team will aim to do the necessary checks as unobtrusively as possible, so as not to interfere with these first moments when you and your partner begin bonding with your baby. If you or your baby needs medical attention after the birth, the medical team will try to reunite you as soon as they can.

If you have decided to breastfeed it is important to offer this to your baby within the first hour. Your midwife will help you to get your baby to latch on. His sucking and rooting reflexes (see p.267) are strong at this time.

Looking after you

Before you leave the delivery room, or before your midwife leaves you if you're at home, she or he will check that your body is beginning to show signs of recovery from the birth. Your midwife will take your blood pressure and temperature, feel your tummy to make sure your uterus has begun to contract, assess your blood loss, and examine your placenta and membranes to ensure they are complete. Your midwife will also ask you if you are happy for your perineum to be assessed to check for any injury – primarily this means checking whether or not you suffered a tear as your baby was born, and if so whether or not this needs stitches.

Your midwife will explain what she or he is doing as the checks are made, and you should be able to continue to hold your baby while you're given the once-over. In fact, your baby can provide the perfect distraction from this final stage in the delivery room.

Your emotions straight after birth

Unsurprisingly, you're likely to feel emotional when you've given birth: not only do you have raised hormone levels, but also the relief and excitement of meeting your baby can be overwhelming. Don't worry if you feel like crying – midwives are used to all manner of emotions in the delivery room and will offer support, encouragement, reassurance, or quietude as your mood dictates.

Q What will be my baby's first reactions on being born?

Your baby's first reaction will be to cry – this is a positive sign that he is able to breathe successfully on his own. Sometimes, babies need assistance and can be given oxygen in the delivery room. Some babies splutter slightly and may need help to clear mucus out of the airways. Your baby will be observed in the first minutes after birth to check his responses.

On first holding your baby, you may notice him turning towards your nipple very soon after birth, displaying the strong instinct newborns have to seek out food immediately.

Next to you Holding your baby skin to skin after the birth can help to get breastfeeding started and promote early bonding.

Q Will I need to have stitches if I tear during the delivery?

This depends on the severity of the tear (see p.217). A first-degree, or superficial, tear will usually be left to heal by itself. A second-degree tear can be stitched by your midwife in the delivery room under local anaesthetic while you hold your baby. A third- or fourth-degree tear needs an obstetrician to repair it in theatre. If you've had an epidural this can be topped up before surgery, otherwise you will be given either a spinal block or a local anaesthetic. Very rarely, a general anaesthetic is given. Your birth partner and your baby may be able to stay with you while you are being stitched.

The stitches are almost always dissolvable so will disappear on their own, within two weeks or so for superficial stitches, and three months for deeper stitches. There is usually no need for a doctor to check them unless you have concerns.

Did you know...

On average, women lose around 5.5kg (12lb) immediately after the birth, as they shed the combined weight of the baby, placenta, and amniotic fluid. However, you will still appear pregnant after your baby is born as your uterus takes time to shrink back down and it takes several days or weeks to lose the excess fluid you carried during pregnancy.

Q I've heard there is some bleeding after birth – how much is usual?

There will be some bleeding straight after the delivery of your baby when the placenta comes away from the wall of the uterus, exposing the blood vessels it was connected to. Normal levels of blood loss can be up to 600ml (1 pint) of blood in the first 24 hours. Once the placenta is delivered, the uterus continues to contract, which helps to close the blood vessels and stem the bleeding. If you have an episiotomy or a tear, that may also cause some bleeding.

Post-partum haemorrhage (PPH) is when you have more bleeding than normal. Heavy bleeding within 24 hours of birth is known as primary PPH, and it affects 5 per cent of women. The main reason for primary PPH is that the uterus isn't contracting efficiently, which can lead to heavy blood loss.

You will also get a bloody discharge known as lochia after delivery as the uterine lining renews itself (see p.259).

Q What if the bleeding is so heavy that it doesn't stop?

Unless bleeding is obviously profuse, your medical team will first try to stem the flow. They may massage the uterus, and/or give you anticoagulant drugs to encourage your blood to clot, or an injection of synthetic oxytocin (see

p.220). If your placenta is incomplete, or the bleeding has no obvious cause, you will probably be taken into theatre, where, under general anaesthetic, an obstetric surgeon will remove the remainder of the placenta surgically, or investigate why you're still bleeding and treat you as necessary. If you have lost a lot of blood, you may be given a blood transfusion.

Q Will I be able to have a bath shortly after the delivery?

Yes. If all is well, you'll be encouraged to wash. You may feel a bit wobbly, so have someone with you. Your birth partner and baby can come with you (you can wheel your baby in the hospital cot). After an epidural, you will be given a bed bath, then once you can walk safely, you can shower or have a bath.

Q I'm anxious about going to the loo after the birth. Will this hurt?

If you are in hospital, your midwife will want to know that you are urinating before discharging you, so you'll need to brave the loo. If you had a tear or episiotomy, passing urine may sting; pouring lukewarm water over the area as you pee can be soothing. To ensure first stools are soft and easy to pass, drink plenty of water and eat lots of fibre over the first few days.

{ Q } How will I know that my newborn baby is healthy?

Your baby's first cries will be a wonderful sound but, understandably, you will want to know she is in perfect health. It is reassuring to know that she will be thoroughly checked immediately after the birth, and have further checks before leaving hospital. The checks are non-invasive and effective in highlighting possible health problems.

The APGAR test

In the early 1950s, American obstetric anaesthetist Virginia Apgar developed a simple five-measure test to assess the health of a baby minutes after birth. The test has been criticized for being too simple, but it remains one of the first assessments your baby will have – at one minute after birth, and then again at five minutes after birth.

THE APGAR SCORE

Virginia Apgar's surname is used as an acronym for the five measures in this test, which is carried out straight after the birth. This is why you will sometimes see it written as APGAR:

>> **Appearance:** Skin and lip colour indicate whether your baby is getting enough oxygen.
>> **Pulse:** Your baby's heart rate is measured with a stethoscope.
>> **Grimace:** Your baby's response to stimuli, such as light or touch, will be checked.
>> **Activity:** Arm and leg movements give an indication of muscle tone.
>> **Respiration:** The rhythm and effort of your baby's breathing is checked.

After both the one-minute and five-minute check, a combined score of seven or more indicates that all is well. Between five and seven can mean the baby needs help breathing, but probably no more than a rub on the chest to kickstart her reflexes. A score of under five can indicate more help is needed, and a paediatrician will be called to examine the baby.

SCORE	0	1	2
Appearance Skin and lip colour	Completely blue skin all over	Pink body with white or blue extremities	Completely pink skin all over
Pulse	No heartbeat	Slow heartbeat	Fast heartbeat
Grimace	Unresponsive	Reacts to stimulation	Crying spontaneously
Activity	Inactive, limp	Slow movements to extend and retract arms and legs	Lots of activity in the arms and legs
Respiration	No breathing	Slow, weak, or very uneven breathing	Strong breaths and crying

Grasp reflex You may be surprised by the strength of your newborn's grip. This is due to the grasp reflex; she will instinctively grasp something that is placed in her palm.

Hands The midwife will place a finger in your baby's palm to check she grasps it

Back Spinal checks are very important as abnormalities can indicate spina bifida

Instant health checks

Your midwife will do the Apgar test so quickly that you are unlikely to notice the checks being carried out. A further top-to-toe check (see right) in the delivery room will highlight if there are any health concerns. If the midwife's checks do highlight any problems, these will be explained to you, and your baby will be given the appropriate care. In some circumstances, the midwife may request that a paediatrician gives a second opinion.

Assuming all is well with your baby, you will be able to take her to the postnatal ward. Within 72 hours of the birth, your baby will be examined again (see p.246), either in hospital or at home. If at any point you are concerned about your baby's health, do inform a midwife or doctor immediately.

Feet Your baby's feet will be checked to ensure she has five toes and that there is no webbed skin

YOUR BABY'S TOP-TO-TOE EXAMINATION

Mouth The roof of the mouth is checked to ensure it is fully formed

Skin The colour of your baby's skin can be checked in an instant. If it is pink all over, that is a sign of good health

Legs The midwife will manipulate your baby's legs to ensure her knee joints have the correct range of movement

1 Head: are the soft spots on your baby's skull (the fontanelles), the head shape, head circumference, and hair texture normal?

2 Facial expression: as your baby scrunches up her face in response to a stimulus, is her expression symmetrical? This is a sign of overall wellbeing.

3 Eyes
» Do the pupils dilate with changes in light?
» Is there "red-eye", indicating cataracts?

4 Nose: is there any mucus blocking the nasal passages, affecting baby's breathing?

5 Cheeks: does your baby turn to the side when her cheek is stroked? This indicates her response to touch and tests for the "rooting reflex".

6 Mouth
» Has the roof of your baby's mouth fully formed?
» Does her tongue move freely, and is it a good colour and size?
» Does your baby suck when the midwife puts his or her little finger inside your baby's mouth?

7 Lips: does your baby "root for food" when a finger is brushed across the top of her lip?

8 Ears
» Does your baby turn her head to a sound?
» Are her ears symmetrical?
» Are there any skin tags?
» Do the ears fold forwards and backwards?
» When the earlobes are gently pinched, does blood flow back quickly to show healthy circulation?

9 Neck: when the neck is manipulated, does your baby's head bend forwards, backwards, and from side to side?

10 Collarbone: was there any injury to the collarbone during birth?

11 Chest:
» Do your baby's lungs sound clear?
» Are the heart position and heartbeat correct?

12 Skin
» Does your baby's skin colour show she is getting a healthy level of oxygen?
» Is there any sign of jaundice (see p.249)?
» Is your baby's temperature normal?

13 Arms
» Are the arms proportionate to the baby's size?
» Does she throw her arms back in the "startle reflex" (also known as the Moro reflex)? If it doesn't happen spontaneously, the midwife will cup your baby's head and safely allow it to seem to fall; this should trigger the reflex.

14 Hands and wrists
» Does your baby open her fingers as if to hold something when the back of her hand is brushed?
» Does she grasp the midwife's finger and hold on when it is placed on her palm? She or he will pull her hand upward, raising your baby slightly, to test grip.
» Are all your baby's fingers there and of the expected length compared with one another?
» Are there any creases in your baby's palms? Some creases can be a sign of Down's Syndrome, but there will be other signs with this condition.
» Do the wrists give the full range of movements?

15 Back
» Do your baby's shoulder blades look symmetrical?
» Are there tufts of hair or fat deposits along your baby's spine line? These can indicate spina bifida.
» Are all the vertebrae there and properly aligned with no unusual kinks or curves?
» Does gently pressing on the spine seem to cause your baby any pain?

16 Tummy
» Are the size and symmetry of the tummy normal?
» Do the organs feel normal? For example, it would be normal to be able to feel the edges of the liver, but unexpected to feel the spleen or kidneys.
» Is the cord stump infected or bleeding?

17 Hips: is there an appropriate range of movement around the hip joints?

18 Genitals
» Has your baby passed any meconium, showing that the anus is open?
» Do genitals look normal and healthy, and have the testicles descended in a boy baby?

19 Legs
» Are the legs the same length as each other?
» Do the knees and ankles have full movement?

20 Feet
» Is the position of the feet at rest normal and are the ankles and the arches of the feet flexible?
» Is there the correct number of toes and are they of the expected length compared to each other?
» Is there any webbing between the toes?

Rooting If anything strokes your baby's cheek, she'll turn her head to root for the object. This reflex ensures successful breastfeeding.

» In this chapter...

The postnatal period

The first few hours, days, and weeks with a newborn can be **challenging, but delightful** at the same time. This chapter will prepare you for what to expect. Read up on **breastfeeding and bottle-feeding** so you're ready to go as soon as your baby is. Once you finally have your **beautiful new baby** to cuddle and love, information on practical baby care will help you get the best out of your precious time together.

A CLOSER LOOK
The first 12 weeks

We talk about babies being fully formed at birth, but of course there are still myriad phases of growth for them to go through, physically, mentally, and emotionally. When you look back in three months at photographs of your baby on the day he was born, you'll barely be able to believe how that tiny, wrinkled, curled-up bundle could become the bouncing, smiling, laughing, grasping, and inquisitive little person you hold now.

1 WEEK OLD Your baby will spend time curled up as he adjusts to life outside the womb. His fists will remain clenched for much of the time.
What you can do: Get your baby to look in a mirror – he loves looking at faces and will seek out yours immediately after birth.

2 WEEKS OLD Your baby may now be able to hold his head up for a few seconds when held to your shoulder.
What you can do: Pull faces at your baby and stick out your tongue. He will try to mimic you.

3 WEEKS OLD You may notice that your baby's movements are less jerky and more controlled. He is gaining control of his muscles. Some of his more primitive reflexes are beginning to fade.
What you can do: Although your days and nights are still a blur, you can help your baby to start to differentiate them by darkening his room at night to help him identify night-time.

4 WEEKS OLD At four weeks, your baby's neck muscles are growing stronger and you may notice him holding his head up a little longer when he is supported on you.
What you can do: Place your baby on his tummy; he will try to lift his head up from the surface. This helps him build more strength in his back and neck.

5 WEEKS OLD Your baby can now focus both eyes and is working his eye muscles hard to focus on objects near and far. He can track a moving object from the side of his vision until it is in front of him.
What you can do: Young babies love black and white patterns. Try placing some where your baby can look at them while he is lying down.

6 WEEKS OLD At around six weeks, you will see something that makes all the hard work worthwhile: your baby's first smile. He is becoming more socially aware and responds to your voice, holding your gaze when you speak.
What you can do: Talk to your baby, it will help him develop his language skills even though he can't respond with words. You may even get a few throaty noises in reply.

FASCINATING FACTS

20–25cm
(8-10in) is the distance your baby can focus on at two weeks old.

4 weeks
At four weeks your baby will be less curled up than after birth.

10 days
The umbilical cord usually comes off naturally 10 days after birth.

7 **WEEKS OLD** Your baby is beginning to discover his hands, you may notice him gazing at them and moving his fingers. This is the start of hand-eye coordination. He may draw his hands towards his mouth to explore them. His eye muscles have developed enough so that his eyes can now move in unison. Cooing and gurgling can start around now, as your baby realizes that he has a voice!

What you can do: Try dangling objects over him – just within swiping reach – as he lies on his back.

8 **WEEKS OLD** Your baby's back and neck muscles are now strong enough for him to hold his head in the midline of his body when he is lying on his back. Try holding your baby under his armpits and letting him bat his feet against the floor. Some babies are able to bear a little weight on their legs at this stage.

What you can do: Give your baby plenty of space to move, stretch out, and build strength in those growing muscles.

9 **WEEKS OLD** Your baby is becoming more sociable. He recognizes his parents and responds to your attention. He is beginning to associate people with fun and playtime.

What you can do: Your baby already loves your voice, but try using varied tones and interesting facial expressions. Copy your baby's coos to help him learn that the art of conversation is better with two!

10 **WEEKS OLD** The ability to calm and soothe himself is an important skill for your baby to learn and it may be developing by around 10 weeks. You may notice that your baby can cope with higher levels of stimulation. He may have worked out how to bring his hands together in front of his face or body.

What you can do: Your baby may enjoy a trip to the swimming pool; not only does it provide new sights, sounds, and sensations, but is also the first step towards learning to swim.

11 **WEEKS OLD** Your baby is beginning to recognize objects, such as his bottle or the movements you make to prepare for breastfeeding, and will show signs of eagerness to feed. He is also able to connect sounds with the object that makes them.

What you can do: Try making a sensory box filled with items of different colours and textures that can make different sounds, such as crinkly paper, rustling foil, and rattles. Put them in your baby's hands so that he can explore them.

12 **WEEKS OLD** By now, your baby is really starting to communicate with you. You may hear coos, squeals, and even a little babbling. Your baby may start reaching out to grab things with intent, rather than simply grasping what's handed to him. Your baby's digestive system is fully matured now. Your baby's giggles begin around now – a sure sign that he thinks you're funny!

What you can do: Try incorporating gentle movement with nursery rhymes.

14–18
The number of hours that your baby will sleep during a 24-hour period.

6 million
There are some six million cells on every square centimetre of a newborn's skin.

4 reflexes
Your newborn baby has four natural reflexes at birth: startle, rooting, grasping, and stepping.

Congratulations on **your wonderful new baby!** Nothing can prepare you for how it feels to become a parent. You are likely to experience a tumult of emotions – joy may be mixed with a sense of **unreality and wonder** as you marvel at this new addition to your family. Enjoy this precious time getting to know this incredible little person.

The first 12 weeks

A new family

As well as bonding with your baby, as a new mother it is crucial that you look after yourself and get plenty of rest. On the following pages, you will find a snapshot of what to expect in the first 12 weeks.

If you gave birth in hospital, you will be transferred to a ward with your new baby. If you have opted to breastfeed and haven't yet done so in the delivery room, you will be encouraged to do this now with support from a midwife. Be reassured that it can take time to establish feeding – both you and your baby are learning – so don't worry if you have some difficulty at first.

Once you are alone with your new baby, the reality that she is actually here may hit you, bringing with it a wide range of emotions. Your baby is likely to be asleep and you may simply spend much of the time staring at her in wonderment. Try to hold her close, preferably skin to skin, and talk to her. You are the one familiar person in this new world, the person whose voice and smell are instantly recognizable to her. If you have had a Caesarean section and find it difficult to hold her, ask your partner to hold her skin to skin instead.

While you will want to share your news with family and friends, contact the key people and then consider turning off your phone. These first hours with your newborn baby are best enjoyed with little interruption. Although you will be allowed visitors to the hospital, it is a good idea to keep the number of people who come to a minimum. There will be plenty of time for everyone to meet the new arrival in the weeks to come.

Going home

Depending on your circumstances, you may be discharged from hospital on the same day as the birth, once the midwives are happy that feeding has been established and your baby has undergone health checks (see pp.238–39). Use the time you are in hospital to ask questions about your baby's care, from nappy-changing and bathing to feeding and sleeping.

Having responsibility for this little person may feel overwhelming, but try to relax and remember you are the best person to care for her. Be reassured that a midwife will aim to visit you at home the day after the birth to check both your progress and that of your baby, and offer advice and support. She or he will visit regularly in the first 10 days to check your baby is feeding well and that you are recovering. Following this, you and your baby will be cared for by a health visitor.

Q Do most people instantly fall in love with their baby?

Some people feel a rush of love, and some don't. If this feeling doesn't hit you straight away, don't worry. For some bonding is a much more gradual process, but the relationship that develops in the end is just as strong and secure.

In the past, experts believed that there was a critical window for bonding shortly after birth, but we now understand bonding as a much more subtle, complex, and long-term process that develops in the days, weeks, and months following your baby's arrival. The deep attachment that comes with a strong and lasting bond is something that happens gradually over time. Holding your baby and caring for her day to day will create a secure attachment, a sense of trust, and a growing mutual love that becomes immeasurable and profound. You may even be unaware that a bond is developing – for many parents, the first time they experience that heart-jumping jolt is the first time their baby smiles several weeks after the birth.

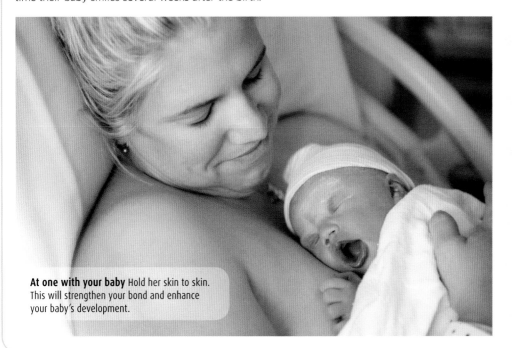

At one with your baby Hold her skin to skin. This will strengthen your bond and enhance your baby's development.

Bonding tips

» **Hold your baby close:** eventually your baby will need to learn to self-soothe and fall asleep alone, but in these early days and weeks cuddle her as much as you want to.

» **Interact:** spend as much time as you can with your baby when she's awake: make eye contact; sing to her; talk to her. She can see you and hear you and this communication will only serve to strengthen the growing bond between you.

» **Make her your priority:** forget the chores and don't be afraid to accept help from others around you. These early weeks are precious so devote as much time as you can to your baby.

» **Limit visitors:** relatives and friends are bound to want to meet your new arrival, but in these early weeks try to stagger visitors. It's important to have time to spend together as a new family.

» **Give yourself time:** don't put pressure on yourself to feel or behave in a certain way. Try to relax and allow the relationship between you and your new baby to develop. If after several weeks you still feel detached, speak to your health visitor.

Q It's a boy! I was sure I was having a girl. How should I adjust to this surprise?

Whether you have had a boy or girl, this is a time of enormous change. The first few days and weeks following childbirth are all about adjusting to the reality of having a small, fragile baby to look after. In addition to this, your baby may look and behave differently to how you might have expected. You will also be experiencing a whirlwind of emotions due to hormone changes, exhaustion from the birth and the hospital environment. Try to focus on bonding and getting to know your new baby.

This can take time, but as the days and weeks roll on, you will develop your own unique relationship, regardless of gender.

Q I am finding the first feeds difficult. Is this normal?

Be reassured that this is normal. Newborn babies are born with reserves and may not require much feeding during this time. Like you, your baby is probably exhausted from labour and birth and will sleep a lot. As a result she may be hard to feed. It may take time for both of you to get the hang of breastfeeding.

However, if you want to breastfeed, it is best to get this underway as soon as possible. Enjoy skin-to-skin contact and put your baby to your breast every few hours, which will aid the production of breastfeeding hormones. If you are struggling, make sure to ask for guidance from a midwife or a feeding specialist.

On average, newborn babies tend to feed around **8 to 12 times a day**, or more, in the first weeks after birth.

Q I'd like to go home soon after the birth, but I know my baby has to be examined first. Why is this?

This thorough top-to-toe check is offered within three days of the birth, and its aim is to identify abnormalities or certain conditions that were missed during antenatal screening.

Your baby will be thoroughly examined straight after the birth (see p.239), but will be checked again within 72 hours, usually by a paediatrician or midwife before you are discharged from hospital. If you leave shortly after the birth, some hospitals arrange for the check to be done by a community midwife or GP at home; for a home birth, a visiting GP or midwife will carry out newborn checks within 72 hours of your baby's birth.

Detecting any health problems this early means that babies can be referred promptly for treatment, which usually leads to better long-term outcomes.

A newborn baby's **heart rate is usually around 110–160 beats per minute.** To begin with, the heart is large in relation to the chest wall.

NEWBORN BABY CHECKS

The checks below are carried out to confirm that your newborn baby is in good health. The paediatrician or midwife may also test your baby's reflexes again at this examination.

» **Skin:** the overall skin colour and any birthmarks are observed.

» **Heart and lungs:** a stethoscope is used to make sure heart sounds and breathing patterns are normal. The pulse is checked.

» **Head and face:** the fontanelles (soft spots) on the head that allowed the bony plates to squeeze through the birth canal, are checked. Your baby's facial features are checked for symmetry.

» **Eyes:** a special torch called an ophthalmoscope is used to check for "red reflex" to makes sure there are no cataracts.

» **Mouth:** the roof of the mouth is examined to ensure there is no split, or cleft, in the palate.

» **Mouth:** the tongue is checked for tongue tie, as restrictions can interfere with breastfeeding.

» **Hips:** the legs are gently bent upwards and rotated at the hips, to check hip joints are not malformed (see p.324).

» **Genitals:** in boys, the position of the testes and the penis is checked. You will be asked if your baby has had a wee and poo.

» **Back:** the spine is examined to ensure it is properly formed.

» **Hands and feet:** the fingers and toes are examined and the creases on the palms of the hands and the resting position of the feet and ankles are checked.

Head The soft spots on your baby's head are examined. Any effects from an assisted delivery will also be checked.

Spine The spine and back are examined to ensure they are straight and free from any abnormalities.

Hips Any signs of dislocation will be found when the paediatrician rotates the baby's hips.

Hearing test This test will usually be done in hospital before you and your baby leave, or alternatively it may be done at home or in a clinic by your health visitor or a specially trained screener.

Q Why does my newborn baby need to have a hearing test in the first 24 hours after the birth?

Around 1 in 900 babies is born with some degree of hearing loss. Being aware of this early on is important for a baby's development as it means he can be given the right support and assistance and have the best chance of developing speech and language skills.

A small earpiece placed in your baby's outer ear transmits clicking sounds down the ear canal; these are received by the inner ear, which responds with an echo. It is a quick and painless procedure, which can be done while he's asleep.

Q What is vitamin K? Why does my baby need it after the birth?

Vitamin K plays an essential role in blood clotting. Some babies are born with inadequate amounts of vitamin K as it doesn't cross the placenta easily, and breast milk contains very little. This puts them at risk of a rare, but potentially fatal, condition – vitamin K deficiency bleeding of the newborn (VKDB), where bleeding can occur in the nose, mouth, and sometimes in the brain. Vitamin K is given as two or three doses of oral drops or a single injection, which works faster and may be needed if you've had an assisted delivery.

Q My baby sleeps all the time. Should I wake him every 2–3 hours to feed?

Rest assured that your baby won't starve himself. After your baby's initial alertness following the birth you may be surprised at how much he sleeps and you may worry that he isn't getting enough to eat. In the first few days, your baby only needs small amounts of the pre-milk colostrum. A teaspoon's worth of this thick and creamy, antibody-rich substance that your breasts produce is perfect for his very small tummy. However, it is fairly good practice to put your baby to the breast every two to three hours at first. This is not to get him into a feeding schedule – it's far too early for this – but to help you both develop your technique, and to stimulate your breasts to produce milk. While your first breast milk arrives on average about three to five days after the birth, the more your baby suckles, the faster your milk is likely to "come in".

Q Why does my baby breathe so noisily when he sleeps?

Your baby breathes in and out through his nose only, which means he can breathe comfortably during a long feed. However it also means that if mucus is blocking his nasal passage, he may snuffle and snort to clear it, or make a wheezing, whistling sound while he breathes. He may gurgle if the mucus makes its way to the back of his throat. As his air passages are still very small, it's easy for them to get blocked.

Babies also spend about half their sleep time in "active" sleep, when dreams occur, so tend to be more restless and noisy. Young babies may also have periods during sleep when they stop breathing altogether for a few breaths, which can be for as long as 10 seconds, then revert to shallow and rapid breathing before resuming normal breathing. This "periodic" breathing is especially common in babies born prematurely, but can also occur in full-term babies, and is a passing phase. Noisy breathing that is intermittent is nothing to worry about, but if your baby is persistently noisy, or his breathing seems very laboured and fast, he flares his nostrils, makes a barking or rasping sound, his breathing pauses for longer than 10 seconds, or he has a blue tinge to his skin, seek medical guidance.

Q My baby has just done his first poo and it was black! Is this normal?

It can be a bit of a shock when you peek inside your newborn's nappy to discover a greenish-black poo. Don't worry – it's a sign of good health.

This greenish-black, tar-like substance is called meconium. It is made up of dead skin cells, lanugo, bilirubin, mucus, and bile that gathered in your baby's intestines while he was in the uterus and which your baby passes in the first 24 hours.

Although meconium looks a little alarming and is difficult to clean, this first sticky bowel movement is quite normal, and its appearance is a welcome sign that your baby's bowels are in good working order. Your baby's poo will change over the first week or so as he settles into feeding. If you are concerned at all, speak to your health visitor.

Bowel movements When you change your baby's nappy it is normal to find stools of differing colours.

WHAT DOES A NORMAL NAPPY LOOK LIKE?

It's often news to first-time parents that baby stools come in a whole range of colours and textures. So knowing what's normal (most of it), and what isn't quite right will stop you worrying each time you look in your baby's nappy. Here's what you can expect:

≫ **In the first couple of days,** your baby will pass meconium, the thick, green-black, tar-like substance that accumulated in his bowels while in the uterus.

≫ **From days three to five,** stools gradually change, turning from dark green through to yellow and light brown.

≫ **Your breastfed baby's** stools will be a mustard-like colour and may be seedy and watery. They are also surprisingly sweet-smelling.

≫ **Your formula-fed baby's** stools tend to be more formed and a slightly darker yellow-tan colour. Some formula can lend a greenish colour to stools.

≫ **In the first few days,** your baby may poo frequently, sometimes after each feed. After about day four, your baby will usually pass around two stools a day for the next few weeks. Breastfed babies sometimes pass stools less often, and may occasionally go several days without a bowel movement. As long as the stools are soft and not uncomfortable for your baby to pass, this isn't a concern.

{Q My baby looks nothing like the pictures in the magazines. Why is this?

First-time parents can be surprised at the appearance of their newborn. The bundle of joy you are handed after birth may not be the picture-perfect vision you had in mind. It is good to understand why and to remember that even though each baby is unique, they all share some physical characteristics at this time.

Whether your baby has been pushed, squashed, and squeezed down the birth canal following a vaginal delivery or has been delivered by Caesarean section, she will have been through an enormous event. Added to this, her appearance bears testimony to the nine months she has spent curled up in your uterus, floating in the amniotic fluid. Given this, it is not surprising that she emerges swollen, bruised, and bloody. Rest assured that many of her newborn features – a larger head in comparison to the rest of her body, swollen facial features, skin covered in a strange coating and enlarged genitals – will settle down after a day or so as she recovers from the birth. Try to enjoy her newborn looks while you can, as they won't last long!

HEAD

Your baby's head is a quarter of her body length. The skull bones are soft and flexible and have gaps between them. These "soft spots" are called the fontanelles – handle these areas gently after birth. They will disappear completely by 18 months old. During labour, the skull bones move and mould the head to help it pass through the birth canal. This can give newborns a cone-shaped head. If you had an assisted delivery, there may be bruising where the forceps were positioned or a swelling where the ventouse suction cup was placed; this goes down in 24–48 hours. Your baby's head will gradually round out and any marks will disappear.

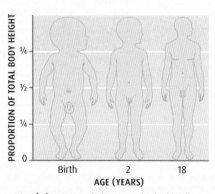

Head size As your baby grows, his body will become more in proportion with his head.

HAIR

Your baby may be virtually bald or have an impressive shock of hair. This hair is often shed in the first few months, and the new hair that replaces it may bear no resemblance to the newborn crop, but look more like the hair you would expect her to have.

SKIN

Your baby is likely to emerge covered in blood, amniotic fluid, and a creamy, waxy substance called vernix caseosa – this coated her skin in the uterus, ensuring that she didn't become waterlogged. If she is born after 41 weeks, she may have shed some of the vernix already, and her skin might be a little dry. Your baby may also have patches of fine, downy hair called lanugo. This would have kept the vernix in place.

While the skin may look purplish at first, once your baby starts to breathe on her own, her colour will settle down. Her skin will also look quite fine, and you may be able to see tiny blood vessels under the surface in certain areas. As the circulation is immature, the hands and feet may appear blue for a day or so.

EYES AND NOSE

Your baby's nose may be quite squashed after a vaginal birth, and that cute, turned up appearance enables your little one to breathe easily while feeding. Your baby's eyes may be swollen and puffy and the whites of the eye may be bloodshot from the pressure of squeezing through the birth canal.

WHEN YOUR BABY HAS JAUNDICE

Jaundice in newborns is so common that it's more unusual if your baby doesn't develop this condition.

It is caused by a build-up in the blood of a yellow substance called bilirubin, which causes the skin and the whites of the eyes to turn pale yellow. All newborn babies can tolerate mild jaundice and monitoring is all that is needed. It tends to clear up naturally within two weeks, and just 1 in 20 babies needs treatment (see p.322).

Jaundiced babies Jaundice improves quickly and often babies don't need treatment.

SPOTS AND RASHES

Your baby may be born with a cluster of tiny, white spots over her nose, cheeks, eyes, and forehead, or these may develop in the early weeks. These are known as milia, and are thought to be caused by underdeveloped glands in the skin. They are harmless and will disappear within a few weeks.

GENITALS

A surge in maternal hormones just before the birth means that both girls and boys may be born with swollen breasts and genitals from the hormones crossing over the placenta. Girls may have a vaginal discharge, which may even have a little blood in it, and there may be a white discharge from the breasts. All of this is normal, and the swelling will die down in the first few days.

BIRTHMARKS

Marks on the skin at birth are common and are usually nothing to worry about. Birthmarks fall into two categories: vascular or pigmented. Vascular birthmarks include:

BIRTHMARK	LOOKS LIKE	DESCRIPTION
Stork marks		Stork marks are also called salmon patches or naevus simplus. These light pink marks can appear on the forehead, the nose, around the mouth, on the eyelids, or the nape of the neck. These usually fade over time until they are hardly noticeable.
Strawberry haemangiomas		These are harmless, raised red marks formed by a concentration of immature blood vessels. They can grow quickly in the first few months, then start to shrink back and disappear. Depending on their size and position, they sometimes require treatment.
Port-wine stains		Port-wine stains, also called naevus flammeus, are flat, red or purple marks caused by a concentration of dilated blood vessels. They darken over time and are permanent. They can appear anywhere on the body, but are usually on the face, neck, or the limbs.

PIGMENTED BIRTHMARKS

	LOOKS LIKE	DESCRIPTION
Café au lait spots		These coffee-coloured patches can appear anywhere on the body. They may be present at birth, and more may appear over the first years of life. While usually harmless, if your child has several, it's worth asking the doctor to have a quick look.
Mongolian blue spots		Mongolian spots are more common on darker-skinned babies. These blue-grey patches of skin typically appear on the back or buttocks, and usually fade of their own accord in the first few years.
Moles		Known as congenital naevi, these are brown or black, and can be flat or raised. These marks are usually harmless, but should be monitored as they carry a risk of becoming malignant later in life.

Umbilical cord The clamped cord will fall off naturally around 10 days after birth.

HANDS AND FEET

Your baby's legs may be "bowed" and her feet curved inwards, reflecting the curled up position she adopted in the uterus. Her limbs and feet will straighten out over time. If your baby was full term, her toes and fingernails may be quite long, and she may even have managed to scratch herself. The nails will be soft, so you can peel them off very carefully or clip them with baby scissors.

Q What checks will be done on my baby once I leave hospital, and in the early weeks?

A community midwife will visit you at home the next day after you leave hospital, and regularly for the following 10 days.

During the visits, the midwife will check how you are recovering from the birth and coping with life at home. She or he will ask how feeding is progressing and also weigh your baby. Community midwives provide an invaluable resource for help and advice and are there to help you in this early period. The visits are a good opportunity to share any worries you may have and to ask for support with anything to do with your health

Weigh-in Once the health visitor is no longer visiting, you will be asked to get your baby weighed at the clinic.

following delivery, and looking after your baby. After the 10 days, you will be handed over to a health visitor (a nurse with specialized training) who will initially come to your home and then you'll go to a local child health clinic. Health visitors can also offer you valuable parenting

support. The health visitor will monitor you and your baby, and will weigh your baby at regular intervals. The health visitor will plot your baby's weight on a growth chart in the red child health record book that will be given to you for safekeeping.

> The average newborn weight is **7lb 8oz (3.4kg) for boys** and **7lb 4oz (3.3kg) for girls.**
> It is normal for babies to lose some of their birth weight in the first week and then regain it.

Q The midwife said she will do a heel-prick test on my baby in the first week. What exactly is it?

This quick procedure, also known as the "blood spot" or Guthrie test, checks for a number of conditions. This test is not compulsory, but it is recommended as the benefits of early screening are enormous. Early treatment can improve the health of your baby and prevent severe disability. You should be given information about this test and the diseases it screens for in advance so you can make an informed decision for your baby.

The test is carried out at around five days after birth. A health professional will prick your baby's heel to collect a blood sample on a piece of card, which is then sent off for analysis. Your baby may feel a little discomfort during this test, which can be upsetting for parents, too. Holding and cuddling your baby and feeding him while the test is being done is thought to minimize any discomfort your baby feels. The

heel-prick test screens for nine conditions: the genetic blood disorder sickle cell disease; cystic fibrosis, an inherited condition; congenital hypothyroidism, a condition that affects growth and mental development; and six inherited metabolic diseases such as MCADD and phenylketonuria (PKU).

You should receive the results by the time your baby is about eight weeks old. If any of the screens are positive, it means your baby is more likely to have one of these conditions and he will be referred for further testing.

Q My baby is hardly gaining weight. Should I be worried?

it's easy to fret if you think your baby isn't piling on the pounds. Watching a baby's weight steadily creep up is a reassuring sign for parents that they are getting it right. However, some babies are just naturally slower at gaining weight. If your baby is happy, alert, responsive,

and reaching milestones, he is probably fine. If you feel uneasy, talk to your health visitor or GP who can check your baby's growth chart. If your baby has gone down two percentiles, or has dropped below the third percentile for growth, further checks and investigations may be recommended.

A failure to gain weight usually happens when a baby isn't getting the calories he needs, or his body isn't absorbing or using nutrients properly. There is often a simple explanation. If your baby has been ill, he may have lost weight and it can take a couple of weeks for his feeding to get back on track. Alternatively, he may not be latching on (see pp.268–69) properly and this can affect his milk intake. If this is the case, seek guidance from a health professional or a breastfeeding consultant.

If your baby is formula fed, ensure the bottle is made up with the right ratio of powder to water so that he gets the nutrients he needs to grow and thrive. Occasionally, slow weight gain is down to a milk intolerance or allergy, reflux, or, more rarely, a medical condition.

Q When should I try to get my baby into a routine?

In the early weeks it is a good idea to begin to teach your baby the difference between day and night, but don't worry about a routine yet.

This can be hard and you may also need to surrender yourself to your baby's world by sleeping when he sleeps, if possible. He has arrived in your world with his own round-the-clock schedule.

Newborn babies sleep for much of the time, around 14 to 18 hours in every 24, but this sleep is broken up into segments. Your baby's tiny tummy can hold only a little food, so he needs to wake every two to three hours to feed. As your baby and his tummy grow, he will be able to go for longer between feeds and a routine will emerge. A degree of flexibility is key, though – accept that sometimes your baby's needs may vary from the routine.

During these first few weeks you can subtly introduce the idea of night and day: dimming lights, reducing activity in the evening, and gradually introducing an end-of-day wind down that will evolve into a bedtime routine. Your baby will need feeds during the night for a while and it is a good idea to give these in a calm, quiet environment. If you can see past the tiredness, try to cherish these first special weeks with your new baby. This time spent cocooned with her is fleeting, and you are likely to look back on it with a sense of awe.

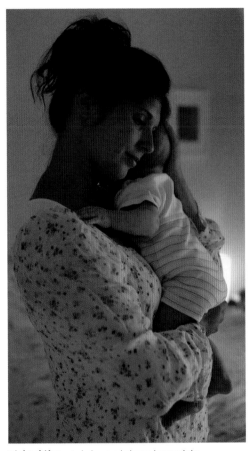

Night shift Try to help your baby understand the difference between day and night by dimming lights.

After **six weeks** your baby may begin to sleep for longer periods during the night and slightly less during the day.

Q Why is my baby often grizzly when I put him down for a nap?

This happens if you miss the naptime window, as overstimulation and overtiredness make it harder for your baby to settle. In the first three months, your baby will start to have longer periods of alertness between naps, but he will still be doing a lot of sleeping around the clock, so it's important that he gets his daytime sleeps.

It can be tricky to time naps as babies can move quickly from being awake and alert to being a little tired, then extremely tired. The moment to put your baby down is that period when tiredness is just starting to kick in, as this is the moment he will be best able to settle down to sleep. Tiredness cues can be as subtle as glancing away or looking a bit glazed. He may become fidgety and make jerky movements, and may clench his fists, tug his ears, or flutter his eyelids. Look out for all these cues.

Q My baby often cries when he's at home with me. Is he bored?

At home, it may often be just the two of you, and the onus to keep your baby entertained and happy falls on your shoulders, which can feel like a burden. Don't try to entertain him every waking minute. He will thrive on the one-to-one attention he gets during 10 minutes of uninterrupted time with you, and he is then likely to coo happily on his play mat for 20 minutes, or be content watching you as you get on with chores.

Moving your baby around the house with you will help him feel secure and confident that you are close by, and this can make him less fretful. Newborns enjoy looking at the world around them so place him by an interesting house plant, a window, or patterned wallpaper to keep him fascinated, and keep changing the view. Remember that your baby knows you are the one who meets his needs, and his cries are his way of communicating with you – when it's just the two of you, he may be more focused on his needs.

Q My friends and family want to visit the baby. How can I manage the visits so I am not overwhelmed?

When you return home from hospital, you and your baby need plenty of time to adjust. Keen visitors need to understand this and their expectations should be managed. It is a good idea to invite them for a short visit and limit visits to one or two per day with gaps between them. Let them know when you are tired and need to rest. Close friends and famiy may want to help so try to think of a task to give them such as shopping or small household chores.

Did you know...

As little as 5–10 minutes of deep relaxation can refresh you. Instead of doing housework, try taking a short nap while your baby sleeps. It is worth learning about different relaxation techniques either online or from your local library.

Q What help is available during the early weeks if I feel that I am beginning to struggle?

Looking after a newborn can be chaotic, tiring, and sometimes overwhelming. Depending on your personal circumstances, you may want some extra, paid help when you return home from hospital.

There are various options available and it is important to remember that paid childcare is generally not cheap. Speak to other mothers for recommendations of good nanny agencies. Magazines and newspapers are also a good source of childcare advertisements. With all forms of childcare, it is vital to follow up all the references.

 Maternity nurse She will help you care for your baby in the early weeks. These are generally the most expensive form of childcare as they usually live in and cover 24 hours a day, six days a week. Most people employ a maternity nurse for approximately four weeks. Their role is to help with daytime care as well as looking after your baby at night, bringing them to you for feeds, and settling them afterwards.

 Night nurse If you need help with night-time duties, this can be a good option. However, the difference between this kind of help and that of a maternity nurse is that they go home during the day and simply come to help with feeding and settling your baby during the night. Night nurses can be useful if your partner cannot share the night feeds. Some people choose to have them a couple of nights a week.

 Doula This is an experienced woman who offers practical and emotional (non-medical) support to a mother during and/or after childbirth. Employing a doula as a caregiver has become popular. The time they spend with you is flexible and can range from a few visits at the start to fixed hours for a period of eight weeks. They provide breastfeeding support, help around the house, and let you catch up on a few hours of much-needed sleep.

Q How should I plan for my baby's first trip outside?

Getting out of the house with a young baby can be nerve racking and challenging. However, with a little preparation and planning you'll be able to make your first trip easier and more enjoyable. The first thing to remember is that you'll need to be able to transport your baby reliably and safely when you are out. If you are going by car, you are legally obliged to have an age-appropriate car seat. Think about whether it would be easier to carry your baby in a sling or use a buggy. If you are using public transport, it might be worth finding out if there are stairs to negotiate. If you are driving, plan the route,

allowing for more stops for feeding and changing your baby. For a first trip outside, try not to be too ambitious. You will still be recovering from the birth so need to look after yourself as well as your baby. Whether you are going for a longer drive or walking to the local shops, preparation is key.

A nappy-changing bag is vital for any trip outside and should contain the following items:
» nappies
» wipes
» muslins
» change of baby clothes
» sunscreen (in the summer)
» spare clothing for yourself in case your baby regurgitates a lot on you.
» a sterilized bottle and formula if your baby is bottle-fed. (See also p.281).

Out and about
Think ahead to what you might need for your baby to help make trips run smoothly.

Q Why do I have to take my baby to see the GP at six weeks?

Your baby's check-up at six weeks old (though it can be up to eight weeks) is an opportune moment to check that everything is on track. It is usually carried out at your doctor's surgery, and you will also be given a postnatal check-up at this time (see p.259). You may have specific questions about your baby's care, feeding, and sleep patterns, or want to discuss any concerns you have. You can also

learn about the immunization programme that begins when your baby is two months old.

The six-week check monitors your baby's progress. The doctor will examine her hips to make sure they are still positioned correctly; listen for any heart irregularities such as a heart murmur; check the alignment of her spine and that there is no dimple at its base that could indicate a nerve problem. For boys, the opening of the penis and the position of the testes will be checked, and for girls, the vaginal area.

Although these things will have already been checked at birth, they are sometimes not detectable until your baby is a bit older. For example, at this point your baby's eyes can be examined to see if she can focus on and follow a moving object. You will be asked whether your baby is smiling and socializing well, and making gurgling and cooing noises as expected. If there are any problems you will be referred to a specialist.

Did you know...

All births in the UK must be registered within 42 days of birth. Some hospitals have the necessary forms, or you can go to your local register office if you had a home birth – or if you need time to decide on a name!

Q My baby is plumper than other babies the same age. Am I overfeeding her?

It's likely that you just have a bonny baby on your hands. Your baby will double her body weight in the first three months. Until she is on the move, her sedentary lifestyle means that her muscles are yet to develop and she will gain a covering of fat.

Some babies are naturally bigger – much is dependent on genetics. Any differences usually iron out by toddlerhood. However, with a global rise in obesity, it's worth being aware of potential pitfalls of weight gain.

Formula-fed babies

A cohort of studies shows that breastfed babies tend to be leaner, largely because they tend to stop drinking milk when they've had their fill. If your baby is formula fed, take care that you are paying attention to her "full-up" cues. It may be tempting to encourage her to finish a bottle, but if she loses interest in a feed before the end, perhaps becoming restless and turning her head, she is signalling that her tummy is full. When parents ignore these natural cues, however well intentioned, they are encouraging a habit of overeating that can continue throughout childhood and beyond.

TIPS FOR A HEALTHY BABY WEIGHT

Don't become too focused on your baby's weight, but do be aware of the following guidelines:

» **Regular checks:** your health visitor or GP can check your baby's weight and length charts and advise you if they think there is a concern. If your baby has moved up two percentiles on her growth chart, this could flag up a weight issue that needs attention.

» **Sleep:** getting enough sleep is linked to a healthy metabolism and weight control; at three months, your baby needs around 15 hours of sleep a day, so putting healthy sleep routines in place is important.

» **Wean correctly:** weaning before four to six months has been shown to adversely affect weight, so don't be in a hurry to get your baby onto baby rice. When you do wean, introduce plenty of fruit and vegetable purées among the rice and cereals.

Little and large Babies' weights can differ by several pounds from birth, and being above or below average weight is perfectly normal.

Q Should I be concerned that my child is lagging behind others of the same age in our baby group?

The rate at which babies reach certain milestones can vary enormously. Socializing with parents who have babies of the same age is beneficial, but it can make you anxious as to whether your baby is doing everything she should be doing for her age and stage.

The truth is that while babies follow the same developmental progression, they do so at their own pace. Your baby develops in four areas: physically; verbally; socially; and cognitively. Learning in one area is often linked to skill acquisition in another arena. But often, a certain skill set takes a back seat while your baby spends time concentrating on something else. For example, while one baby may tirelessly swipe at objects on her play mat, another may be concentrating on the new noises she can make, fascinated by the coos and gurgles she is producing. Eventually both babies will build muscle strength and develop their communication skills.

As long as your baby has the opportunities and stimulation to learn new skills, often the actual learning of a new skill is more important than the time frame for when the skill is mastered. For example, if a developmental chart suggests your baby will walk between 12 and 15 months, and she doesn't take her first step until 17 months, this doesn't mean that there is a problem. If you are concerned about any aspect of your baby's development, always seek advice and reassurance from your health visitor or GP.

If you have **twin babies,** try not to compare their development too closely. Remember, **they are individuals** and will each develop at their own rate.

Q When will my baby have to be immunized?

Your baby's immunization programme starts at two months of age, and he will have boosters and additional vaccinations at three, four, and 12–13 months. You will be sent reminders when your baby is due for his immunizations.

IMMUNIZATION PROGRAMME

As well as newborn jabs, further vaccinations are given in early childhood and in the adolescent years. A detailed breakdown of the immunization programme is given in this table.

AGE	VACCINE RECEIVED	REASON
2 months	The 5-in-1 vaccine (DTaP/IPV/Hib)	A combined vaccine. Protects against diphtheria, tetanus, whooping cough (pertussis), polio, and Haemophilus influenzae type b (Hib), a bacterial infection that can lead to pneumonia and meningitis
	Pneumococcal (PCV) vaccine	Protects against infections that lead to pneumonia, septicaemia, and meningitis
	Rotavirus vaccine	Given as an oral drop. Protects against diarrhoea and sickness caused by the rotavirus
	Meningitis B vaccine	Protects against a particular type of meningitis
3 months	The 5-in-1 vaccine (DTaP/IPV/Hib)	Second dose
	Meningitis C vaccine	Protects against meningitis and septicaemia
	Rotavirus vaccine	Second dose
4 months	The 5-in-1 vaccine (DTaP/IPV/Hib)	Third dose
	Pneumococcal (PCV) vaccine	Second dose
	Meningitis B vaccine	Second dose
12–13 months	Hib/Men C booster	Two second doses combined in a single jab
	Measles, mumps, and rubella (MMR)	Three vaccines combined in a single jab
	Pneumococcal (PCV)	Third dose
	Meningitis B	Third dose
2, 3, & 4 years	Children's flu vaccine	Protects against influenza
3 years & 4 months	Measles, mumps, and rubella (MMR)	Second dose
	4-in-1 (DTaP/IPV) pre-school booster	A single jab that protects against diphtheria, tetanus, whooping cough, and polio
12–13 years (girls only)	HPV vaccine	For protection against cervical cancer – two injections are give between six months and two years apart
13–15 years	Meningitis	Booster
13–18 years	3-in-1 (Td/IPV) booster	A single jab that protects against diphtheria, tetanus, and polio

Q What exactly do immunizations do and why are they needed?

Being immunized protects your baby from developing potentially serious illnesses. Immunity is a natural, learned process in the body; once we are exposed to an infection, our body creates antibodies to resist it in the future. A vaccine is a very diluted version of a disease, usually given by injection, designed to let your baby develop immunity to the disease without actually catching it.

All new babies have some immunity from their mother, but this effect wears off after about two months, which is why immunizations begin after this age.

Q My friend said my baby doesn't have to have immunizations. Is it true that I can refuse them?

Your consent will be asked before any of the routine vaccines offered for your baby (see chart, left) are given. If you decide against allowing your baby to have a vaccination, the healthcare provider should report this in your baby's records.

Do, however, carefully weigh up the benefits against potential risks before deciding not to immunize your child. Vaccination programmes have successfully managed to significantly reduce or eliminate many serious and fatal diseases. If you don't vaccinate your child, you are not just increasing your child's risk of contracting a disease, but you are also affecting what's termed "herd immunity" – an effect of vaccination that makes it difficult for a disease to pass around the general populace when enough people have been immunized.

Side effects

The side effects of vaccinations tend to be mild (see opposite) – more serious side effects are rare. Some parents worry that having several vaccinations in one go could weaken their young baby's immune system. However, just a tiny fraction of the immune system is involved in creating the antibodies against live vaccines. In reality, your baby is exposed to many bacteria and viruses that are far stronger than the weakened bacteria and viruses given in vaccines, and his body handles these perfectly well.

Q How can I prepare for my baby's injections and comfort him after?

Like most new parents, you may feel ill at ease about taking your baby for his immunizations but rest assured it is a very quick and efficient procedure.

Your young baby will be unaware that he is being immunized, but he may pick up on your tension if you feel stressed. While it's a natural instinct to be concerned, try to stay as relaxed as possible and remember that being immunized is in your baby's best interests.

Try not to plan anything else for that day, before or after the immunizations, so that you don't feel rushed and have proper time to focus on your baby's needs afterwards.

What happens

When you take your baby to the clinic or surgery for his immunization, the nurse may suggest that you sit him on your lap while the injection is given. He will be soothed by your presence, touch, and voice, so talk to him gently, and give him a reassuring cuddle as he is immunized. You may also wish to breastfeed your baby while he is being injected, which will be comforting for him and provide a distraction from the jab. Be aware, though, that you may have to interrupt the feed if you are in a busy clinic or GP's surgery. Most clinics and surgeries have a set time allocated to immunizations so there may be several babies there for their jabs at the same time.

Giving pain relief

If your baby develops a fever and seems uncomfortable, you can give the recommended dose of infant paracetamol or ibuprofen, and continue with his regular feeds to keep him well hydrated.

It's very important that you do not give a dose of pain relief before an immunization, in anticipation of your baby developing a fever, as doing this could compromise the effectiveness of the vaccine.

Aftercare Following his immunizations, give your baby infant pain relief to help lower any fever and ease discomfort.

Did you know...

Vaccination programmes have been extremely effective around the world. For example, in 1914 in England and Wales there were approximately 60,000 cases of diphtheria, which caused 5,800 deaths. Following the introduction of the vaccine in 1942, there were 41,404 known cases and 1,827 deaths from the disease. By 1946, the diphtheria death rate had fallen to just 472.

In Japan in 1974, around 70 per cent of Japanese children were being vaccinated against whooping cough and there were only 393 cases in the whole of Japan. When immunizations rates began to drop, only 10 per cent of children were being vaccinated. The result was that more than 13,000 people developed whooping cough in 1979, of which 41 died. When children began to be routinely vaccinated again, the cases of whooping cough fell again.

Q Will there be any side effects from the immunizations?

It's natural to worry about possible side effects from vaccinations, but these tend to be mild and short-lived if they occur at all. There may be some local swelling and redness, and possibly a small lump at the injection site (usually the top of the thigh), all of which are harmless and disappear within a couple of days.

Occasionally babies develop a fever after an injection, in which case infant paracetamol can be given. It's very rare for babies to have an allergic reaction to a vaccination. If it does happen, it is treatable.

Premature babies have immunizations at the same age as other babies – **their immunity** from their mother lasts the **same two months**.

Q My baby has eczema. Can he still have his immunizations?

Having an allergy, such as eczema, asthma, or any type of food intolerance, does not prevent your baby from being immunized. The only reasons for not immunizing your baby on a particular day would be if he had a fever, in which case the appointment would be rescheduled. If you are concerned that your child is not well enough on the day, seek advice from the GP's surgery or clinic. If your child had a previous bad reaction to an immunization, (although this is rare) again, seek advice from the health professionals.

Q Is it true that I can't take my baby swimming until he has had his jabs?

It is a common myth that babies can't go swimming before they have their jabs. You can take your baby swimming at any time before or after he has been immunized.

Building strength By 12 weeks your baby has learnt a certain degree of head control. Some babies can lift their head up at this stage when lying on their front. Spending short amounts of time on his tummy helps to strengthen your baby's neck, back, and core muscles.

It's really important to **take care of yourself** as well as your new baby. Being in labour will have left you exhausted, or you might have had a C-section. Either way, you will need time to recover as well as adapt to your new life. Your body will also undergo an **enormous amount of change** as you return to your pre-pregnant state.

Birth recovery

Physical impact

Whatever type of labour and birth you had, you will be feeling the physical effects. You are likely to be exhausted, especially if you had a long labour. If you tore or had an episiotomy (a cut to the vagina and perineal area), you will be sore from the stitches, which can make sitting uncomfortable and may sting when you urinate. If you had a Caesarean section, you will be recovering from major abdominal surgery, which takes several weeks. You will need to take it easy and draw on all the support you can.

Your body has done an amazing job in the past nine months, and now it will begin to return to its pre-pregnancy state, which will involve some dramatic hormonal changes. Your breasts will start to fill with milk to feed your baby.

Emotional roller coaster

Your emotions after birth can swing wildly: one minute you feel intensely happy, imbued with the joy of motherhood as you nestle in with your new baby, but the next moment you may feel anxious and weepy as exhaustion sets in. Hormones play havoc with your emotions, and you may feel an odd sense of emptiness as, bereft of your bump, you have lost the intimacy of carrying your baby around with you. Most women experience "the baby blues" a few days after the birth. In the middle of this physical and emotional upheaval, you are having to get straight on with one of the most important tasks of your life: looking after your new baby. This is the time to accept all the support you can get. The most significant being from your partner, who is there to hold the helm in the first few days while you recover, and give you the emotional and physical support you need.

Help from family and friends over the coming weeks will make a real and valuable contribution and each gesture will make all the difference – whether it's having meals cooked, ironing done, or simply letting someone care for your baby for an hour or two while you sleep. Be honest with those close to you about what you need.

Give yourself time

While six weeks is often talked about as the period of time it takes to recover from birth, this figure is somewhat arbitrary. A recent study found that women need a year to recover completely and get back on track after birth, so it's vital to go slowly. Give yourself time to put your feet up, and to concentrate on you: eat well, find ways to relax, and gradually regain your activity levels, eventually returning to a gentle exercise regime. All of these things will help you to recover well.

Q I'm experiencing what feel like mild labour pains. What's happening?

Your uterus doesn't stop working straight after the delivery. Having stretched ten-fold during pregnancy, it begins the job of returning to its pre-pregnancy size – a process known as involution.

As your uterus shrinks back down, you will experience cramping pains, like mild labour contractions, commonly called "afterpains". These are generally quite manageable, especially in a first pregnancy, when the previously unstretched muscles are stronger and able to contract back down more easily.

If you do find the pains too much to bear, seek advice from your midwife. You can take paracetamol for the pain and you can also try using the breathing techniques you used in labour. You may notice that the pains are stronger when you breastfeed; this is because the hormone oxytocin released during feeding to let down your milk is the same one that encouraged uterine contractions. While you may not welcome the stronger sensation, breastfeeding helps your uterus to contract back down more quickly. It takes up to six weeks for your uterus to get back to its pre-pregnancy size. Pains are usually felt most strongly in the first week or so, and many women find they are barely noticeable after this time.

YOUR SHRINKING UTERUS

Within a couple of days of the birth, your uterus will be the size it was about midway through your pregnancy. It will then rapidly reduce in size, until at about six weeks after birth it is no bigger than a plum (the size it is pre-pregnancy).

One to two days after birth By this time, the uterus is about the size of a cantaloupe melon and weighs around 450g (1lb).

Seven days after birth A week after giving birth your uterus is approximately the size of grapefruit and weighs around 300g (11oz).

Six weeks after birth Some weeks after the birth the uterus is no bigger than a plum and weighs around 100g (3½oz).

Q I'm shocked by the heavy bleeding. Is this normal?

It's completely normal: as the uterus shrinks, it sheds blood and tissue called lochia. At first it's like a heavy period, but then tails off. Lochia changes from red to a watery pink colour, and then becomes a yellowy discharge. Wear a sanitary towel as a tampon could infect the uterus. Heavy bleeding can last up to two weeks. Seek medical help if: the bleeding becomes heavy and red again after having lightened; is so heavy that you need more than one sanitary towel an hour; you pass large clots of blood; the discharge is smelly; or you feel feverish or dizzy. Excessive bleeding anytime from 24 hours to six weeks after the birth is known as secondary postpartum haemorrhage (PPH). This may happen because part of the placenta is still attached to the lining of the uterus.

Q When is my follow-up appointment and what will the GP check?

Your "six-week check" can take place six to eight weeks after the birth, usually at the same time your baby is checked (see p.252). The GP will check your blood pressure and examine your abdomen to make sure that your uterus has returned to the correct size. Your GP may examine any stitches or scars to check everything has healed. Make an appointment sooner if you have any physical effects of breastfeeding (e.g. blocked milk ducts or mastitis) that need treatment. Your GP will also advise you about contraception. This is a chance to talk about how you're feeling, so be honest with your GP, who can direct you to support.

It is possible to become pregnant while you are still breastfeeding, so don't rely on it as a form of contraception.

Q Why is my Caesarean section scar sensitive to touch and painful?

It's normal for your scar to feel tender to the touch while it's healing. You have had a major incision and your body is undergoing the complex job of knitting back together the layers of muscles and fibres to seal the wound.

As the wound site heals, it's common to experience some pain, especially if you move in an awkward way and "catch" your scar. Be careful how you move around. Gradually building up your activity levels will give the wound time to heal. It may not be glamorous, but for comfort, wear big pants (or your partner's boxer shorts). Smaller pants are likely to rub against your scar, causing discomfort.

Apart from the first couple of days after a Caesarean section, when even the slightest movement can be extremely painful and you have to make careful, small steps, often with support, the pain should be fairly manageable, albeit with some soreness. If you take your painkillers regularly, you should feel quite comfortable, perhaps experiencing occasional twinges if you overdo things or are especially tired. If after the initial couple of days pain feels extreme, constant, or seems to be getting worse, and if the scar is red and inflamed, talk to your healthcare provider.

The collagen that makes up scar tissue tends to be less elastic than the original tissue, and when the new collagen fibres form, they often do so in a haphazard fashion, which can cause hardness and restrict movement in surrounding tissues.

Adhesions can also develop, where the scar tissue sticks to surrounding tissues and other organs, which can cause discomfort. Once your scar is well healed, usually at around six weeks, some gentle fingertip massage can help to soften scar tissue, break up adhesions that may be forming, and also improve circulation, which in turn promotes good healing. Rubbing in some vitamin E oil can also help. In addition, a healthy lifestyle will help your scar to heal well and reduce discomfort. Gentle walking is perfect exercise after a Caesarean section.

Time to heal To begin with the C-section scar, which is usually along the bikini line, will look very red. As it heals, the redness will fade. It is normal to experience some itchiness as the scar heals.

layers of muscle and skin slowly knit back together. As with any major surgery, trying to do too much too soon can set you back. At six weeks, your scar may look fairly well-healed, but there is still internal healing taking place.

If you feel a sharp twinge while attempting something strenuous, such as picking up a heavy bag, it's a sign to rest. Continue to take care with how you move around, for example get out of bed by rolling on to your side, and avoid lifting heavy weights for two to three months after the birth.

Some women experience pain from trapped gas after a Caesarean section. Eat a fibre-rich diet, drink plenty of fluids, and chew food slowly. The trapped air can irritate the diaphragm and cause shoulder-tip pain; drinking peppermint water or peppermint tea can help. While rest is essential, gentle activity is also important for improving circulation, which reduces the risk of conditions such as deep vein thrombosis and also promotes healing.

Q I feel disappointed that the birth didn't go as I'd planned. How will I come to terms with it?

All pregnant women are encouraged to write a birth plan (see p.88), but this may not come to fruition on the day. Events might have unfolded very differently to how you had hoped, you might feel that you lacked control throughout labour, and birth may not have been the joyous occasion that you envisioned it to be. However, with time you will come to terms with your feelings of disappointment.

The best way to deal with your experience and help yourself to resolve any feelings of disappointment or failure is to talk to people about what happened – to your partner, family, and, in particular, the obstetrician or midwife. If this doesn't happen before you leave the hospital, make an appointment to speak to him or her at a later date. If you fall pregnant again, discuss what happened with your midwife so that you can, if possible, avoid the same experience again. You can also speak to friends about your experience or read online forums. You will soon feel that you're not alone and that it's completely normal to feel disappointed, upset, or even angry at how things went.

Try not to blame yourself or your baby for what took place and speak to your GP if you are feeling anxious or depressed.

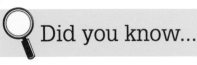

Did you know...

After a C-section, you can begin doing pelvic floor exercises (see pp.66–67) as soon as you feel ready. If those feel comfortable, you can go for short walks to work your lower abdominal muscles. After six weeks, you can begin light sit-ups, and gentle cycling, walking, or swimming – build your pace up slowly in periods of 10 minutes at a time. Stop if you are in pain and consult your GP.

Q I'm still getting pains four weeks after my C-section. Is this normal?

It's very common to feel twinges as your body heals. The incisions through your abdominal wall, the underlying muscles, and your uterus understandably need time to join back together. The recovery time varies, but it is often six to eight weeks before you feel back to normal after this major surgery.

Women usually experience an improvement after a few days, but while it becomes easier to move around, there may be considerable tenderness at the incision site as the various

Q How long will it take for my body to get back to normal?

Once you've had your baby, it's understandable that you want to feel like your old self again. It may, however, take several months for your body to return to normal so be patient and don't expect too much too soon.

There is no such thing as a **miracle cream** to get rid of stretch marks, but using moisturizer will keep your skin **smooth and supple**.

BODY CHANGES

Your body has been affected by growing and carrying your baby, so some physical changes are perfectly normal.

» **Breasts:** your breasts become swollen and hard, and may be sore as your milk comes in a few days after birth. This usually eases as breastfeeding becomes established.

» **Skin:** most women are left with some stretch marks. These are caused by the collagen beneath your skin tearing as it stretches to accommodate your growing baby. They may not go completely but they will fade with time.

» **Pelvic floor muscles:** you may have temporary urinary incontinence, so find that a little bit of urine seeps out when you laugh, sneeze, or cough. Do pelvic floor exercises (see p.67) to strengthen the muscles.

» **Hair:** due to changes in oestrogen levels, it's normal to experience some hair loss for six to 12 months after the birth.

» **Abdomen:** your tummy and pelvic muscles will be slack. If you had a vaginal delivery, you can do gentle abdominal exercises in the first few weeks. If you had a C-section, wait until after your six-week check.

» **Bladder:** the trauma on the bladder can put you at risk of a urinary infection. Drink plenty of water to reduce the risk of this happening.

» **Anus:** many women develop haemorrhoids, or piles (see p.132), in late pregnancy. Eat plenty of fibre and drink lots of water to ease bowel movements. Use an over-the-counter ointment on the affected area.

Q I had stitches because I tore during the delivery. What can I do to ease the discomfort?

It's normal to feel discomfort and soreness as this area heals and there are several ways to ease the discomfort. Using painkillers will help you feel less pain. It can also help to apply towel-wrapped ice packs to your perineum, no longer than an hour at a time, in the first couple of days. Keep the perineum clean to avoid an infection, washing your hands before touching the area and bathing or showering regularly. Two or three drops of pure essential oils added to bath water can soothe perineal discomfort; lavender, geranium, and chamomile are recommended. Pelvic floor exercises help blood flow to the perineal area, which promotes healing. Pouring a jug of warm water over your vulva or using a water spray can be soothing and reduce the stinging sensation when you pass urine. Going to the toilet in a warm shower has the same effect. Squatting over rather than sitting on the toilet seat, or sitting with your feet and knees raised a little, can reduce stinging. Avoid getting constipated. Drink plenty of water and eat fibre-rich foods. If you had a bad tear or are constipated, you may be prescribed a mild laxative to soften your stools. Don't hold off going to the loo as it increases the risk of a UTI and constipation. Talk to your healthcare provider or doctor if the area is still sore after a few weeks.

Q I'm exhausted and can hardly get out of bed. Is this normal?

It's normal to feel exhausted in the early weeks and months. Give your body time to heal. The hormone relaxin lingers in your body after the birth. In pregnancy, it makes your ligaments more elastic to cope with labour, but after the delivery, it can exacerbate complaints such as backache and joint pain. If getting out of bed feels like an achievement, it is because it is! Sleeping when you can, eating well, and slowly becoming more active are key to recovery.

As soon as you are able, get up and **move around** as **activity** can help with many things, including getting your digestive system working.

Q I should be happy now my baby's here, so why am I weepy and overwhelmed?

Your wonderful baby may be everything you dreamed of, and yet the challenges of new parenthood can be difficult to handle. The days following your baby's birth are intense, and emotions tend to sea-saw as your hormones surge and you grapple with adjusting to your new role while feeling exhausted from the birth.

A touch of the blues

The "baby blues" are experienced by women shortly after giving birth (usually around day four). The blues tend to last a day or so. During this time women feel weepy, irrational, and generally a little overwhelmed by everything.

There are various reasons for the baby blues. After birth, your body undergoes dramatic changes as it returns to its pre-pregnant condition. The hormones progesterone and oestrogen that helped sustain your pregnancy plummet and breastfeeding hormones rapidly rise. While these hormonal swings alone can play havoc, you are also recovering from the after-effects of the birth, including exhaustion, stitches, and perhaps major surgery. If you had a difficult birth experience, you may be struggling to process this. In addition, your breasts feel tender as they fill with milk, and your sleep is disrupted. Not least, you are adapting to your new role as a parent.

Feeling depressed

If, like 1 in 10 women, you still feel low and weepy beyond the baby blues, or find that negative feelings develop around one to two months after the birth, you may have postnatal depression (PND) and should seek medical help.

SHORT-TERM BABY BLUES

There's no need to seek treatment for the baby blues as they will pass naturally as your hormones settle down, but getting adequate rest, feeling supported, and giving yourself time can make them more bearable. All these things will help with postnatal depression, too, although you will also need medical treatment.

» Getting adequate rest: we all struggle to cope when we are overtired and when you have a new baby to care for this can be exacerbated. After the exertion of the birth and delivery, you need quiet, restful time, which can be hard for new mothers to come by. Being inundated with visitors, coping with a noisy hospital ward, and dealing with a crying newborn and disrupted sleep are not conducive to good rest. Don't feel that you should "do it all" – putting your feet up while your baby sleeps isn't lazy, but crucial as it allows your body to recover from the birth and builds your energy back up.

» Love and understanding: partners and loved ones play a crucial role, both practically and emotionally. They need to encourage the mother to rest as much as possible while they hold the fort; be patient; allow the mother to cry and listen to her concerns; make sure she is well-nourished; and reassure her that her feelings are natural and that she will feel better soon. In turn, be honest with those around you about what you need.

» Time to adjust: having a baby may be the most life-changing event of your life, and yet it's a role that is hard to prepare for in advance. This is a period of adjustment. You need to shift your priorities and take life at a slower pace for the moment. Give yourself time and be kind to yourself.

Approximately **70 per cent** of new mothers experience a form of mild depression, called the "baby blues" around four days after birth.

POSTNATAL DEPRESSION (PND)

Be aware of the risk factors and warning signs of PND and don't hesitate to seek support. Speak to someone as soon as you notice any of the warning signs.

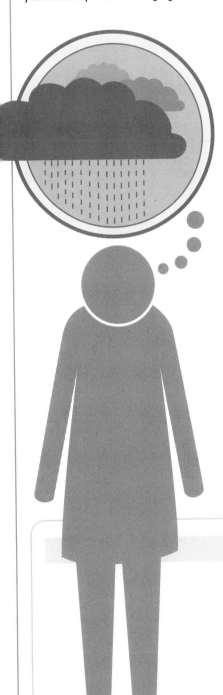

Risk factors

The risk factors listed below make it more likely you will suffer with PND. If any of them apply to you, take steps to reduce your chances of developing the condition; it's easier to take preventative action than to motivate yourself to find help once you are depressed.

» You have been depressed before or during your pregnancy.
» You had a traumatic delivery.
» You had a recent stressful event, such as a bereavement.
» You generally have little support.

Warning signs

» You find it hard to sleep, have fitful sleep, or wake too early feeling anxious.
» You feel low-level anxiety, or perhaps feel very anxious and suffer from panic attacks.
» You feel irritable and lack concentration.
» You struggle to feel enjoyment or pleasure in life, and lack humour.
» You feel guilty and generally miserable.
» Your appetite is poor, or you overeat.
» You feel lethargic, tired, and unmotivated, and you aren't managing to look after yourself properly.
» You feel isolated.
» You have little interest in your baby.

Support

Talk to your partner, or other loved ones, and consult your GP or health visitor if you experience any of the warning signs more than a week after the birth. Don't ignore these feelings as they are easily treatable – if left they can affect your relationship with your baby, partner, and others.

If you have suffered from depression before, the symptoms will feel familiar, although with PND there is the added factor of how your illness impacts on your baby and your relationship with him. Getting help may make all the difference to your experience of motherhood.

GETTING HELP

There is help available to treat PND, so make an appointment to see your GP as soon as possible.

Many women recover from PND without treatment, but up to a quarter of women still have PND after a year. In this time, their relationship with their baby will have suffered, which might affect the baby's social development.

Your doctor may refer you for talking therapy, prescribe antidepressant medication, or do both. Antidepressants may help to lift your mood to enable you to explore the root causes of your depression. There are antidepressants that are compatible with breastfeeding. Antidepressants take around two weeks to start working and need to be taken for six months to deal with the depression effectively.

Your thyroid function may be tested, as levels of the hormone thyroid can drop after pregnancy, which can cause some of the symptoms of depression.

A CLOSER LOOK
Skin to skin

Skin to skin is when you place your naked baby (bar her nappy) directly on to your bare chest. Take time to relax in each others' quiet company – time spent doing absolutely nothing other than being together is valuable bonding time, especially if you choose to do it skin to skin. Pull a sheet over you both to keep snug. Allow yourself to enjoy your baby's physical presence: her warm weight on your chest, her small hand curling round your finger, and her soft head against your cheek.

Getting acquainted The more time you spend skin to skin the quicker you will get to know each other in the early days and weeks. It's a way of communicating your love for your baby and feeling confident that you can provide for her as you have done during your pregnancy.

Skin-to-skin contact This provides immediate benefits straight after birth. Direct contact can help you and your baby feel close throughout the first hours of her life. It's a perfect transition from the warmth and protection of your womb to the coziness of your body.

Calm your baby If your baby is upset or hungry or generally unsettled then holding her against your skin can help her to relax. The technique is particularly useful if you are struggling to breastfeed as it gets your baby used to being close to your breast.

FASCINATING FACTS

One hour of skin-to-skin contact immediately after birth makes a baby significantly less stressed after the trauma of the birth experience.

During skin-to-skin contact, your baby's **heartbeat and breathing** are more regular and stable.

Babies who have regular skin-to-skin contact tend to **cry less**.

Babies who have skin-to-skin contact **digest their food better**.

37°C (98.6°F) is the normal body temperature. During skin-to-skin contact your body helps to regulate your baby's temperature and keep it at the right level.

Skin-to-skin contact helps your baby pick up friendly bacteria from your skin, which **protect her from catching infections**.

Skin-to-skin contact **helps establish breastfeeding** because your baby can see and smell the nipple, which encourages her to feed.

Skin-to-skin contact helps **trigger your breast milk** to flow.

Skin-to-skin contact helps to make you feel **more confident** that you can look after your baby.

Family bonding Your partner can use skin to skin as a way to bond with your newborn. Encourage your partner to spend time alone with the baby to help build a closeness with the new addition to your family. It will give you a chance to get some sleep or rest.

The milk you make for your baby is **uniquely tailored** to meet all his **nutritional needs** for around the first six months, and provide **immunity protection** at birth and beyond. The composition of this dynamic fluid constantly adapts and changes to give your baby **exactly what he needs** at each stage of his development.

Breastfeeding

Tailor-made nutrition

From the moment your baby is born, your breasts are primed to feed him, first with the pre-milk colostrum made during pregnancy and ready for your baby straight away, and then, after about three days, with your breast milk. The production of breast milk is triggered by a surge in the hormone prolactin at birth.

Your milk production works on a supply-and-demand basis, so each time your baby feeds, your breasts are stimulated to produce more milk for his next feed. During growth spurts, your breasts respond to increased sucking by producing a greater quantity of milk, and in this way, your baby grows and thrives. Even if you manage only a handful of feeds in the first few days, your baby will receive concentrated nutrients and immunity-boosting antibodies that can't be obtained from formula milk, and that will give him the best possible start.

Benefits for you and your baby

As well as being free and nutritionally perfect, countless breastfeeding studies point to health benefits. Breastfed babies have fewer ear, chest, and gastrointestinal infections in the first year, and later on a lower incidence of childhood obesity and diabetes. Breastfeeding is thought to offer some protection against childhood eczema, and

there are fewer incidents of cot death in breastfed babies. Several studies have looked at the link between breastfed babies and higher IQs. Studies have found that breastfed babies do better at school and beyond, regardless of wealth or class, which may be due to the high number of special fatty acids in breast milk that promote healthy neural development.

Mums also benefit from breastfeeding, often losing weight more quickly as breastfeeding burns additional calories, and the oxytocin released during breastfeeding helps the uterus to contract after birth. Breastfeeding mums are also less likely to develop postnatal depression, or in the long-term, breast, ovarian, and endometrial cancers, or osteoporosis.

Getting started

Although breastfeeding is a natural process, it does not necessarily come naturally to new mums. It takes time and practice to perfect, and it can feel uncomfortable at first. Advice and support can make a real difference, so take advantage of any help provided by the hospital, and ask your midwife, health visitor, or a breastfeeding consultant for advice when you're back home. You will soon find that you get better at reading your baby's hunger cues, which makes the feeding experience calmer and easier.

Q I've heard that "breast is best" but what exactly is in breast milk?

Your breasts won't fill with milk until three to five days after the birth. Before that time, they contain the "pre-milk" colostrum, a highly concentrated, thick, creamy-yellow substance that has countless health benefits for your baby.

Colostrum is the perfect first food, delivering vital nutrients as well as protective antibodies that give your baby an instant immune boost. Colostrum is made in very small quantities, with your baby receiving no more than a few teaspoons worth in the first few days. This amount is exactly right for your baby, whose tiny stomach is the size of a walnut.

Colostrum is protein-rich, providing amino acids for growth and development; high in carbohydrates and fat-soluble vitamins and minerals; and low in fats, which are difficult

for your baby to digest at first. Key nutrients in colostrum are essential for the development of the brain, heart, and the central nervous system. Colostrum provides a high concentration of disease-fighting white blood cells, and immunoglobulins that protect against germs. It also acts as a natural laxative, triggering your baby's bowels to excrete meconimum (see p.247).

As well as giving him colostrum, getting your newborn to suckle will stimulate your breasts to produce milk. The composition of breast milk is also highly remarkable, as outlined below.

Magic milk Breast milk contains the perfect balance of nutrients, as well as protective antibodies.

FAT 3.8%

Fats make up nearly 4 per cent and are essential for growth, the development of the brain and nervous system, and easy absorption of vitamins. Breast milk is rich in long-chain polyunsaturated fatty acids, key to eye and neural development.

WATER 88.1%

Mature breast milk is just under 90 per cent water. At the start of a feed, your baby receives a more watery hydrating foremilk; then, as he continues sucking, the creamier, more calorie-dense hindmilk, essential for weight gain, is released from the fat cells and makes its way more slowly up the milk ducts to the nipple. So each time your baby feeds, he receives a complete meal that both hydrates and nourishes him.

PROTEIN 0.9%

The main proteins in mature breast milk are whey and casein. Other specific proteins include secretory IgA, the main antibody in mature milk, which protects against ear, nose, and throat infections.

LACTOSE 7.0%

The principal carbohydrate in breast milk is lactose, which provides energy. It prevents the growth of harmful bacteria in the gut, in turn helping the absorption of essential nutrients such as calcium and phosphorus.

OTHER 0.2%

Vitamins and minerals reflect your intake. The exception is vitamin D, so it is recommended that you take a daily 10mcg vitamin D supplement if you are breastfeeding.

Q I've been told that breastfeeding is natural, but how do I start?

If your birth is straightforward, you will be encouraged to latch your baby on straight away. Hold him skin to skin, so that he can seek out your nipple. He will do so naturally if he is given uninterrupted time. Try not to rush and remember it is a new experience for him, too. Stroke his cheek to trigger his rooting reflex, talk to him, and make eye contact. If he makes mouthing and sucking movements, gently guide him to the nipple. He may suck intermittently while he gets used to the mechanics of feeding. At birth, your baby's tiny stomach holds no more than about 15ml (1 tablespoon) of milk so he needs to feed at regular intervals.

Q Sometimes I'm feeding for an hour. How long should a feed take?

Breastfeeds can be anything from a few minutes to an hour or more. Once feeding is more established, you will probably find it becomes more efficient and quicker. The length may be down to a baby's temperament. While some suck enthusiastically for a short period of time, others prefer to take it a little more slowly, perhaps pausing for a break mid-feed.

It's important that you don't limit your baby's time on the breast as this could stop him getting the fattier, nourishing hindmilk that is released from the ducts towards the end of a feed, which satisfies his hunger and ensures healthy growth.

Q Did you know...

The general guideline is that newborn babies should feed at least eight to 12 times in a 24-hour period, with feeds given evenly throughout the day and night. If your baby is very sleepy after the birth, you may need to stir him every two to three hours to offer a feed, stroking his cheek to stimulate his rooting reflex. Feeding frequently in these first few days allows your baby to practise latching on and sucking while your breasts are relatively empty, before your milk comes in after around three days.

How can I make sure my baby is latched on to the breast correctly?

The key to successful breastfeeding – feeding that is comfortable for you and ensures your baby gets sufficient milk – is to position your baby well at the breast. There is an art to getting your little one "latched on" properly. You may not get it right until you have breastfed a few times, but give yourself time and seek support if necessary.

Why a good latch is important

When your baby isn't latched on correctly, she will drag on your nipple rather than massage your breast tissue with her sucks. The result is sore and cracked nipples and possibly problems with milk supply, as your baby's weak suck may not be stimulating your breasts to make enough milk. If your baby isn't emptying your breast properly, this also increases your risk of developing complications, such as mastitis (see pp.274–75), as breast milk can stagnate in the ducts and become infected.

The midwives at the hospital, and then community midwives once you are home, will help and advise you. There may also be help available from breastfeeding consultants.

A STEP-BY-STEP GUIDE TO LATCHING ON

Get as comfortable as possible before you begin a feed. Choose a chair that supports your lower back, and use cushions for additional support of your back and arms if this helps. Specially designed U-shaped feeding cushions that support your baby can be helpful, especially after a Caesarean section, as they bear the weight of your baby and thereby avoid putting pressure on your scar.

1 HOLD YOUR BABY NOSE TO NIPPLE
Position your baby facing you ("tummy to mummy") with her nose opposite your nipple. Gently support her head and shoulders with one hand. Her head and body should be in a straight line so that she doesn't have to twist to get to the nipple. Bring your baby close to your breast: her head should tilt back slightly, her chin touching your lower breast, and your nipple should be aimed towards the roof of her mouth, far closer to her top lip than the middle of her mouth. You can gently stroke her cheek with your finger or brush her nose/upper lip with your nipple, which will trigger her to open her mouth wide.

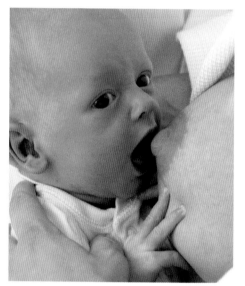

2 WAIT FOR AN OPEN-WIDE MOUTH
Hold back until your baby's mouth is open very wide, as though she is yawning, before latching her on to your breast. This is crucial because she needs to suck on a good mouthful of your breast tissue. If she is sucking only on your nipple, it will be painful and cause breastfeeding problems.

3 LATCH HER ON
Once her mouth is open wide, swiftly bring her on to the breast, drawing her whole body to you so she isn't craning forwards. Aim your nipple towards the roof of her mouth, making sure it is well back in her mouth. If she has difficulty latching on, try using your thumb and forefinger in a U-shape to compress the nipple area a little, but don't press on the breast tissue too much.

Successful feeding A correct latch ensures your baby feeds efficiently and will feel most comfortable for you.

Space under the nose Your baby's nostrils are clear of the breast so that she can breathe easily.

Ear and jaw movement Look for the correct muscle movements in her face.

Nipple position Her mouth covers the areola so she isn't sucking only on the nipple.

IS SHE WELL LATCHED ON?

Make sure your baby's bottom lip is curled backwards, with her chin resting on your breast; her nose is free so that she can breathe easily; her lower lip covers more of the areola than her upper lip. She will settle into a rhythmic sucking-swallow pattern. Her bottom jaw and ears will move as she feeds. You may hear swallowing noises and lip smacking. When she comes off the breast, your nipple shouldn't look compressed.

SIGNS OF A POOR LATCH

A little discomfort is normal at the start of a feed, but this shouldn't persist, and you shouldn't feel pain. A clicking noise also indicates that your baby isn't latched on properly as this is produced when your baby sucks only on the nipple.

TAKING HER OFF THE BREAST

If the latch doesn't feel right, don't carry on feeding. Gently break the suction by putting your little finger into the corner of your baby's mouth, and start again. Don't remove her without breaking the suction as this will pull on your nipple.

EARLY HUNGER SIGNALS

It will be much harder to latch on a hungry baby, so learn to read her hunger cues:

» Her eyelids flutter as she stirs from sleep.
» She opens and closes her mouth and may make sucking actions and stick out her tongue.
» She puts her hand to her mouth and may suck it.
» She clenches her fist.
» She turns her head side to side and "roots" or nuzzles towards your nipple.
» She makes jerky leg and arm movements.

Tasty hand If your baby is sucking her hand, it is quite likely she is ready for a feed.

THE LET-DOWN REFLEX

As your baby starts sucking at your breast, nerves in your nipple are stimulated, which in turn triggers the release of hormones.

The hormone prolactin sends a signal to your breast tissues to produce more milk. The hormone oxytocin stimulates cells in your breast to release milk, which is pushed through the ducts towards the nipple, a process known as the "let-down". This can create a tingling sensation when your baby starts sucking. Some women feel a slight pain that quickly passes, or discomfort and a sensation of pressure.

Milk ducts Breast milk is pushed through the ducts

Milk flow The milk released by the let-down reflex flows towards the nipple to feed your baby.

Q How should I prepare for a feed and what are the best positions?

Make sure you are comfortable and well supported when you settle down to a feeding session. This is key to ensuring that breastfeeding goes smoothly. If the session is likely to be fairly lengthy, make sure you have a drink and snack to hand.

As you will be spending a considerable amount of time sitting still while your baby feeds, you need to make sure that your upper back, shoulders, and neck aren't strained, and that your lower back and arms feel supported. If you are slouched, this can lead to back and shoulder pain and make it harder for your baby to latch on well, which in turn can result in sore nipples and other breastfeeding problems. Tension resulting from bad posture could impede your flow of milk.

Sit in a firm-backed chair, or use cushions to support your lower back so that you can hold an upright posture throughout the feed. Try not to hunch your shoulders, which we tend to do when we are tense; instead, consciously draw them down, which is instantly relaxing.

It is possible to breastfeed twins at the same time, for example by using the rugby hold position (see below). Seek advice from your midwife or a breastfeeding consultant about breastfeeding twins.

FEEDING POSITIONS

How you position your baby at the breast can help him to feed effectively and prevent sore nipples. If your breasts feel a bit tender or your nipples are sore, alternating positions from one feed to another will ensure pressure is more evenly distributed around the nipple area (areola).

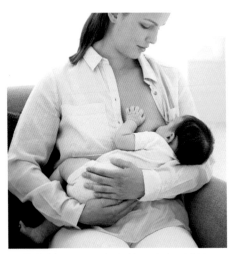

Cradle hold Sitting upright, hold your baby with his tummy facing your tummy, supporting his back and bottom. You may find it helpful to place a cushion on your lap to support your arm and your baby's weight throughout the feed.

Reclining Hold or cradle your baby so that he is completely supported by you. You may find that this is a good position for night feeds. Support your back with pillows or cushions so that you are comfortable as you recline in this semi-upright position.

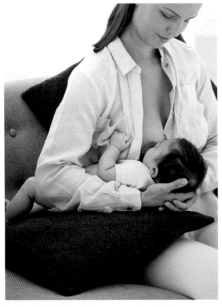

Rugby hold This position can work well after a C-section, as it prevents pressure on your scar, or for feeding twins. Position your baby on a cushion, placed on the side he will feed from, that supports his whole body. Support his head with your hand.

Side by side Lie on your side with your baby facing you. You may want a pillow behind you for support or to raise your body by lying on a folded blanket or towel. Prop yourself up on your elbow, or rest your head on your forearm, then use your free hand to support your baby's head and upper body and gently guide him to the breast. This relaxing position is ideal for a first feed following a Caesarean section, and while recovering from a C-section, as it avoids putting any pressure on your abdomen, and of course is perfect for nighttime feeding.

Q Should I always offer my baby both breasts at every feed?

There are no hard and fast rules – it's best to be guided by your baby and watch out for signs that he is full up. You may find that when your milk comes in, sometime during the first week, your breasts are very full and your baby may be satisfied feeding from one side only. This is fine and you just need to remember to start the next feeding session on the other side so that

your milk supply is even, and so that one nipple doesn't become sore from overuse. If you struggle to remember which side you last fed from, try swapping a bracelet or hair band from one wrist to the other, or simply make a note of which side you fed from.

You may find that your baby continues to be happy feeding from just one side. Or, as your milk supply settles down, your baby may want to feed from both sides in one feeding session. If he seems unsettled when you take him off the breast, try offering the second side.

It's important that your baby stays on one breast long enough to get both the watery hydrating foremilk, and the creamier hindmilk, so don't move him to the other breast too soon.

When your baby has growth spurts, which are frequent in the first weeks and months, you may find that he is dissatisfied for a day or so after just one side and needs to feed from the second breast. If he is very hungry, you may even need to return to the first breast and feed until he is satisfied. Your breasts will increase their supply in line with your baby's needs.

Q How do I wind my baby and is it always necessary?

It is good practice to wind your baby after a feed as this will release any trapped air that he has swallowed along with his milk that could make him fussy, uncomfortable, and hard to settle.

If your baby appears to be fussy mid feed, perhaps squirming and coming away from the breast unsettled, he may need winding to release trapped air before he can carry on. Bottle-fed babies (see pp.278–81) tend to take in more air when they suck on a teat.

As your baby grows, you will become accustomed to his needs, and you may find that you need to wind him routinely, or that sometimes he settles without being burped.

Your baby may bring up, or posset, a little of his feed when he burps – this is quite normal. Having a muslin at the ready to catch any milk spews can save your clothes.

If your baby suffers quite a bit with wind, try keeping him upright for around 20 minutes after a feed as this can help to bring up trapped wind, easing his discomfort. If he's having trouble burping, try switching positions or applying a little more pressure.

WINDING POSITIONS

There are a few positions for winding. As with feeding positions, you and your baby will probably settle on the winding technique you both find most comfortable and effective.

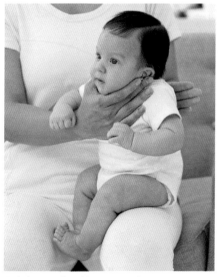

Hold baby over your shoulder A newborn suits being held upright with his head supported over your shoulder, while you gently rub or pat his back. Place a muslin over your shoulder to protect your clothing in case your baby regurgitates some milk.

Lay baby face down Hold your baby face down across your arm or your lap, with his head a little higher than his body. Make sure his head is properly supported, then gently rub or pat his back to help release the trapped air in his tummy.

Sit baby upright, chin supported When your baby's neck muscles are a little stronger, try sitting him on your lap, your palm supporting his chest and your thumb and forefinger spread out to support his chin. Rub or pat his back.

Q What does "expressing" breast milk mean and why should I do it?

Expressing your breast milk involves extracting milk from your breasts without your baby sucking, and it is done for a whole range of reasons.

If your baby is premature or unwell and unable to breastfeed, expressing means she can be fed breast milk and get the health benefits. If your breasts are full and uncomfortably engorged in the early weeks, your baby may find it tricky to latch on (see pp.268–69) to a very full breast. Expressing off a little milk can reduce the fullness and make latching on easier. If your baby has a weak suck, expressing can help to stimulate your milk supply and keep this at a good level.

Expressing your breast milk also allows you to delegate feeding to someone else. Having a supply of breast milk in the freezer can be handy if you're feeling unwell, or need to be away from your baby. If you are returning to work, putting in place an expressing regime means your baby can carry on enjoying your breast milk. If you are still breastfeeding by the time you start weaning your baby onto solids, you may want to express milk to mix with her baby rice or purées.

How to express

You can express breast milk with your hands or by using a pump. As you get used to expressing, you may combine methods, perhaps using your hands to stimulate the release of milk, and then a pump. Electric pumps are available to hire if you want to express for a short period, for a premature baby for example. Speak to your midwife or health visitor about hiring one.

EXPRESSING WITH A BREAST PUMP

Before expressing, make sure that your hands are clean and that all the equipment you use has been washed and sterilized (see p.279).

Expressing with a manual pump This is a bottle with a pump mechanism and a shield that creates a vacuum over your breast. Place the shield over your breast with the nipple area in the middle, then start pumping. Manual pumps are lightweight, but the action of pumping can be tiring.

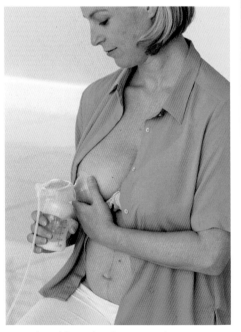

Expressing with an electric pump An electric motor does the pumping. You can usually adapt the strength of the pump to find a comfortable suction level. These pumps can be more fiddly to sterilize than manual ones, but they extract milk more quickly so are a good option if you plan to do a lot of expressing.

HOW TO EXPRESS BY HAND

Have a sterilized container ready to collect your expressed milk. It can take a bit of practice to express your milk by hand, so if you manage to squeeze out only a few drops on the first attempt, try not to give up.

Manipulate the milk Support your breast with one hand and place the other hand above your areola to manipulate the milk towards the nipple.

Squeeze and release Gently squeeze your breast and then release. Repeat this action, gradually building up your speed.

Catch the milk It can take a couple of minutes before milk appears and starts to flow. Catch the expressed milk in a sterilized container. You may need to move the position of your thumb and fingers around your breast to milk all areas.

Q How soon can I start expressing and giving my baby a bottle?

This can depend on your reasons for expressing. If you want breast milk for your premature baby, you can start expressing straight away in the hospital. If you are breastfeeding, you might want to wait until it is well established.

Waiting a few weeks before giving your baby expressed milk in a bottle will allow her to develop her sucking technique, which for breastfeeding involves co-ordinating her tongue and jaw movements in a unique action. Feeding from a bottle is very different, as gravity rather than your baby's sucking brings the milk to your baby, and the milk flow tends to be faster.

Introducing a bottle (and by the same token a dummy) in the early weeks of breastfeeding can lead to the phenomenon known as "nipple confusion", whereby your baby loses the sucking action needed for breastfeeding and, together with frustration at the slower flow of milk, shows a preference for feeding from a bottle. However, not all babies experience nipple confusion – some happily take to a bottle and are happy to switch between a breast and a bottle.

Giving expressed milk Once breastfeeding is well established, you should be able to feed your baby from the breast and give her expressed milk in bottles.

Q Should I be expressing my breast milk at a particular time of day?

There are no set rules about when you should express. Some experts recommend expressing after a feed, so that you don't remove milk your baby would have fed on, but if you are confident that your supply is plentiful, you can express either before or after a feed.

If you express before a feed, do this away from your baby so that she doesn't smell your milk or see your breasts and then want to start feeding. Women often find their supply of milk is most abundant in the morning after a night's sleep, so after your baby's first feed of the day can be a good time to express.

Once you grow more confident expressing, you can pump one breast while your baby is feeding from the other one. Your breasts will replace whatever milk is removed so you don't need to worry about your supply running out.

Did you know...

Breast milk contains substances that either relax or stimulate your baby depending on the time of day. Relaxing nucleotides are present in the evening and stimulating ones found earlier in the day.

Q I can express only a few millimetres of milk at a time. Does this mean I'm not producing enough breast milk?

Your breasts are almost certainly producing enough milk. Don't judge your overall supply on how much milk you manage to express. While some women fill bottles effortlessly, others don't find it as easy. Perhaps expressing works best for you by producing smaller amounts more frequently. Each woman is different.

Some women who find that expressing is unproductive have thriving, growing babies and are clearly producing enough milk. Your baby's sucking is by far the most effective way of extracting milk, so even if you aren't producing much when you express, she is almost certainly extracting more when she feeds.

There are ways to help stimulate your let-down reflex (see p.269). Tension can hinder the let-down of your milk, so get comfortable and relaxed. Having a warm shower or putting a warm flannel on your breast can help. Choose a time when you are less likely to be interrupted, pick a quiet spot, have a hot drink, and listen to some music if this helps. Massaging your breasts can help your milk to start flowing – use circular movements and then stroke downwards towards your nipples. Try to think about your baby when you start to express – imagine you are feeding or cradling her – as this can trigger the let-down reflex.

It is normal for the smell, colour, and consistency of **expressed breast milk** to vary depending on what you have eaten.

Q Are there any guidelines on how breast milk should be stored and how long I can keep it?

Always refrigerate or freeze your expressed milk straight away. Decant the breast milk into a sterilized container – a plastic bottle, specially sterilized breast milk bag, or ice cube trays (these smaller quantities are very handy for quick defrosting). Always make a note of the date on the container.

Your milk can be stored in a refrigerator kept at 4°C (40°F) or lower for up to five days. Place it at the back of the fridge as the temperature can fluctuate near the door. You can also store it in the freezer compartment of a fridge for two weeks, or for up to six months in a main freezer section kept at 18°C (0°F).

Defrost your milk in the fridge or at room temperature and don't refreeze it. Your baby can drink the milk cold, or you can warm it safely by putting the bottle in a bowl of warm water if she prefers to drink it that way.

Q I've been breastfeeding for two weeks and my nipples are sore and cracked. What can I do?

Your breasts and nipples are not used to doing the job of breastfeeding so it is common for discomforts to occur, especially in the first few weeks.

It is important to address any physical discomforts early on, so that breastfeeding becomes a positive experience for you. If you dread any discomfort it causes, this won't be good for your wellbeing and it may affect how your baby feeds.

Sore and cracked nipples are a common discomfort, but should not be an ongoing problem once your baby is latching on correctly and feeding efficiently. Not least because shorter feeds will mean your nipples have a break from feeding.

Problems such as cracked nipples can prevent your baby feeding efficiently and lead to other discomforts. If milk isn't properly drained, it can cause blocked ducts and, in a worst-case scenario, mastitis. Both can be painful and make you feel unwell so should be treated without delay.

Comfortable feeding Any physical discomforts of breastfeeding should be addressed early on.

BREASTFEEDING: COMMON CONCERNS

Understanding the causes of breastfeeding discomforts can help to prevent them becoming worse. Take action as soon as possible to resolve any problems so that efficient feeding can be established.

PROBLEM	DESCRIPTION	CAUSES
Sore, cracked, and bleeding nipples	It's normal for your nipples to feel tender as your baby's sucking stretches them, but sore nipples that last beyond the first week can indicate a problem that needs addressing. If the nipples become cracked, you may experience sharp pain for a few seconds at the start of a feed. Cracked nipples may also bleed, and your baby may swallow some blood. Streaks of blood may appear in your baby's stools or when he possets. Although alarming, this isn't harmful for your baby.	If your baby isn't latched on correctly, he may suck on your nipple, rather than your breast tissue. This makes the nipple increasingly tender, and the pressure of the sucking can cause the nipple to crack, and sometimes bleed. As your nipples are often moist when breastfeeding, it is hard for the cracks to heal. If nipples suddenly become red and sore after a period of being fine, you may have thrush, a fungal infection that can pass between you and your baby. You will both need medical care.
Blocked milk duct	A blocked duct can result in a lump with swelling and inflammation, and the area may be tender. The swelling may be alleviated slightly after breastfeeding. If bacteria reach the blocked duct, this can lead to mastitis (see below).	Milk ducts form a series of channels that carry milk to your nipple. A milk duct can become blocked if your breast isn't drained completely, often because your baby has a poor latch or weak suck. In the early days, when your breasts are producing a lot of milk, they may become engorged, leading to a blocked duct. A poorly fitting bra can put pressure on a part of the breast and cause a blockage. If you have redness, swelling, and lumps, contact your midwife or GP. Early treatment can help to avoid further complications, such as mastitis.
Mastitis and breast abscess	If you have hardness, swelling, and redness, and your temperature is slightly raised, you may have mastitis. If the infection worsens, this can become very painful, your temperature may escalate, and you may have flu-like symptoms. Occasionally, pus forms in the area and an abscess develops, which feels like an extremely painful lump. Mastitis is most common in the early weeks of breastfeeding when your milk supply hasn't settled down.	Problems can stem from your baby having a poor latch or weak sucking, which leads to a blocked duct or an area where there is a build up of milk, referred to as milk stasis. If bacteria present on your skin travel to a blocked milk duct, this can cause a mastitis infection. If you are anaemic, or very run down, your resistance may be lowered, making you more susceptible to infection.

Placing **Savoy cabbage leaves** on the breast helps soothe and cool down the affected area.

WHAT YOU CAN DO

» Check your latching-on technique (see p.268).

» At the end of a feed, allow the air to get to your nipples so they dry naturally. Try rubbing a couple of drops of breast milk into them, as breast milk has anti-bacterial properties.

» Apply a little purified lanolin cream, which is safe to use even before a feed.

» Avoid breast pads as these keep moisture in.

» Nipple shields can help but only use them for a short time as they can affect your baby's latch.

» Don't stop feeding from the sore breast.

» Continue to feed your baby, checking that he is latched on properly to ensure effective sucking.

» Babies often suck most strongly at the start of a feed, so putting your baby on the affected side first may help to drain the milk.

» Warmth can help your milk flow, so placing a warm flannel on your breast at the start of a feed may be helpful, and gently massaging your breast can help to reduce swelling.

» Contact your midwife or GP. They can put you in touch with a breastfeeding consultant who can help to improve your baby's latch.

» Contact your GP straight away if you think you have mastitis. If infection has set in, your GP will prescribe antibiotics that are safe to take while breastfeeding. It's important to keep breastfeeding so that milk is removed regularly and your breasts don't become engorged. You may need to feed more often than usual, and express milk so that the breast is sufficiently drained.

» Many women find placing a cold flannel or chilled Savoy cabbage leaf against the breast soothing as these remove heat from the breast.

» It's important to get plenty of rest.

» Mild pain relief can help. Ibuprofen also acts as an anti-inflammatory.

» An abscess that doesn't respond to antibiotics may need to be surgically drained.

Q My breasts feel as though they're about to burst. Will this last?

This feeling of fullness, or engorgement, should subside within one or two days. It's common for women to feel that their breasts have gone up a cup size or two when their milk "comes in", around three to five days after the birth.

As well as filling up with milk, blood flow to the breasts increases during breastfeeding and apart from feeling very full, breasts may feel hot, hard, lumpy, and tender. This engorgement is usually relieved when you feed your baby and the milk supply starts to settle down.

If the engorgement is uncomfortable, or your baby is finding it hard to latch on, you can hand express or pump a small amount of milk (see p.272) to reduce the fullness just enough to make latching on easier. Be careful not to express too much, though, as you don't want your breasts to make even more milk.

Massaging your breasts a little while your baby feeds may help the milk flow. Or try putting a hot flannel on your breast or having a hot shower before a feed to help trigger the let-down reflex. After a feed, a cold flannel or compress, or a chilled Savoy cabbage leaf, can be soothing and take any heat out of the breast. A properly fitted nursing bra will support your breasts and make them more comfortable; you may want keep a bra on at night, too.

Q My breasts keep leaking milk. How can I cope with this?

An over-abundant milk supply can mean that breasts leak. This leaking can also happen when your let-down reflex (see p.269) is triggered unexpectedly. Leaking may occur in one breast while you're feeding your baby on the other side, or when you're in a warm environment, such as the shower, or when you hear your baby cry, or even just think about your baby.

Expressing a little milk before or after a feed may reduce leaking, and feeding frequently will ensure that milk is regularly removed and milk production falls into sync with your growing baby's needs. If you sense that you're about to leak milk, discreetly crossing your arms over your chest so that you are putting gentle pressure on your nipples may stem the flow. Placing breast pads inside your bra can contain leaks. Bring spare clothes when you go out.

Q My baby falls asleep during feeds. What should I do?

If your baby nods off during a feed you should gently wake him. Your baby may come off the breast on his own once he is full, but sometimes babies can fall asleep while on the breast, or carry on comfort sucking. If his jaw is no longer moving, or his sucking has become lighter and quicker, but he doesn't appear to be swallowing, he may be full. If this happens, or he falls asleep, gently rouse him and wind him, then check if he wants to continue with the feed before bringing the session to a close.

Q My baby cries when he comes off the breast. Am I making enough milk?

If you feed your baby regularly you will almost certainly be able to make enough milk for him. Your baby may need more milk for a day or two because he is going through a growth spurt. He may cry as soon as he finishes a feed, or shortly after one, and you may feel like you're feeding continuously.

If you meet your baby's increased demands, your supply will increase to meet his needs. Offering both breasts at each feed will help your milk supply to increase more rapidly, and you might even need to keep swapping breasts until your baby seems completely satisfied.

The clearest sign that your baby is feeding well and thriving is that he is gaining weight. Being nice and alert when awake, and having more than six wet nappies a day are also sure signs that your baby is well-nourished. Talk to your midwife or GP if you have any concerns.

Q I have inverted nipples. Will this prevent me breastfeeding?

It is possible to breastfeed if your nipples are inverted, but you will need some guidance. A breastfeeding consultant can check how you are managing to feed. She may recommend using a breast pump to draw out the nipple before you begin feeding, or using a nipple shield to help the baby latch on. Pulling the breast tissue back as your baby latches on will also help the nipple to protrude. Seek advice from your midwife if you are finding it hard.

Q I'm still finding it tricky to get my baby latched on properly. Where can I get more support?

There are numerous avenues of support. In the early days, you may be able to access support from a breastfeeding consultant in your hospital or birth centre. In hospital, midwives on the postnatal ward can check your technique and community midwives or your health visitor can help once you're home.

If you need to talk to someone quickly, there are breastfeeding organizations that have helplines allowing you to chat to an experienced mother or breastfeeding consultant trained to offer advice and support. While chatting on the phone can be very helpful, sometimes it isn't a substitute for sitting with someone while they watch your feeding technique. Organizations such as La Leche League and The Baby Café provide drop-in meetings where you can meet other mums, and often get one-to-one help from healthcare professionals such as health visitors and breastfeeding consultants.

You may have been given details of local breastfeeding drop-in centres when you were discharged from hospital, or your midwife or GP practice can provide information of where you can go, or check out centres online. The camaraderie and support these facilities provide can be invaluable.

Feeling supported by your partner is important, too. Having your partner's full backing can give you the encouragement to overcome problems and carry on with feeding.

Don't delay in seeking help if you're encountering a problem, as if you don't get on top of an issue, it can quickly escalate. Most breastfeeding problems can be resolved with the right advice and support.

Around **75%** of new mums **seek help with breastfeeding.** Most work through their problems and go on to breastfeed successfully.

Q Breastfeeding is so convenient, but I feel anxious about doing it in public. How can I gain confidence?

Knowing your rights and thinking ahead can help counter initial jitters about public breastfeeding. It is normal to feel self-conscious in the beginning, but in time you will grow in confidence and it will become second nature.

One of the joys of breastfeeding is that you can feed your baby any time or place as soon as she is hungry. Your breast milk is always available at the right temperature in the exact amount your baby needs, so when you start to venture out with your baby, you don't have to do preparation such as sterilizing bottles and measuring out the formula you will need.

Breastfeeding is simply extremely convenient. Most mothers find that it's easy to choose a spot where they can feed their baby discreetly, and that actually the majority of people barely notice, or if they do, they are entirely respectful.

Your right to feed in public

Occasionally, you may get a disapproving look or comment, which makes you feel self-conscious and perhaps even a little humiliated, even though feeding is the most natural thing in the world. So it's good to know that you do have rights in such a situation. The Equality Act of 2010 states that in England and Wales it is sex discrimination to treat a woman unfavourably because she is breastfeeding. This applies to public places such as parks, leisure centres, cafés, restaurants, hotels, theatres, cinemas, public buildings, and on public transport. In Scotland, the Breastfeeding Act of 2005 makes it an offence to try to stop a woman breastfeeding in a public place. So if you do encounter any opposition, knowing your rights can help to reassure you that it is definitely the other person who is in the wrong, not you.

Planning ahead

Think about what you are wearing: loose tops you can lift up a little to let your baby latch on help to make breastfeeding discreet. Apart from an initial flash of flesh, it's pretty hard to see anything other than your baby. Wearing a loose vest under a T-shirt means you can pull this down to hide your postnatal tummy, and often, your arm cradling your baby will do this job. Practise undoing your nursing bra with one hand, too.

Some women use a muslin cloth or a breastfeeding scarf for a bit of extra cover, but others feel that this actually draws attention to the fact that they're feeding. Go with whatever feels best for you – if covering up a little more feels reassuring, that's fine, but you shouldn't ever feel that you have to hide yourself when you are breastfeeding your baby.

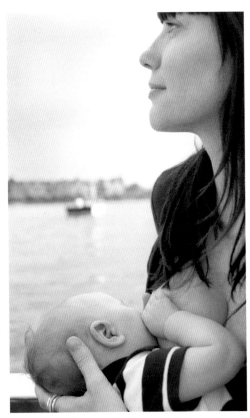

Confident feeding Breastfeeding your baby is natural and not something you should have to hide or be embarrassed about.

Q I want to continue breastfeeding, but I'm struggling. Is it really worth persevering?

Breastfeeding is time-consuming, tiring, and, in some circumstances, leads to physical discomfort. For these reasons, it's not uncommon for mothers to reach a point where they are unsure if they can carry on.

Like many new mums, you may be surprised at the demands of breastfeeding. After all, unless you have started to express milk, you are the only one that can feed your baby. It's natural to want to share the feeding and consider putting your baby on formula, not least so that you can have a break and a night of undisrupted sleep while your partner bottle-feeds the baby.

Give it time

Be reassured, though, that once you have settled into breastfeeding, it becomes easier. Your baby will feed more efficiently, meaning that feeds are likely to be shorter and less time-consuming. You will also, hopefully, have overcome initial breastfeeding discomforts (see pp.274–75). Don't forget, rather than using formula you can also begin to express your milk (see p.272), which can give you a break while ensuring your baby is still getting all the benefits of breast milk.

Reaping the rewards

Most women who persevere with feeding are incredibly glad they did so as they reach the stage when breastfeeding becomes a real joy – convenient, easy, and a wonderful bonding experience. So yes, it is worth persevering because breastfeeding can be such a mutually rewarding experience. But if you really feel that breastfeeding isn't for you, there is no shame in giving it up.

For many women **breastfeeding becomes pleasurable,** which more than compensates for any initial difficulties.

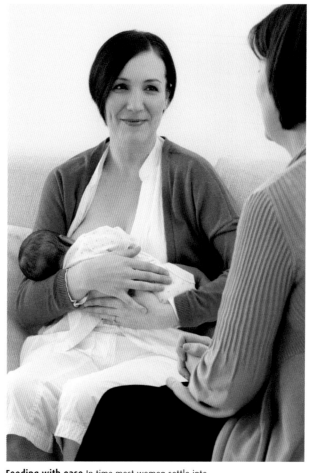

Feeding with ease In time most women settle into breastfeeding and find it mutually rewarding.

Q Will introducing a bottle of formula for one of our baby's feeds affect my milk supply?

It depends on when you decide to do this.
Giving your baby a bottle of formula allows you the occasional break and your partner a chance to feed your baby, and perhaps to help with night feeding. However, if you want to continue breastfeeding for a while, albeit on a reduced schedule, it's advisable to wait for around six to eight weeks before you introduce your baby to a bottle.

In the first few weeks, your breasts are adapting to feeding your baby and your milk supply is becoming established. If you introduce a bottle of formula, it might reduce your milk

supply, as it works on a supply and demand basis. Introducing a bottle and teat also means that your baby has to learn a new sucking technique, which could lead to "nipple confusion" (see p.273).

After six to eight weeks, your milk supply will have settled down and you can try to introduce a bottle. However, this will reduce the amount of breast milk you make, and it can be hard to reverse this decision, so be certain this is what you want to do before you introduce the formula feed.

It's also worth bearing in mind that if you are hoping to have a break from night feeds, preparing a bottle of formula at night can be a lot more time-consuming than breastfeeding, and your partner may not be able or willing to do every night-time feed.

Did you know...

It is recommended that you breastfeed your baby exclusively until you start introducing solid food at around six months. This means only giving your baby breast milk – no other food or drink until then. Once you start weaning, you can continue to breastfeed and use your breast milk to prepare foods. It is quite common for women who return to work to continue to breastfeed or combine breastfeeding with formula milk. Expressed milk can be given to your baby by the person caring for her.

You might be **bottle-feeding** your baby if you are **combination feeding**, moving on to formula **after breastfeeding**, or perhaps breastfeeding just hasn't worked out for you. Either way, it's reassuring to know that you can raise a healthy baby on **formula milk**.

Bottle-feeding your baby

Why bottle-feed

There is a lot of pressure put on new mums to breastfeed, but some women are uncomfortable with breastfeeding, or are unable to breastfeed. It's important that your baby gets the right amount of food to grow, so try not to worry about where her nourishment comes from; you will give her a good start in life with formula milk. Feeding your baby from either the breast or a bottle is a wonderful bonding experience. Some mums express breast milk from the start and their baby drinks it from a bottle, while others combine breast and bottle-feeding. There are some advantages to bottle-feeding your baby. Firstly, someone other than you can prepare and give a feed, allowing you time to rest. Secondly, bottle-fed babies tend to have fewer feeds. Thirdly, they generally sleep better at night (after the first few weeks) as they're less likely to wake up for a feed – cow's milk forms a more solid curd that takes longer to digest than breast milk. If you bottle-feed from the start, it will take around seven to 10 days for the milk your breasts produced after the birth to dry up, during which time your breasts may feel heavy and full.

First feeds

Your newborn needs to feed little and often, so offer her the bottle when you notice her hunger cues (see p.269). Young babies are especially vulnerable to germs while their immunity builds up, so be meticulous about hygiene rules when preparing feeds and sterilizing bottles and teats. Bottle-fed babies take in more air during feeds (their mouths form less of a seal around a teat compared to a nipple) so wind your baby regularly.

Switching to bottle-feeding

If you want to wean from breast to formula feeds, or to give bottles of expressed breast milk, you will need to get equipped with bottles, teats, and a sterilizing system (see p.191). Some bottles boast a similar feel to a nipple to help a baby make the switch from breast to bottle. If you wish to continue breastfeeding while trying a bottle, called combination feeding, start with one bottle a day, so that your baby gets used to the different taste and the feel of a teat. It can help if your partner does the first few bottle feeds until your baby gets used to the bottle.

Q What is the best way to sterilize bottles and teats for my baby?

It's good to know that there are a few different safe methods you can use to sterilize baby feeding equipment, rather a single correct way. Before sterilizing, wash bottles, teats, and the equipment used to make up your baby's formula thoroughly in hot, soapy water to remove all traces of milk residue. This is easier to do soon after a feed, and using a bottle brush to clean the crevices. Rinse off the detergent. Parts from breast pumps should be washed this way after each use and then sterilized according to the manufacturer's instructions.

Washing alone does not kill harmful bacteria and viruses, so the bottles, teats, and related equipment need to be sterilized. Cold-water sterilization involves submerging the equipment in cold water treated with a chemical agent, which comes in tablet or liquid form. Leave the equipment covered in the solution for at least 30 minutes before use, to keep it sterile.

Steam sterilizers range from quick-to-use microwave steamers to electric sterilizers. Place the openings of bottles and teats face down so that the insides are sterilized by rising steam.

To boil feeding equipment, immerse the items completely in a large, lidded pan of water. Boil for at least 10 minutes to kill germs, and keep the lid on the pan until the equipment is needed. Boiling teats can wear them out quicker, so check for signs of damage before using them.

Q How much formula does my baby need each day? Does it depend on his appetite, or should I stick to a set amount?

In the first week or so, just like a breastfed baby, your baby will probably manage just small amounts of formula at each feed. After this, and until around six months of age, the rule of thumb is to give 150–200ml (5–7fl oz) per kg (2lb 3oz) of your baby's weight each day.

Q Is there a certain way I should make up my baby's feeds?

There is a particular method that you must follow each time you make up a powdered formula milk feed for your baby (see below).

Special care needs to be taken when making up formula for two reasons. One is that cartons of formula powder, although sealed, are not sterile (unlike ready-to-drink cartons of formula milk, which are), so could contain bacteria such as salmonella that could make your baby extremely unwell. This means that meticulous hygiene is paramount when making up bottles. Secondly, the ratio of powder to milk needs to be exactly right to make sure your baby is getting the correct balance of nutrients. Too little powder can mean that your baby isn't getting enough nourishment; and too much powder could make your baby constipated and dehydrated. Always read the manufacturer's instructions carefully before you begin and make up a feed using the scoop provided.

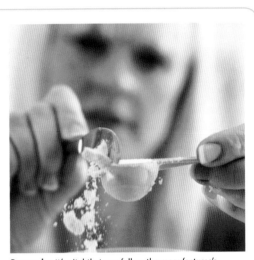

Be precise It's vital that you follow the manufacturer's instructions when making up powdered formula milk.

STEPS TO MAKING UP POWDERED FORMULA

Here are the steps to follow each time you make up a feed. You'll soon get the hang of it and will be able to follow the steps effortlessly. However, you must continue to be stringent with the process.

1 Start by boiling 1 litre (1³/₄ pints) of fresh tap water (rather than water already sitting in the kettle). Leave the water to cool for no more than 30 minutes so that it is at least 70°C (158°F) – hot enough to kill off any bacteria present.

2 Wash your hands thoroughly and make sure the surface where you are preparing the bottle is scrupulously clean. You can spray the area with anti-bacterial spray and wipe it down before you start to make up a feed.

3 Put the water in the bottle first, pouring in the exact amount recommended by the manufacturer on the packaging. Don't dilute or strengthen the formula as it can affect your baby's digestive system.

4 Using the scoop provided, loosely scoop out some formula, then level this off with a clean, dry knife, or with the leveller provided, and add the specified number of scoops to the water. Always use the scoop that came with the formula.

5 Holding the teat by its edge, push it through the retaining ring, screw the ring on to the bottle, and cover with the cap. Shake the bottle so that all the powder dissolves. Leave the formula to cool before you give it to your baby.

6 Test the temperature on the inside of your wrist to help you gauge whether it's ready for your baby: it should be just warm, but not hot. To cool it down, place the bottle in a bowl of cold water or run the bottom half of the bottle under a cold tap.

Q What's the best way to give my baby his bottle?

First, get comfortable yourself, sitting upright with your back straight and supported. Feeds can take a while, so you don't want to strain your back.

Hold your baby close to you, cradling him against your body and facing you, so you can talk and make eye contact during a feed. It's a wonderful chance to bond with your baby. Keep him upright holding him at your chest height, as this will help him to swallow at a steady pace. Allow your baby to pause during a feed if he wishes (as he would naturally when breastfeeding), then resume the feed. If he squirms or seems restless mid-feed, remove the bottle and try winding him, then continue once he is settled. It's important that you never leave your baby with a bottle propped up in his mouth as he could suffocate or choke.

HOW TO BOTTLE-FEED STEP BY STEP

By following these simple steps you will soon become a natural at giving a bottle. It will quickly turn into a familiar routine that you and your baby both enjoy.

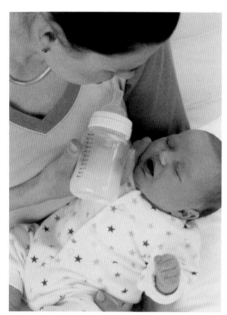

1 Gently rub his cheek to encourage the rooting reflex. Then place the teat so that it is touching his top lip. Don't push the teat into your baby's mouth, wait for him to open his mouth to take it, or gently nuzzle it against his lips to encourage him to take it.

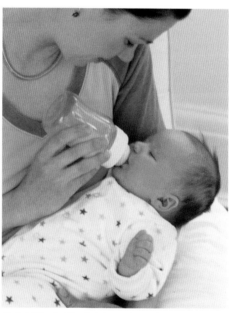

2 Hold the bottle slightly upright, making sure the milk covers the opening of the teat and the neck of the bottle. This will help to ensure that your baby isn't taking in too much extra air during a feed. Support your baby's head with the cradle of your arm.

3 Tilt the bottle up a bit more as the bottle empties so that the milk continues to cover the teat. At the end of a feed you can put your little finger (make sure it's clean) into your baby's mouth to break off the suction and remove the bottle.

Q I am breastfeeding and plan to introduce a bottle. Any tips on making this switch?

While some babies switch from breast to bottle without a hitch, others go into a screaming meltdown. If your baby protests loudly whenever a bottle comes near him, there are a few tactics you can try. Getting your partner to give a bottle means that your baby can't smell your milk. Choose a time when your baby isn't very hungry, perhaps an afternoon feed, so that he is less likely to get distressed if he isn't getting the milk he wants. If you're not in a rush to get him on to formula, you could try giving expressed milk first, as he may be more willing to try a bottle if the contents are familiar.

Bear in mind, too, that breastfed babies need to suck harder to get their milk, so starting off with a slow-flow teat can help ensure your baby isn't overwhelmed by a fast flow of milk. Conversely, if your baby is very hungry, a slower flow may frustrate him. Experiment to find the teat that suits him. Let your baby play with and get used to the bottle, and don't carry on trying if he refuses after about three attempts. Take a break, offer a breastfeed after about 10 minutes, then try the bottle again in a few days time.

Q Should I make up each bottle of formula fresh when our baby needs it?

Yes, in recent years the guidelines on making up and storing feeds have been revised. You should always freshly make up each bottle of formula milk.

It used to be common practice to make up feeds for one day and keep them in the fridge until needed. However, bacteria are still able to multiply in a fridge (and at room temperature this can happen very quickly), so this increases the risk of harmful bacteria reaching a baby. Each bottle should be made up fresh and any remaining milk, or unused formula that has been left at room temperature, should be discarded. Bacteria also multiplies in saliva left on a teat, for which reason you should not reuse them after a feed or share bottles between babies.

WHAT YOU NEED TO KNOW

» **Make up feeds fresh** as and when your baby needs them.

» **Make the feed within 30 minutes** of boiling the kettle. Always use fresh water.

» **Put the correct amount of water** in the bottle before adding the formula powder.

Travelling with formula Pack sterilized bottles. You can purchase travel containers with in-built dividers to keep powdered formula in pre-measured quantities.

Feeding on the go

If you are away from home, there are a few options for bottle-feeding. Think about your day and how long you will be out as you don't want to get caught short.

» **Take a sterilized bottle** and a carton of ready-made formula, then decant this when needed. This is by far the easiest solution. You might need to bring a pair of clean scissors as opening ready-made cartons of formula isn't always that easy.

» **Put the correct amount of formula** in a clean, plastic container and pack this along with a flask of just-boiled water and a sterilized bottle, then make up the feed when needed, allowing the water to cool before you give the feed to your baby.

» **If someone else needs to give your baby a feed** when you are not present, for example a childminder or grandparent, make sure they know how to make up the formula correctly. If your baby is looked after with other babies, make sure his sterilized bottles are labelled with his name.

Q Can I put my bottle-fed baby on a feeding schedule?

No, bottle-fed babies should be fed on demand just as breastfed babies are, as your baby's small tummy means he needs to feed more frequently at first. Although bottle-feeding can feel more structured as you make up bottles according to your baby's weight and know exactly how much milk your baby takes each day, it doesn't follow that bottle-fed babies adapt well to a schedule. Formula manufacturers suggest giving larger feeds at more spaced apart intervals, but this may not suit even your older baby, who may need smaller, more frequent feeds, especially if he brings up a lot of milk after feeds. Feeds that are too large can make your baby overfull, possibly sick, and could lead to him becoming overweight.

Q Which formula should I choose? Do I have to give my baby cow's milk formula?

Choose a formula that is appropriate for your baby's age. First infant formula is recommended from birth (and your baby can continue to enjoy it until his first birthday). First formula milk replicates the same of ratio of 60:40 whey to casein proteins that is in breast milk, to ensure it is digestible for your baby and provides the right balance of hydration and nutrition. "Follow-on" formulas contain a greater percentage of the thicker casein protein, but they are harder for your baby to digest and are not suitable in the first six months.

Cow's milk formula is the recommended choice for your baby. It has been formulated to strict nutritional guidelines to ensure it is a suitable food for a growing baby. Unless your doctor or midwife say otherwise, your baby should have formula derived from cow's milk in his first year. Some babies react to the proteins or the sugar lactose in cow's milk formula. In this case, your doctor can prescribe a special type of formula called "fully hydrolyzed", where the protein is broken down and the lactose removed. Soya-based formula is seldom recommended because babies who react to proteins in cow's milk often react to proteins in soya milk, too. There are also concerns that phytoestrogens in soya formula may affect the reproductive organs, and some soya products have glucose added, which could affect your baby's emerging teeth. Soya milk formula should not be given to babies under six months old, and then only if your doctor recommends it, which might be the case for vegan families, or if your baby won't drink other alternatives.

For such a little person, your **amazing new baby** requires a lot of looking after. If this is your first time caring for a newborn, you may feel you lack the full qualifications for the job. Rest assured that, while it's very natural for new parents to feel a little nervous, your **confidence will grow** in the coming days and weeks.

Caring for your baby

On-the-job training

So much of parenting is about learning on the job, and you will find that your baby is naturally forgiving of any initial awkwardness. What he needs from the outset is your love, attention, and reassurance that you are there to meet his needs. The rest of your parenting skills will soon fall into place: where those early cries perplexed, before long you will be able to decipher what it is your baby is asking for, and from those first tentative holds, you'll become adept at handling and holding your baby just the way he likes while you wash, dress, and soothe him.

Caring for your baby every day

An important part of caring for your baby is ensuring that he is kept clean and comfortable and that he is safe in his environment. From preventing nappy rash to ensuring good sleep hygiene – making sure your baby's sleep environment is safe and conducive to rest – the everyday care you give your baby helps him to feel content. Many of the practices you put in place in these early days will instill good habits for life. As well as your baby's everyday practical care, he also needs stimulation and interaction with you and his environment. At first, this may be as simple as making eye contact, copying facial expressions, and exchanging smiles. Then, increasingly, play will involve activities, toys, and exploring other environments. All of the time you spend together, both in play and with simple caring tasks, helps to strengthen your bond.

Young babies are vulnerable to infection, so it's worth avoiding contact with germs in the first few weeks. However, your baby will inevitably be unwell at some point. Knowing what signs indicate that your baby is unwell, and when to seek medical help, can reassure you that you will give your baby the care he needs.

Looking after you

These early weeks and months caring for your little one are amazing and all-consuming. Getting the right amount of rest, being mutually supportive with your partner over your baby's care, and paying attention to your diet and lifestyle will ensure you have the energy and resources needed to give your baby your very best care.

Q I've never changed a nappy before! Where do I start?

Pick a warm, draught-free spot – babies can object to the feel of cold air on their skin – and lay your baby down on a wipe-clean nappy mat or a towel.

Changing your baby's nappy at floor level is safest for your baby, but it can be tough on your back. A purpose-made changing table is convenient and easier for you, but you need to keep an eye on your baby at all times. Have everything you need to hand: the quicker and more efficient the nappy change, the less likely it is that your baby will become distressed.

YOU WILL NEED

» **A clean nappy**, and nappy liner if you are using disposable nappies.

» **Cotton wool and warm water**. Baby wipes can be harsh on your baby's skin, so limit their use and avoid them for newborns.

» **Nappy sacks or bin**, for disposal

» **Barrier cream** (optional)

CHANGING YOUR BABY'S NAPPY

Remove the old nappy. If it's soiled, use the front of the nappy to wipe away faeces. Fold the nappy in on itself, seal with the tabs, and dispose of it (or flush a disposable liner if using reusables). When removing a boy's nappy, hold it over his penis for a moment so you don't get sprayed by urine.

1 **Clean the nappy area** with wet cotton wool, a flannel, or wipes. Wipe girls from front to back to stop bacteria reaching the vagina. Clean carefully around a boy's testes and penis, and don't pull the foreskin.

2 **Once you've finished cleaning**, let the air get to the nappy area for a few minutes as this can help to prevent, or soothe, sore nappy rash. If you wish, you can apply a thin layer of barrier cream to the skin.

3 **Gently lift up his legs** by the ankles, then slip a clean nappy under his bottom, bringing the side tabs level with the waist. Check a boy's penis is facing down before bringing up the front of the nappy.

4 **Bring the nappy** up between the legs, and secure with the side tabs. You should be able to fit a finger between the nappy and tummy. For a reusable, put a liner inside the nappy, and add an outer wrap if using.

Q How often should I change my baby's nappy? It's hard to tell when it's wet.

It goes without saying that you should change your baby's nappy each time he has a bowel movement. With today's super absorbent disposables, it can be hard to tell if a nappy is wet. To get an idea, pour four tablespoons of water into a dry nappy – this is what a soaked one feels like. You'll change your baby's nappy at least six times a day after the first week.

Q Do I always need to change a nappy after a night feed?

Use common sense and judgment when it comes to night-time nappy changes. Some parents worry that the extra disruption this causes will make a sleepy, satisfied, and ready-to-settle baby suddenly very awake. Check the nappy. If it feels fairly dry and your baby doesn't have uncomfortable nappy rash, it's probably okay to leave it. You may prefer, though, to be on the safe side and change his nappy so that he doesn't wake again shortly afterwards feeling wet and uncomfortable.

Q What's the best way to treat my baby's sore bottom?

While nappy rash is common, when your baby's bottom becomes red, take this as a prompt to check that you are practising good nappy hygiene. Spending time in wet and soiled nappies irritates your baby's skin. Babies usually let you know when they're soiled – or you can smell it! – but they don't always complain when a nappy is wet. Keep an eye on the state of his nappies and change them frequently. Baby wipes can be irritating on your baby's delicate skin, so avoid these while his bottom looks sore, and use just warm water and cotton wool for cleaning. Let your baby go nappy-free for a short while each day so that air can get to his skin to speed up healing. Before putting a new nappy on, apply a thin layer of zinc oxide barrier cream to protect his skin. If you have reusable nappies, make sure they are rinsed thoroughly after washing so that all traces of detergent are removed.

Q What's the best way to keep my baby clean each day?

Until your baby is on the move, crawling around and picking up dirt, a daily bath isn't vital, but you do need to give her a thorough clean, or "top and tail", each day.

This involves washing her face, bottom, and in the skin creases where dirt and posseted milk accumulate. Get organized first, so you don't have to root around for nappies or cloths in the middle of cleaning, and instead can give your baby your full attention so she doesn't become anxious and restless. See page 186 for the equipment you'll need for bathing your baby.

YOU WILL NEED

» **A bowl, or sink, of warm water.**

» **Some cotton wool** and a flannel.

» **A clean nappy,** and nappy liner if you are using disposable nappies.

"TOPPING AND TAILING" YOUR BABY

Wash your hands before you start. Lay your baby down on her changing mat in a draught-free room. Put a towel on top of the mat for added comfort if you wish. Then either undress your baby down to her vest and nappy, or if it's a bit chilly, keep her sleepsuit on and undo the top and bottom half separately, keeping one half of her covered while you clean the other half.

1 **Using a separate piece of damp cotton wool** for each eye, gently wipe your baby's eyes from the inner to the outer edge. Use a new piece of cotton wool to clean behind (not inside) the ears and around the neck, cleaning out milk residue from skin creases.

2 **Gently lift up your baby's arms** and clean in her armpits; then clean the palm of your baby's hand and uncurl her fingers to clean in between each one. Wash your baby's feet, again gently cleaning between the toes, and clean her legs, wiping the creases under the knees.

3 **Use a clean damp flannel** to clean around the umbilical cord area. You can use plain water, or mild baby wash if the area is soiled by faeces. Pat the area dry and let the air get to the skin. Then clean the nappy area (see p.283) before putting on a new nappy.

Q How can I dress my baby so that she isn't too hot or too cold?

Generally, the advice is for your baby to wear one more layer of clothing than you are wearing, which may just mean adding a vest under a sleepsuit and cardigan, or placing a blanket over her in the buggy. You should regularly check, though, whether your baby seems comfortable. Young babies aren't good at regulating their body temperature, and so rely on you to make sure they are just right. By dressing your baby in several lightweight layers, you can quickly adapt her clothing when you are moving between indoors and outdoors, perhaps adding a cotton blanket, or removing a jacket, as required. It's important, too, not to leave your baby sleeping in outdoor layers when you get home, however tempting it may be not to disturb her, as she may overheat.

Gauge your baby's temperature by feeling her tummy, chest, or the nape of her neck – if these areas feel hot to touch, remove a layer, or add a layer if they feel cold. Bear in mind that babies' hands and feet are often on the cool side, so don't use these to judge temperature.

On sunny days, make sure your baby's shoulders are covered up and put a wide-brimmed sunhat on her. Your baby's skin is very delicate and can burn quickly, so as well as keeping her covered, keep her out of direct sunshine during the hottest part of the day. Use a sunshade on her buggy, and apply a sunscreen that is specially formulated for babies, with a minimum of SPF 30.

Q What's the easiest way to put on my baby's vest and sleepsuit?

Vests with envelope-style necks can be pulled wide, making them easy to pass over a baby's head. Lay your baby down, gently lift the back of her head, then pull the neckline over, lifting the fabric off her face. Pull each vest arm out to pop her hands through, then smooth the vest over her body and do up the poppers.

Lay the sleepsuit out, poppers opened, and place your baby on it. Gently bend her legs and place them in the sleepsuit legs, then do up the poppers around the legs and nappy area. Gather the fabric on an arm and pass her hand through the sleeve, putting your hand through the other end to guide it. Do up the remaining poppers.

Q Why is my baby crying? Should I assume she is hungry?

Crying is a natural state for your baby, and is her first and main means of communication. Your baby may not know why she's upset, she just knows that something is wrong. Your job is to work out what that thing is. In the first days and weeks, hunger is often the reason for her cries; you may want to offer a feed if it has been a couple of hours since she fed. As your baby grows and feeds become more spaced out, you may not want to offer a feed instantly – in fact, if you do so, she may expect a feed each time you pick her up.

As you get to know your baby, you'll notice clues as to what's wrong. If your baby is grizzly, perhaps rubbing her eyes, yawning, and looking glazed, she probably needs a nap. Babies can cry when over-stimulated, whether they are feeling tired or because there is too much going on. Other reasons include wanting to change position, needing a nappy change, or feeling too hot or too cold. If she's been asleep, she may cry because she needs reassurance that you are close by. If she's uncomfortable, she may simply be craving the comfort and reassurance she feels when held in your arms.

If your baby is crying intensely (three hours a day or more) and won't be soothed, often at the same time each day, and maybe looks flushed, is clenching her fists, and drawing her legs up to her tummy while crying, she may have colic – the term used when otherwise healthy babies cry excessively. You should see your GP so that he or she can rule out any other cause for your baby's crying.

Q I love carrying my baby in a sling, but will it make her too clingy?

Carrying your baby in a sling, or "baby wearing", is comforting for mum, or dad, and baby. This closeness makes your baby feel secure and loved, and in turn confident you're there for her, so fears about clinginess are ungrounded. The sound of your heartbeat relaxes your baby, and you'll quickly pick up on feeding cues. Make sure your baby is safe in the sling. It should be tight enough to hold her securely and support her back, her face should be visible at all times and not obstructed, her head should be close to yours, and her chin should not rest on her chest.

Q How can I comfort my grizzly baby?

Sometimes comfort and closeness to you can be enough to soothe your baby and reassure her that all is well.

When you respond to your baby's cries with soft words, a gentle touch, and by keeping her close, she learns that she can trust you to recognize her needs and that the world is a safe place for her, and in the long run she is likely to become more independent and confident. There's no right or wrong way to soothe your baby, and you and your baby will find techniques that work for you both.

SOOTHING TECHNIQUES

Experiment with different comforting methods to find the ones that work best for you and your baby.

» Rhythm and motion is naturally soothing to your baby, perhaps reminding her of her time in the womb. Gently rocking or swaying your baby, or carrying her in a sling, is reassuring, and being close to you makes her feel safe and secure. If crying is persistent, a trip around the block in the buggy or car may lull her to sleep, though you may not want her to become too dependent on these methods of soothing.

» Sucking is inherently comforting for your little one, so if hunger isn't the problem, she may enjoy sucking on your finger or a dummy (though you may be avoiding dummies in the early weeks to avoid nipple confusion, see page 273).

» White noise can help your baby to switch off and zone out when she is over-stimulated. The sound of the washing machine cycle may remind your baby of swooshing noises in the uterus and prove a comfort.

» Whispering, talking gently, singing a soothing lullaby, and smiling can all help to calm a grouchy baby, especially one who is just in need of a bit of company.

» Rubbing your baby's back while held upright, or while gently swaying her as she's held face down along your arm, may help if she has wind or is colicky.

» Physical contact is essential to your baby's wellbeing. Stroking her head and gently patting her back or bottom can be soothing, and if your baby has colic, a baby massage can help her to relax if she's receptive. Stroke her arms and legs, her palms, and the soles of her feet; then stroke her brow and, if comfortable for her, stroke her tummy in a clockwise motion.

If crying is persistent, occurs around the same time each day, and your baby is inconsolable, she may have colic. Talk to your doctor or health visitor about ways to ease this.

Close to you Snuggled close, listening to your heartbeat, is naturally soothing for your baby.

A calm hold Older babies often enjoy being held upright as you move around.

Face down Some babies love to be held face down and gently rocked back and forth.

Q How much sleep does my baby need?

On average, babies sleep 14–18 hours per day in the first few weeks. This time spent in slumber is vital for their growth and development.

Babies grow at a tremendous rate in the first few months. The time they spend asleep allows their bodies to focus on growing (growth hormone is released during sleep), and for them to process all the new information they receive each day. Newborns can manage only brief periods of sleep before their tiny tummies need feeding again, so their sleep is spread over both night and day and they will wake as frequently at night as they do in the day. Apart from needing to wake often to feed, your baby has short sleep cycles of 45–60 minutes, and when he stirs from a cycle, he finds it hard to drop back off to sleep naturally. All of this means that in the first six to eight weeks, you will need to feed your baby around the clock, waking every two to three hours in the night to tend to him. At around two months (later for some, earlier for others), your baby will start to manage slightly longer stretches of sleep at night, and slightly shorter stretches during the day: his tummy has got bigger and his awareness of night and day is kicking in.

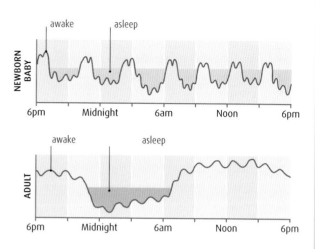

Amounts of sleep A newborn baby spends on average 16 hours asleep each day (this can range from 12 to 20 hours). The average adult requires half this amount of sleep.

AVERAGE SLEEP BY AGE

While each baby has different needs, the following is a rough guide to what you can expect for your baby's sleep over the first three months of life:

NEWBORN	ONE MONTH	TWO MONTHS	THREE MONTHS
As a new baby: he sleeps around 14–18 hours in every 24, with around 7½ hours in the day, and 8½ hours at night. **In the daytime** sleep is divided into 3-4 periods of sleep. **In the night-time** your baby will wake up every two to three hours for a feed.	**At one month:** your baby sleeps around 15½ hours in every 24, with around 6-7 hours of sleep in the day, and 8½ hours sleep at night. **In the daytime** sleep is divided into around three nap times. **In the night-time** your baby will still wake around two to three times.	**At two months** your baby will sleep around 15½ hours in every 24, with around 5½ hours sleep in the day, and around 10 hours at night. **In the daytime** sleep is divided into around three nap times. **In the night-time** your baby may manage slightly longer periods of sleep.	**At three months:** your baby will sleep around 15 hours in every 24 hours, with around 5 hours in the day. **In the daytime** sleep is divided into 3 nap times. **In the night-time** your baby may sleep for around 10 hours, with perhaps just one or two night-time feeds.

Q Where is the best place for my baby to sleep? Should I put him in a cot?

In the first six months of life, it's recommended that the safest place for your baby to sleep is in a Moses basket, crib, or cot in a room with you during the night-time and for daytime naps. Keeping your baby nearby means you will be aware quickly of his needs, and he will feel comforted to be close to you. If you wish, you can place your baby in a cot from the outset. However, a full-sized cot can be too big for a newborn baby, and he may be more comfortable in a Moses basket or crib for the first few weeks. It mimics the feeling of being cocooned in the womb, and is portable. You may find that at

around two months, your baby is looking a bit cramped in his Moses basket. He should be able to sleep with his arms out to the side, or flung up by his head, without touching the side or top of the basket.

Q Can I co-sleep with my newborn baby? What are the risks?

Sharing a bed with your new baby can feel like the most natural thing in the world. If you are breastfeeding, being in the same sleeping space means you can feed your baby as soon as he stirs, minimizing sleep disruption. Some studies also suggest that co-sleeping could actually help

to regulate babies' breathing, and that generally the sleep patterns of mother and baby become more synchronized. The mother may be more responsive to the baby's needs. Your baby is also likely to feel very secure being so close to you, and may settle back down to sleep more easily. However, experts believe that you shouldn't co-sleep with a baby under three months old, and the general advice is to avoid this practice if your baby was premature or was a low birth weight. If you do decide to co-sleep, be aware of the risks. There shouldn't be a duvet or pillow anywhere near your baby, and you should never co-sleep if you have been drinking, smoking, have taken drugs, or taken medication that makes you sleep very deeply and slows down your reaction time.

Q How many daytime naps should my baby have? Will it prevent him sleeping at night?

In general, you should be aiming to let your baby have three naps during the day to ensure he does not get overtired. He will probably get himself into a pattern of having a nap in the morning shortly after he has woken up and fed, another nap over lunch-time, and then a third nap late afternoon. The third nap should not be too close to bedtime or he might struggle to fall asleep later on. It is also important to make sure he does not sleep too much during the day, as this can affect the quality of his night-time sleep. As he grows, he will start dropping his naps, usually the late afternoon nap goes first.

Q What is a good bedtime routine for my young baby and is it too early to try to establish one?

After six weeks, as part of helping him learn the difference between day and night, it can be helpful to set up a regular bedtime routine. Following the same steps every bedtime means your baby will become familiar with the routine, and in turn associate the process with bedtime. If you follow the same pattern every night, your baby will feel safe and secure, and learn to differentiate between daytime naps and bedtime. A relaxing bath, followed by a long feed, and a story will help your baby unwind. Even if you just point out the pictures, your baby will love hearing your voice and having

your undivided attention on him. If your baby is really tired, a bath will revive him to allow him to have a good feed before bed. Many parents find this a special time of day when they share a quiet cuddle with their baby.

> Night-lights can **trick your baby's** brain into perceiving daylight and staying awake. Try using a **red light bulb** instead (which our brains don't see as daylight) to find your way during night feeds.

Q What is SIDS and how can I prevent it? Are there any key risk factors?

There are several steps you can take to keep your baby safe while he sleeps. Most important is that you are always in the same room as your baby while he is asleep.

Very rarely, a baby dies in his sleep, known as Sudden Infant Death syndrome (SIDS), or cot death. While the causes still aren't completely understood, there are a number of factors that have been shown to increase the risk of SIDS significantly, and the greatest risk occurs in the first six months of life. Low birth weight and premature babies, as well as male infants, are also more at risk.

PRECAUTIONS AND PREVENTION

The following will help to ensure that your baby sleeps safely:

» **Put your baby down** to sleep on his back with his feet at the very end of his cot ("feet to foot") so that he can't wriggle down under bedclothes.

» **For the first six months,** it is safer to put your baby to sleep in a cot or Moses basket, in the same room as you.

» **Avoid pillows,** baby duvets, and soft toys in the cot for at least the first year.

» **Keep the room temperature** where your baby sleeps around 16–20°C (60–68°F).

» **Don't smoke** near your baby, or allow anyone else to. Never sleep in the same bed as your baby if you have smoked, drunk alcohol, or taken drugs or medication that makes you drowsy.

» **If possible, breastfeed** your baby. There is a lower incidence of SIDS in breastfed babies.

» **Never sleep on a sofa or chair** with your baby.

» **Using a dummy** (after one month if you're breastfeeding) may reduce the risk of SIDS.

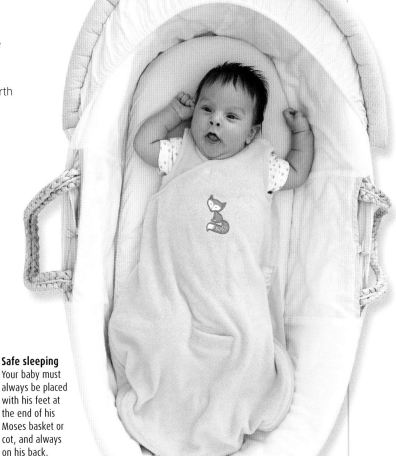

Safe sleeping
Your baby must always be placed with his feet at the end of his Moses basket or cot, and always on his back.

{Q How can I interact and play with my new baby? She's too young to do very much!

Your baby may seem to do little but feed and sleep in the first few weeks of life – she is very busy growing after all – but she is also primed for interaction and discovery. Play and stimulation are essential for your baby's development, helping her to learn about her world, about you, and how she fits in to this new place.

Early learning

You are your baby's first playmate – your play and responses guide your baby and give her the confidence to try new things. In the early months, your baby interacts with you and her surroundings in simple ways: looking, cooing and gurgling, making facial expressions, touching, and grasping. By providing stimulation suitable to her age and stage, you enable your baby to practise and learn new skills that will take her forward to the next stage of development. You can dedicate some one-on-one time to playing, perhaps five minutes playing peek-a-boo, 10 minutes settling down to explore a book with fun textures, or a few moments showing her a new object or toy. Equally, much of your interaction will be weaved into the fabric of your day: chatting during a nappy change, pointing out objects around the home, or spontaneously blowing a raspberry on her tummy as you dress her. Each interaction is intrinsically valuable.

Playmate and teacher Even small interactions, such as gazing into your baby's eyes, mimicking her facial expressions, and beaming back when she smiles, create new connections in her brain and increase her understanding of the world.

HOW YOUR BABY DEVELOPS

Being aware of your baby's pattern of development in these early months can also help you to target play to enhance her development, and ensure that you aren't frustrating her with activities beyond her capabilities.

 ## Physical skills

Your baby will need some time to learn control of her limbs. Her movements are uncoordinated in the early weeks; she is slowly unfurling and stretching her limbs after being curled up in your uterus. As her muscles strengthen, however, you can provide opportunities for her to practise moving her limbs and body.

» **Place your baby on her back** to allow her to get used to moving her limbs around, waving her arms, and kicking her legs. This gentle exercise will develop and strengthen her muscles.

» **Join your little one on the floor** and talk to her about what she is doing, or place her under a play gym so she can swoosh and bat at the dangling objects.

» **Put your baby on her tummy,** when she is a little stronger. As your baby gets older, she is likely to become increasingly excited and to kick and wave enthusiastically. A few moments of "tummy time" each day will help to strengthen her back and neck muscles, and will set her on the path to rolling and crawling.

» **Give your baby an incentive to reach out** once her strength and coordination grows. Place your baby on her tummy on the floor with a colourful toy just in front of her so she can practise reaching out. Always supervise tummy time when your baby is very young, and don't leave her on her tummy if she becomes frustrated.

 ## Social and cognitive skills

Reading, singing, and chatting to your baby all help develop her language skills. Your first "conversations" – responding to your baby's coos and gurgles with ones of your own – enable her to watch the shapes your mouth makes, learn about sounds, and copy the noises you make. These interactions also teach important social skills: how conversations involve turn-taking and listening.

 ## Your baby's senses

Stimulating your baby's senses is incredibly important in these early months. Your baby learns about the world around her through touch, and also derives comfort from cuddles, caresses, and skin-to-skin contact. Although she can focus her eyes only a short distance at birth, she will soon be taking in everything she sees.

» **Provide a feast for your baby's eyes** with bold patterns, mirrors, and bright objects.

» **Fabric books** with different textures help teach concepts such as smooth and bumpy, soft and hard, furry and crinkly.

» **Talk about and identify textures** and point out contrasts in everyday objects.

» **Comment on different noises** that you can hear inside the house or outside, and talk about the aromas in the kitchen.

 ## Outdoor Exploration

Day trips out with your baby can keep you both feeling fresh. A walk to the shops, a longer trip to the park, or just some time in the garden all provide a change of environment and new stimulation for your baby. Talk to her about the sights and sounds outside: look at the leaves blowing in the breeze, at the pattern of clouds or shadows on the ground, and at the buses, trains, and planes passing by.

WHEN YOUR BABY HAS HAD ENOUGH

Rest time Even low-key family visits can feel full-on for a baby, especially if she's passed around.

Each day your baby is absorbing and enjoying new sights, sounds, and information, but she also tires easily. If she doesn't have an opportunity for some downtime, she can feel overwhelmed by too many new noises, activities, and sensations.

Try to plan your baby's day so that there are times when activities are downscaled, and be alert to signs that your baby has had enough. Symptoms of over-stimulation and tiredness include:
» Becoming fussy and cranky.
» Turning her head away from you and from toys and activities.
» Appearing withdrawn.

If your young baby has been awake for around two hours, she probably needs to be put down for a nap. Or she may just benefit from some quiet time in her cot, or being cradled in your arms.

Q My baby isn't her usual self, but there's nothing specific I can put my finger on. Should I call the GP?

As a new parent, it can be hard to judge when your baby needs medical attention, or whether you are overreacting to a harmless sniffle.

Perhaps your baby hasn't been feeding well for a couple of days, or isn't quite as alert as usual. As young babies often don't show many symptoms when they are ill, sometimes it can be hard to tell whether a baby is just a little under the weather or if there is something a bit more serious going on. For this reason, it's always best to listen to your voice of doubt and trust your instincts and get her checked over by your doctor. The chances are that there is nothing seriously wrong, but doctors are always happy to see young babies – and often prioritize them – and would rather that you erred on the side of caution. For example, a slight fever is usually nothing to worry about in an older child, but a fever is relatively unusual in a baby under three months old, and is sometimes the only sign of a more serious infection, so it's vital not to ignore it. Because a baby's immune system is still immature, they can be more susceptible to a secondary bacterial infection, and can deteriorate quite quickly. It's most likely that your doctor will be able to put your mind at rest, but he or she will also reassure you that you did the right thing by making an appointment.

Keeping calm Try to stay calm as your baby will respond to how you are acting and will pick up on any stress.

Q Which symptoms always require medical attention?

There are certain symptoms and signs that should not be ignored and that should be dealt with quickly. Some signs (see bottom) need urgent attention.

SIGNS OF A SERIOUS ILLNESS

The following signs could signal that your baby has an illness and needs to see a GP. Do not hesitate to call and make an appointment if you notice:

» **Behavioural changes** are often the first sign that something isn't right. If your baby is lethargic, drowsy, hard to rouse for feeds, or persistently irritable for no reason, this may indicate that she isn't feeling well.

» **Changes in crying patterns** or sounds, for example a lack of crying or unusual high-pitched cries.

» **Changes in feeding patterns** and feeding poorly, or if your baby refuses several feeds in a row.

» **Severe vomiting or diarrhoea** that lasts for longer than 12 hours (see p.295), or that is streaked with blood or mucus should be assessed.

» **Signs of an eye infection,** or a discharge from the eyes.

» **Your baby isn't responding to sounds** or has a discharge from the ears.

» **A temperature of 38°C** (100.4°F) or more if she is under three months old; or of 39°C (102.2°F) or more if she is under six months old.

» **A sunken or bulging fontanelle,** the soft spot on your baby's head should be checked. Usually, this should be firm to the touch and may dip in a little. When your baby cries, lies down, or is sick, the fontanelle can bulge, but it should return to normal when your baby is upright and calm.

» **An unexplained rash,** especially if it accompanies a fever or diarrhoea.

» **Signs of dehydration** (see p.294).

» **Signs of constipation,** such as hard, small stools, with fewer bowel movements than usual.

 ## CALL AN AMBULANCE

You should always call an ambulance if you notice that your baby is displaying any of these symptoms:

» **Stops breathing** or is struggling for breath.

» **Is unconscious** or unaware of what's going on.

» **A seizure,** even if she recovers.

» **One or more symptoms** of meningitis (see p.295).

 ## GO TO ACCIDENT & EMERGENCY

Go straight to Accident & Emergency if you spot your baby showing any of the symptoms and issues listed below:

» **Has a fever and is persistently lethargic,** despite taking medication.

» **Is having difficulty breathing,** including fast or panting breathing, or is very wheezy.

» **Has severe abdominal pain.**

» **Has a cut that won't stop bleeding** or is gaping open.

» **Has a serious fall or bump to the head.**

» **Is turning blue.**

Did you know...

When looking after an ill baby it's important that you keep her fluids up, keep informed (know the signs and symptoms), let go of routines, don't overdress her, keep her room draught-free (but not too stuffy or warm), and remain calm so as not to alarm her.

Q What might I need to ask or tell the doctor?

To make the most out of the possibly limited time you have with your GP, think about the information your doctor might need to know, and have questions at the ready. Taking a notepad and pen means you can have questions written down so that you don't forget to ask anything, which is easily done when you're busy listening to what the doctor has to say.

Jot down any instructions or suggestions your doctor gives you for caring for your baby at home. Be ready to give your doctor information about your baby's symptoms and when they started; about whether your baby has been feeding well and has had wet nappies; and about changes in your baby's temperature, and the time you checked her temperature. If you have given your baby any medicine, let your doctor know what you have given, how much, and when. Have your baby's immunization history at the ready.

Q What are the signs of a fever and how should I treat it?

If your baby looks unusually flushed, her skin is clammy and sweaty, and if her forehead, the back or her neck or her tummy feel hot to touch, she may have a raised temperature that needs checking (see p.292). Your baby may also be cranky and drowsier than usual.

Most babies and infants work through a fever in a matter of days. If your doctor has seen your baby and is happy for her to be cared for at home, continue to monitor her for as long as she isn't her normal self. Keep her fluid intake up and be on the look out for signs of dehydration, such as fewer wet nappies than normal or a sunken fontanelle (see p.294). Once your baby starts to rally, don't launch straight back into normal activities

– your little one may still be tired and need a bit of time to get back to her normal self. Having said that, babies often bounce back surprisingly quickly from minor illnesses. If at any point she deteriorates, perhaps becoming drowsier or clearly dehydrated, or if she develops a rash, or you just feel concerned, listen to your instincts and go straight back to the doctor, or to the hospital if you are very worried.

HOW TO TREAT A FEVER

Follow these methods to help reduce your baby's temperature. You can also talk to your baby soothingly and reassure her that you're there to help.

» **While the first port of call** is to get medical advice when your young baby has a fever, you also need to ensure that she doesn't become dehydrated. A fever makes your baby sweat more, so she loses water as it evaporates on the skin. Keep topping up her fluids with frequent breast or formula feeds, and for formula-fed babies, give top-ups of water (fresh water that has been boiled and cooled).

» **Make sure** that your baby's environment isn't too hot – it should be around 18°C (64°F).

» **If your baby is distressed** by the fever, is over two months old, and weighs at least 4kg (9lbs), you can give the recommended dose of infant paracetamol – and if she is over three months old and weighs more than 5kg (11lbs), she can have a recommended dose of infant ibuprofen. If she doesn't seem to be responding to one medicine, you can try the other. They can be spaced out, or given one after the other if the fever isn't calming down.

» **There is no need** to sponge your baby with tepid water, or remove layers of clothes – check, though, that your baby isn't uncomfortably hot with too many layers of clothing. You can strip her down to her nappy if she is incredibly hot.

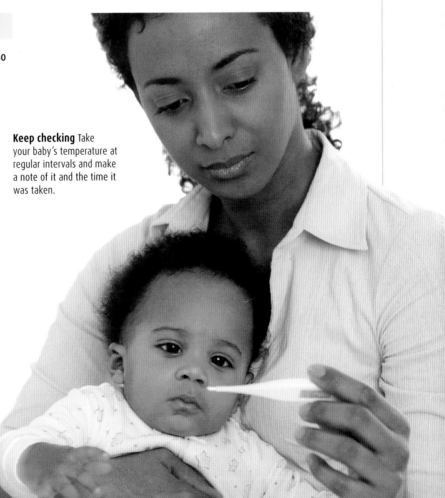

Keep checking Take your baby's temperature at regular intervals and make a note of it and the time it was taken.

Q How do I take my baby's temperature, and what is a normal reading?

A normal temperature for your baby is around 37°C (98.6°F), with slight variations being usual between children.

If your baby's temperature is higher than 37.5°C (99.5°F), then she has a fever. If your baby is under three months and her temperature reaches 38°C (100.4°F) or higher, or she is under six months with a temperature of 39°C (102.2°F) or more, then consult a doctor straight away.

Is a fever always a concern?

In babies over six months and toddlers and children, a fever in itself isn't such a great concern, and other signs of illness are used to gauge a child's wellbeing. In older infants, a raised temperature is actually a positive sign that her body is fighting off an infection, as it is harder for bacteria and viruses to survive in a hot environment.

Fevers in young babies are less common, and because with young babies it can be harder to spot other signs of illness, or to tell if there is a potentially serious underlying infection, a raised temperature should always be taken more seriously as it may be the only clear sign that something is wrong. You should therefore consult your doctor straight away or go to the accident and emergency department if your young baby has a high temperature and you can't contact your doctor.

TAKING YOUR BABY'S TEMPERATURE

While you may be able to gauge if your baby has a fever by looking at or touching her, taking her temperature lets you know exactly what her temperature is, which is important in young babies. There are several types of thermometer you can use.

THERMOMETER TYPE	DESCRIPTION	
Strip thermometer	Very convenient and easy to use, especially if your baby is fidgety, you simply hold the strip on your baby's forehead. However, they are not very accurate as they measure skin, rather than body, temperature.	**STRIP THERMOMETER**
Digital underarm thermometer	These are cheap and fairly accurate. Place the bulb of the thermometer under your baby's arm in her armpit, then gently hold her arm alongside her body. You need to hold the thermometer in the armpit for a set amount of time - some beep when they are ready to read. Often the trickiest part of taking a baby's temperature with this type of thermometer is getting her to stay still. Hold and soothe her before you start, and talk to her calmly while you take her temperature. Never place a thermometer in the mouth of a child under five years of age.	**DIGITAL UNDERARM THERMOMETER**
Digital ear thermometer	Although more expensive, these take a reading quickly. However, if they aren't placed correctly, they may not be that accurate.	**DIGITAL EAR THERMOMETER**

In the US, young children and babies with a high temperature account for around **20 per cent** of the admissions to the children's emergency department at hospital.

Q Can a high temperature increase my baby's risk of having a seizure?

Yes, febrile seizures or fits are brought on when a baby or child has a raised temperature. However, although they can look alarming, they are usually harmless. Seizures most often occur between six months and three years of age, and are fairly unusual in babies younger than six months old. During a seizure, a baby or child may become stiff, and may lose consciousness and shake her limbs. If your baby has a seizure, hold her on her side and remove anything from her mouth that she could choke on, such as a dummy. Make sure her head is turned to the side so that she doesn't choke if she is sick. Stay with her, and time how long the fit lasts. A baby who has had a first fit should always be checked by a doctor at hospital. If your baby has had a fit before and a subsequent one lasts longer than five minutes, she should be checked by a doctor, and if a subsequent fit lasts less than five minutes, call your doctor for advice.

Q How do I give medicine to a wriggling baby?

Getting a baby to take medicine or tolerate drops being put in her eye can be one of the most exasperating tasks for parents. As far as possible, try to stay calm.

Your baby's distress coupled with your concern about helping her to get better means that it is easy for both of you to end up in a tight ball of stress. Even if you don't feel calm, try to sound reassuring and be matter of fact. Time medicine for when your baby is most receptive, perhaps after a cuddle, or before a feed, when she's a little hungry and happy to swallow something.

ADMINISTERING MEDICINE AND DROPS

Before you give medicine or drops, always check that they haven't passed their use-by date, and after using, store the medicine or drops as recommended by the manufacturer or pharmacist.

>> **Giving oral medicines:** these can be given via the syringe or dosage spoon provided by the manufacturer. For a very young baby, a syringe can be the easiest way to get the medicine into her mouth as the contents are less likely to be spilled. Also, up until about four months, your baby has a thrust reflex, which means she automatically pushes things out of her mouth, so it's easier to use a syringe. Draw up the correct dosage of medicine into the syringe. Hold your baby close to you in an upright position, and, if it helps, stroke her cheek to encourage her to open her mouth, then place the syringe in your baby's mouth. Let your baby suck on the syringe if she seems willing to do so, or squirt the contents slowly, or a little at a time, into the side, rather than the back, of her mouth, so she doesn't choke. If you use a spoon, gently tip the medicine into the mouth, giving small amounts at a time if this works best.

>> **Administering eye drops:** if possible, get someone else to help you do this, with one of you holding your baby while the other gives the drops. You may also find wrapping your baby in a blanket helpful, if this doesn't distress her, so that she isn't able to thrash her arms and legs around. Wash your hands. With your baby laid flat or in a reclined position, gently pull down the lower eyelid, then squeeze one drop into the lower lid, taking care not to touch any part of the eye with the dropper. Once you let go of the lid, your baby should blink, which helps to disperse the drop. If your baby won't allow you to pull down her lid, place the drop on to the side of the closed eye nearest the nose. Although not as effective, some of the fluid will hopefully make its way into the eye once open.

>> **Administering saline nose drops:** your doctor or pharmacist may recommend these if a blocked nose is interfering with your baby's feeding or breathing. Wash your hands. As with eye drops, recruit a helper if possible. Wipe away any mucus. With your baby lying flat, place the dropper just inside the nostril and squeeze the right amount of drops into the nostril. Try to hold your baby in this position for a minute or so to help the drops spread through the nose.

>> **Giving ear drops:** the sensation of liquid going into her ear may upset your baby and she may wriggle, so wrapping her in a blanket can help to keep her still while you give her the drops. Wash your hands. Lay your baby down and try to tilt her head to one side. Gently pull the ear lobe down to open up the ear canal, then squeeze the correct number of drops into the ear. Keep her in this position for a couple of minutes so that the drops can work their way into the ear.

Administering eye drops Do this as swiftly and calmly as possible, talking to your baby constantly during the procedure to reassure her.

Q Did you know...

Breastfed babies have a lower incidence of infections and illnesses during the first year of life, including gastrointestinal infections that lead to diarrhoea and vomiting, respiratory tract infections, and recurrent ear infections. Studies also show that when breastfed babies do catch an infection, this is likely to be less severe than in infants who aren't breastfed. For example, breastfed babies are far less likely than formula-fed babies to be hospitalized for respiratory illnesses.

Q How can I help protect my baby from catching bugs?

Infections are inevitable in babies and young children as their immune system builds up its resistance over time. However, there are a few things you can do to limit the number of infections your little one picks up. Breastfeeding for as long as possible is one of the best ways to keep your baby well, as your milk passes on protective antibodies. When your baby is very young, it's also worth limiting, or avoiding, contact with people with colds and bugs. At two months, she'll be offered her first vaccinations, so keeping up with her immunization programme from this point protects her against a range of serious infections.

Q How can I best comfort and care for my baby while she is ill?

Caring for a sick baby is a new experience for many parents, and understandably, anxiety can take hold. Bear in mind that your comforting presence is an important factor in keeping her calm, which in turn helps her body fight illness. Your baby feels less secure when she is ill, so staying close by, giving plenty of cuddles, and talking soothingly will all help reassure her.

While young babies can go downhill quite rapidly, with the right attention they usually recover quickly, too. Knowing what to look out for, when to seek medical help, or when to tend to her at home, gives you the confidence that you're equipped to give her the right care.

{Q} How can I identify common illnesses and complaints?

Often it's clear when your baby is unwell – he may be irritable, off his feeds, and lethargic. A fever is a clear sign that he is fighting infection (see p.291), and a snuffly nose and cough are easy to spot, as are tummy upsets. Other signs are less obvious: perhaps your baby is clingier than usual or isn't feeding well. Trust your instincts: if you think something isn't quite right, call your doctor.

☾ Dehydration

» Symptoms:

Fewer wet nappies than usual, dark yellow urine, hard stools, and constipation are all signs of dehydration. Other signs include lethargy, crying without producing tears; a dry, sticky mouth; and/or a sunken fontanelle (the soft spot on his head).

» What you should do:

If your baby is suffering with vomiting, diarrhoea, or has a temperature (see p.292), try to keep up his fluid intake to prevent dehydration occurring in the first place. Offer frequent breast or formula feeds (you may need to give small feeds more often). Offer oral rehydration solution (available from pharmacies) between feeds; cooled, boiled water may be given instead if your baby refuses the solution. If your baby has any of the above symptoms of dehydration, contact your doctor.

Frequent breast feeds Feeding your baby often ensures that his fluid levels are maintained.

☾ Cradle cap

» Symptoms:

Scaly patches on the scalp that may be thick and crusty. These may be caused by overactive sebaceous glands in the first months, which then settle down. Cradle cap is usually harmless and doesn't cause itchiness or discomfort.

» What you should do:

Cradle cap typically clears up within weeks or months, and can usually be managed at home. For mild cradle cap, wash your baby's hair regularly with a baby shampoo to prevent scales building up, and use a baby brush to loosen flakes. Massaging a little olive oil into the head and leaving this overnight softens the scales before brushing in the morning. Don't pick the scales as this could damage skin and cause an infection. If cradle cap is persistent, ask your pharmacist about stronger shampoos to loosen cradle cap. If patches spread to the face or body, self-help measures don't work, or there's bleeding or inflammation, consult your doctor.

☾ Eczema

» Symptoms:

Red, dry, and itchy skin on the face, and in areas where the skin creases, such as the elbows, knees, and in the neck. The condition often starts in babies between two and four months old and may be connected to an allergy to milk.

» What you should do:

Talk to your doctor about managing your baby's eczema. He or she can advise you on treatments such as emollient moisturizing creams, and may prescribe a topical corticosteroid. Scratch mittens can stop your baby damaging his skin further, and keep your baby's nails short. Avoid bath products if your baby has a flare up, and use non-biological washing detergent for your baby's clothes. If the eczema is stubborn and sore, talk to your doctor about other remedies, such as wet wraps, which can help the skin to heal.

☾ Thrush

» Symptoms:

If your baby has oral thrush, a condition caused by the yeast fungus *Candida albicans*, he may have a white coating on his tongue and white patches around the mouth with a curd-like texture. These don't rub off easily and, if sore, can interfere with feeding. Your baby may also have a nappy rash caused by the same infection. If you are breastfeeding, the infection can be passed between you and your baby and can make your nipples sore and painful.

» What you should do:

Make an appointment with your doctor. While the condition isn't usually serious, he or she may prescribe an antifungal medicine or gel for your baby. If you're breastfeeding, your doctor may prescribe an antifungal cream for your nipples.

☾ Conjunctivitis

» Symptoms:

This eye infection causes an inflammation of the thin membrane (conjunctiva) covering the white of the eye. The eye is red, inflamed, itchy, sticky, and watery, and there may be a discharge. The eye may be crusted over after sleep. It is caused either by an infection, or an allergy or irritant, such as cigarette smoke. In newborns, conjunctivitis may be contracted from bacteria in the birth canal.

» What you should do:

Use cotton wool soaked in cooled boiled water to remove the crust and goo from your baby's eye, using a separate piece of cotton wool for each eye so you don't pass infection between them. Wash your hands after touching your baby and use a separate towel to stop the infection spreading to others. If your baby is under 28 days old, or the infection is severe or doesn't clear after a week or so, contact your doctor as your baby may have a bacterial infection that needs treating with eye drops.

Diarrhoea and vomiting

» Symptoms:

Watery, loose stools, that may be mucus-stained and smelly, indicate diarrhoea. Vomiting is when your baby brings up a sizeable quantity of milk (rather than a few teaspoons' worth). Causes include gastroenteritis, reflux, and allergy.

» What you should do:

Replace the fluids your baby is losing to prevent dehydration. Offer frequent breast or formula feeds; give oral rehydration solution in addition, or cooled, boiled water if your baby refuses the solution. Consult your doctor if your baby has had diarrhoea six or more times, or has vomited three or more times, in the last 24 hours. Consult your doctor too if your baby also has a rash, fever, signs of dehydration, or blood in his vomit or stool.

Reflux

» Symptoms:

Frequent regurgitation of milk and stomach acid. (Some spitting up is normal – the muscular valve that closes the stomach doesn't fully develop until 12–18 months of age.)

» What you should do:

Feed in smaller amounts more frequently, and burp often. Avoid overfeeding; for bottle-fed babies, try a teat with a smaller hole. Hold your baby upright after feeding to ease reflux. See your doctor if your baby has frequent reflux with coughing, gagging, persistent crying, or poor weight gain.

Colds and flu

» Symptoms:

A runny nose, a cough, red eyes, and sometimes a raised temperature. Cold symptoms combined with a sudden fever of 38°C (100.4°F) or more may indicate flu. Other signs of flu are lethargy, lack of appetite, vomiting, and diarrhoea.

» What you should do:

If your baby is under three months of age, call your doctor. Meanwhile, make sure your baby gets plenty of fluids (see Dehydration, left). If your baby has a blocked nose and feeding is difficult, try raising the humidity levels to loosen his mucus: place a bowl of warm water in the room or sit in a steamy room. You can buy saline nasal drops to help thin the mucus from pharmacies. Your baby will also need to sleep more while he is recovering from a cold.

Ear infections

» Symptoms:

It can be hard to tell if a baby has an ear infection, but if he rubs or tugs on his ear, is irritable, off his feeds, vomits, doesn't respond to quieter noises, and has a temperature a few days after the onset of a cold, he may have an ear infection. Pus may appear if the eardrum is damaged.

» What you should do:

Ear infections usually clear up in around three days without treatment. If your baby is under three months old and has a temperature of 38°C (100.4°F) or more, or is under six months old with a temperature of 39°C (102.2°F), consult your doctor. Your doctor may give antibiotics if your baby is under three months of age. A warm flannel placed over the ear can be soothing. Repeated infections may be treated with grommets – tiny tubes inserted into the ear to drain fluid.

Bronchiolitis

» Symptoms:

Symptoms are similar to a cold with a fever. They may worsen after a few days and include a dry, rasping cough, noisy or fast breathing, brief pauses between breaths, vomiting, feeding less, and having fewer wet nappies.

» What you should do:

Symptoms usually clear in a couple of weeks. If your baby is under three months and has a temperature of 38°C (100.4°F) or more, or is under six months with a temperature of 39°C (102.2°F), consult your doctor. Keep your baby hydrated, and upright as much as possible to ease congestion. An air humidifier, or bowl of warm water in a room keeps the air moist. Call your doctor (or an ambulance if you're very concerned) if your baby is having difficulty breathing, is breathing rapidly, isn't feeding well and hasn't had a wet nappy in the last 12 hours, or is unresponsive or is irritable.

Croup

» Symptoms:

Difficulty in breathing and a distinctive barking cough. Croup most commonly affects children aged between six months and three years, but can occur in younger babies.

» What you should do:

Mild croup can be managed at home. Keep your baby hydrated, hold him upright to ease breathing, and comfort him, as crying worsens symptoms. Your doctor may prescribe an oral corticosteroid to reduce swelling in the throat.

Whooping cough (pertussis)

» Symptoms:

A dry, persistent cough with prolonged bouts of coughing, interspersed with gasps for air. There may be a runny nose, fever, and vomiting. Coughing may last for months.

» What you should do:

Get a vaccination against the virus between 28 and 38 weeks of pregnancy to protect your baby at birth, and have your baby vaccinated at two months of age. If your baby has symptoms, consult your doctor at once, who may give antibiotics. If he has trouble breathing, call an ambulance.

Meningitis

» Symptoms in babies:

Meningitis is a viral or bacterial infection of the membranes surrounding the brain and spinal cord. Symptoms include a bulging fontanelle; a fever with cold hands and feet (although young babies may have a normal or low temperature); sleepiness; rapid breathing; grunting; a high-pitched or moaning cry; shivering; stiffness and jerking or floppiness; irritability from muscle aches – perhaps not wanting to be picked up; diarrhoea and vomiting; a stiff neck; dislike of bright lights; blotchy skin; and convulsions or seizures. A purple "pin prick" rash or purple bruises that don't disappear under a pressed glass, may indicate blood poisoning – a medical emergency. Symptoms can occur in any order.

» What you should do:

Don't wait for a rash to appear before getting help. If you suspect meningitis, call an ambulance immediately and say that you suspect meningitis.

The glass test A rash that doesn't disappear under a pressed glass indicates blood poisoning.

Life with your **new baby** is full of novel experiences, intense emotions, and **positive changes**. It also brings with it many new **responsibilities** and considerations, and you will find that you need to **plan ahead** far more than you did in the past.

Planning for the future

Thinking ahead to work

One of the main considerations when taking time off with your baby is when, or if, you plan to return to work after the birth. You may have already set a date with your employer, though you might change your mind about this date once you are on leave – perhaps wanting to return earlier for financial reasons, or to take an extended period of time off. In the UK, most employed women can take up to 52 weeks maternity leave, some of which will be unpaid (see pp.110–11). Individual employers may have their own terms and offers, so discuss these with yours. If you are planning a return to work, getting organized early on with childcare means you can relax and enjoy your precious time with your baby.

A growing family

After a certain period of time, and once you feel settled with your new family unit, you and your partner might start to think about adding a new addition to the family, providing a sibling for your baby. There are so many reasons for and against different age gaps between siblings, and you may feel that some of these are worth considering. Essentially, though, if you and your partner feel ready emotionally, physically, and financially for this step, then the time could be right to try for a new baby. Keep discussions open with your partner so that you are aware of each other's feelings and expectations, and any differences of opinion can be talked through.

Changes to the home

Now you are three, it's natural to re-evaluate your home setup and consider how well this works for your new family unit. Perhaps you are thinking about a move to a new area where you can get a larger home for your money, which is something many parents consider in the preschool years. Or if a move isn't on the agenda, you might think about changes that can be made to your existing home. Bear in mind that your child will feel happy wherever she is as long as she is surrounded by love and has good care, so don't feel you have to make changes to your home if it is likely that these are going to be stressful or financially challenging.

Q What things could I be putting in place now that will benefit my child's future?

There are a number of issues that may not have worried you too much until you had a baby and became a responsible parent. The issues discussed below are worth considering and prioritizing.

While many of these are financial, such as whether you want to start a savings account for private schooling or university, some are practical, such as leaving a will and assigning guardians to your new child should anything happens to you and your partner. You may also like to consider "legacy" issues such as family stories, letters, heirlooms, and cultural matters (particularly if there are varied nationalities in the family) you would like your child to read or know about in the future. Here is a checklist for some of the things you may want to put in place.

PLANNING FOR THE FUTURE

| SAVINGS ACCOUNTS AND FUNDS | INSURANCE | WILLS AND GUARDIANSHIP | PENSIONS AND RETIREMENT |

Whether starting to save now for her future education or first home, or a trust to safeguard your child from having to pay large tax bills in the future, you may like to consider setting up a bank account now.

Look at life and health insurance as you may want to increase your plans now that a child is in the picture, so you are financially covered should something happen to you or your partner. If you have private health or dental plans, you should add the name of your baby.

Set up a will to avoid leaving the fate of your child's guardianship and your assets in the court's hands. Assign a guardian who would be able to step in to raise your child, should the worst happen, and help her with her education, health, and keep her safe and looked after until she is an adult.

It may seem a long way off but you will want to ensure that there is sufficient money in the pot for you later in life, so that the burden of old age and what it may bring with it doesn't fall on your child.

Q We definitely want to try for another child. Is there an ideal age gap between siblings?

There are pros and cons for different age gaps, and your decision on when to try for another baby is likely to be influenced by how you both feel about managing family life. You may feel that having a second baby while your first child is still very young means that you will be able to deal with the full-on baby and toddler stages all in one go. Your children are likely to be natural playmates and develop a strong bond, and can be companions once at school. Also, if you are planning to have a big family you may not want to wait too long before you have a second child. Some suggest, though, that siblings very close in age may squabble more when competing for toys and attention. Conversely, you may want to wait until your first child is out of nappies before considering another baby,

so that you have more time to dedicate both to your first child's early years and then to the new baby. Physically, this may also be more appealing, giving your body plenty of time to recover from the birth of your first baby, so that you have more energy for the new arrival. Financially, a bigger age gap means you may not need to invest in items such as a double buggy or an additional cot, and you can spread the cost of childcare out over a longer period.

Q Healthwise, is there an optimal time to wait before getting pregnant again?

Both you, and your future baby, can benefit from having a suitable space between pregnancies. Pregnancy and breastfeeding can deplete your reserves of essential nutrients such as folate and iron, so giving your body

some time to build up these stores before you conceive again can benefit both your own and your unborn baby's health. Furthermore, recent studies have shown that women who gave birth again within 18 months of having a baby were considerably more likely to have a premature delivery than those who waited longer to get pregnant again. Waiting at least 12–18 months after having a baby before conceiving again is thought to eliminate the increased risk of premature birth.

There are **factors** other than age, such as **personality** and **gender**, that will determine how well or not your **children get on.**

Q I'm undecided about whether or not to return to work. What should I consider?

For many families, one of the deciding factors about returning to work is the financial situation and balancing salaries with the cost of childcare.

The most important thing is doing what is right for you and your partner. Both of you need to review your job circumstances, the long-term and short-term salary implications, and feelings about staying at home to make sure the appropriate person is the main carer. Whatever you decide, be prepared to be flexible. What you imagined might work for you when you were pregnant might not turn out to be the case once your baby arrives. Well-thought out plans can change, and you

may feel you want to take a bit more time off than planned, or that an earlier return will suit you. If you adore being at home, then it's likely that you will find this a fulfilling option. Your feelings may change later on. You may find that you are missing your work environment and that you are keen to pursue your career. If parents are happy and fulfilled, and you feel completely comfortable with your childcare of choice, then the whole family is likely to thrive.

DISCUSSION POINTS

If you have a choice between staying at home and going back to work it's a good idea to communicate with your partner and ask yourself a few key questions:

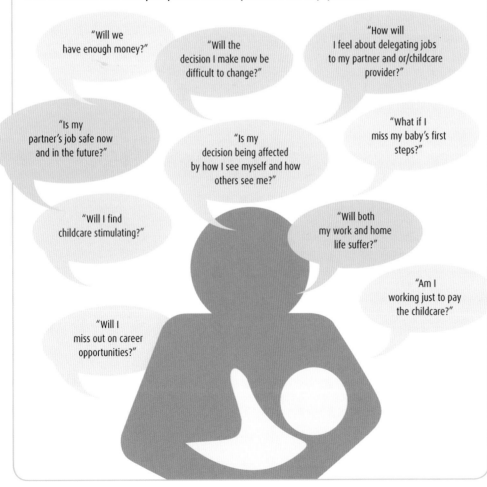

"Will we have enough money?"

"Will the decision I make now be difficult to change?"

"How will I feel about delegating jobs to my partner and or/childcare provider?"

"Is my partner's job safe now and in the future?"

"Is my decision being affected by how I see myself and how others see me?"

"What if I miss my baby's first steps?"

"Will I find childcare stimulating?"

"Will both my work and home life suffer?"

"Am I working just to pay the childcare?"

"Will I miss out on career opportunities?"

Q I will be returning to work when my baby is one year old. When do I need to start organizing childcare?

Though your return to work may seem a long way off, and handing your baby over to a carer is probably the last thing you want to think about at the start of your maternity leave, it is definitely worth looking into this now. You may have already given some thought at the end of pregnancy to the type of childcare you would favour – if not, start considering what you think would suit you as a family. What will your finances allow? Start making enquiries locally, look online, contact the Children's Information Service at your local council for lists of childminders and nurseries in your area, ask any local parents you know for recommendations, and chat to friends with older children, who will have some good advice.

Q My partner and I are thinking about dividing childcare between us and another carer. Is this a good idea?

If you are all on board and you are happy with your choice of childcare, this can be a good solution. Often, fathers can feel regretful that they aren't spending enough time with their child, and many find that taking over one or two days a week can be extremely fulfilling. For yourself, returning to work part-time allows you to achieve a satisfactory work/life balance, and your baby gets quality time with both parents. It is worth checking that you are all following a similar naptime and feeding routine, and that you agree on things like discipline and potty-training methods so that your baby doesn't become confused and unsure as to what's expected of him.

72%
of two-parent families and **60 per cent** of single mothers **are in work**, an increase of one-fifth since the mid 1990s.

Q How can I help my baby adjust to a new childcare arrangement?

Make sure that you have chosen a carer that you are happy with, so that you can be as relaxed as possible. Your baby will pick up on your anxieties.

Give your baby plenty of time to get used to the new person and routine and try to start the settling in process well before – preferably a few weeks – you go back to work. Babies are far more adaptable than we give them credit for and, with time and patience, can get used to any new arrangements. Initially, it is helpful for you and your baby to spend time with the new carer before introducing short periods of time when he is alone with the carer. Gradually build up the time he spends away from you with the carer so that by the time you go back to work you are all used to the situation and he is completely happy to be left.

Gentle hello Be as relaxed as possible when introducing your child to a new carer.

SETTLING IN TIPS

Here are a few pointers to make the transition easier for you and your child:

» **Keep calm:** however anxious you might feel about leaving your baby, try to be as relaxed as you can; your baby will pick up on any nerves. Think positive!

» **Home visit:** your baby probably feels more relaxed and confident in his own surroundings so it can be useful for a childminder, or member of staff from the nursery you are considering to visit you both at home in order for you both to get to know each other better.

» **Take a toy:** it can be helpful for your baby to have something familiar with him, such as a favourite toy or comforter.

» **Keep it brief:** try to make a clean break when you say goodbye to your baby, even if he cries. However upsetting this can be, if you go back to him repeatedly it may simply prolong his distress (and therefore yours). Most babies are easily distracted once you have gone. You could ask the carer to call you later to let you know he has settled down happily.

» **Communicate:** while this is a challenging new experience for you and your baby, your carer has probably been through this many times. Share any worries and concerns that you have. Your carer will want to listen and talk through how best to deal with any distress that you or your baby is experiencing. Remember that you are all working towards the same goal: a happy baby.

Q I'm worried about putting my baby into childcare. Will he miss me or will he love his carer more than me?

Be assured that your baby will benefit from forming new relationships with different adults who he will indeed form a strong bond with and grow to love – but this doesn't mean that he will love you any less. Leaving your precious baby with a carer can cause a whole range of emotions from guilt, to sadness, not to mention some relief that you have a little time to yourself. He will be thrilled to see you each time you go to collect him and you will cherish these moments. Your baby has more than enough love for you, his family, and his carers.

Q The future feels unknown, but very exciting! How should I cope with not knowing what lies ahead?

Parenting constantly presents new challenges, and just when you think you've got the hang of things, your child reaches a new developmental stage, and you need to catch up. Deciding the right work/life balance and choosing childcare are big decisions. At times, being a parent can seem terrifying – will you be able to do the very best for your child, and will he be happy and fulfilled? There aren't many things you can do in life that have such a profound effect on you as when you become a parent. However, the best way of coping is to try to be as organized as possible, to enjoy your child, and to be as flexible as you can. Things can and will change. Highs and lows can be intense (not helped by exhaustion in the early years), but mostly, becoming a parent is pretty exhilarating as you experience a totally new and heart-stopping kind of love, and feel a renewed sense of purpose.

> **The more people who care for your baby**, and that he forms lasting bonds with, **the more loving he will become himself.**

{Q What do I need to think about when choosing childcare?

Choosing a person or nursery to entrust with the care of your baby is a hugely important decision, and one that you will want to consider carefully. Think about your priorities, which things you consider important and what you want for your baby, and look for childcare that meets these requirements.

Personal choice

Talking to other parents can be useful, but bear in mind that the right childcare for one family may not suit another. So while getting personal recommendations can be invaluable, you may have quite different views. For example, while one family may think the social setting of a nursery is advantageous, you may prefer your child to be in a more homely environment. Aim to visit a few different types of settings rather than ruling anything out too early on. When you visit, watch how carers interact with your child and other children. Are they responsive and caring, is the environment clean and welcoming, are there plenty of planned activities and toys for the children, and is there dedicated down time? Do the children seem happy and relaxed, and is there outside space? Ask to see copies of any policies, procedures, or certificates – any reputable carers will be happy to share these. Consider speaking to some parents who currently have their child attending the setting.

DIFFERENT CHILDCARE OPTIONS

Here is some information on different settings and options for childcare. The logistics and prices vary so it is a good idea to do as much research as possible so that you make the right decision.

Nursery

The set-up: usually privately run, a nursery offers all-day childcare for young babies through to four to five years of age. Staff are trained in the Early Years Foundation Stage, and there are strict guidelines on ratios of staff to children. Babies and toddlers should have separate areas or rooms where the facilities are appropriate for their age.

 What to think about: your baby should get plenty of stimulation, and will have lots of other children to socialize with. One-to-one time may be seldom. The cost can be high, the opening hours are set, and there may be times when the nursery is shut. There will be an illness policy, so you will need a back-up plan if your child is unwell.

Childminder

The set-up: these are individuals who look after a small group of children in their own home. They should be registered with either Ofsted or a childminder agency. They can look after up to six children under eight years of age. Three can be under the age of five, and normally only one baby at a time can be cared for (exceptions can be made for siblings).

What to think about: your child will be in a home environment, will have a few other children to socialize with, and will receive plenty of attention. Childminders care for children for an extended period of time, which gives continuity, and your child is likely to form a close bond with them. If your childminder is unwell, you will need to have a back-up plan.

Nanny

The set-up: a qualified individual who will look after your child in your own home.

What to think about: your child will receive one-to-one care in her own home. Nannies can become a significant part of the family and can stay in touch for years to come. They may be more flexible, occasionally being available for babysitting or weekend care. Nannying is usually the most expensive childcare option, and you are the nanny's employer so will need to pay tax, National Insurance, and holiday pay. Some nannies ask for extras such as the use of a car. Your child will be on her own unless your nanny organizes meet-ups with other nannies and their charges.

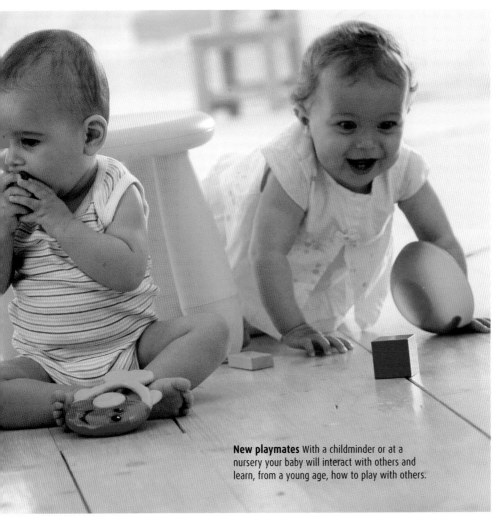

New playmates With a childminder or at a nursery your baby will interact with others and learn, from a young age, how to play with others.

 ## Family care

The set-up: grandparents, uncles, and aunts take on the responsibility of carer. This can also take on the form of shared care between the parents.

 What to think about: depending on whether you pay your relatives, this can be one of the more cost effective options and is particularly appropriate if the family members live close by. Your child will be looked after by those who love her and will be in a familiar environment. Care can also be divided between parents. In all instances of shared family care, it is vital to establish a consistent routine and rules of behaviour.

Au Pair

The set-up: these are generally young people who have come to the UK to improve their language skills and who live with you. They have their own room and receive board and lodging, as well as some money.

What to think about: they are classed as a member of the family and as such, live in your house, have meals with you, and accompany you on outings. In return they undertake household and childcare duties, but generally for not more than 30 hours per week. Many do not have any training or previous experience of childcare and you may not have the chance to meet them before they start.

QUESTIONS TO ASK

When visiting a nursery or meeting a carer, it is a good idea to note down a few questions beforehand. Here are some issues you might want to ask about:

» What will my child's daily routine be? Usually a childminder will be happy to adopt your baby's current routine or they might be able to suggest an alternative one. At a nursery as there are so many babies, they may encourage her to fit in with the others.

» What will my baby be fed and where will she sleep? A nursery will provide milk and nutritious food for your baby. You will need to let them know about about any allergies. All care providers should have a quiet room for babies to nap in.

» How will you keep me informed of my child's progress? Both childminders and nurseries should keep a developmental record of your child's progress. You should be able to have access to this at any time and it may be sent home to you so that you can review and add to it yourself.

» How do you deal with challenging behaviour? All children need boundaries to keep them safe, but make sure you are happy with how the potential carer disciplines children and ask to see their policy document.

» What is the sickness policy? Most childcare settings are happy to accept children with minor coughs and colds, but your child will need to go home and be kept off if she has a fever, sickness, or anything more serious. Ask to see the policy document regarding illness.

» What are your qualifications? It can be reassuring to know that the person caring for your baby is fully qualified, so do check that nursery staff, childminders, or nannies have the relevant recognized childcare qualifications and up-to-date certificates for first aid. Always follow up on references.

Special situations

Unexpected events can take place during pregnancy and birth, and your health professional will always advise you on your particular circumstances. In this chapter we answer some of the questions that commonly arise in different situations. **Support and expert guidance** can be invaluable to help you understand your options and enable you to cope and move towards the future with a positive outlook.

Between 15 and 20 per cent of pregnancies in the UK result in miscarriage, most of which occur during the first 12 weeks of pregnancy. Being **aware** of the possible causes, **symptoms**, and procedures involved in miscarriage can help you to feel more in control if this happens to you, and to enable you to make **informed choices**.

Miscarriage

What is a miscarriage?

A miscarriage is the spontaneous loss of a pregnancy during the first or second trimester, before a baby has reached 24 weeks gestation. After 24 weeks, a baby is considered "viable", which means that she is developed enough that if born this early she might be able to survive with specialist medical care. The loss of a baby after 24 weeks is known as a stillbirth (see p.309).

While some miscarriages have a specific cause, such as a structural problem with the uterus or the cervix (see opposite), most miscarriages that occur in the first trimester are thought to be due to a one-off chromosomal abnormality in the fetus. Your risk of miscarriage falls the further into your pregnancy you are, and by the beginning of the second trimester, the risk of miscarriage is around just one per cent.

The symptoms of miscarriage can vary and may depend on the type of miscarriage (see box, opposite). You may have a dull ache and a bloody discharge or some spotting, or experience severe period-like pain, which may be accompanied by heavy bleeding and clots. Sometimes a miscarriage can be symptomless and a woman may be quite unaware that there is anything wrong until a routine ultrasound scan reveals that the fetus has stopped developing in the uterus.

Investigating miscarriages

Each miscarriage is distressing, but it can be some consolation to know that, even if no cause is found, the majority of couples go on to have a healthy pregnancy in the future. Around one in 100 couples experience three or more successive miscarriages, known as recurrent miscarriage. If this happens, you are likely to be offered tests to try to establish a cause (see p.306). If a cause is found, there may be a treatment that can increase your chances of a successful pregnancy next time. Sometimes no cause is found, and the miscarriages are unexplained. Though upsetting, statistically you are still more likely than not to have a healthy pregnancy in the future.

Moving forwards

Following a miscarriage, couples need time to grieve and recover. It may take a while before you feel ready, physically and emotionally, to consider trying for another baby, or you may feel that you want to try again as soon as possible. If you're undergoing tests or treatment, these can influence when you can try for another baby. If there are no complications and the bleeding has stopped, you and your partner can try again once you feel able. It may be worth reviewing your lifestyle to maximize your chances of a healthy future pregnancy (see p.29).

Q What are the types of miscarriage?

There are different terms for different types of miscarriage, which can be confusing at a time when you are likely to be feeling vulnerable and upset. Being familiar with these terms can help you to feel more informed, which in turn can help you to cope.

The two main types of miscarriage are inevitable and missed miscarriages. With an inevitable miscarriage, the cervix begins to open up before the baby is viable, and once this happens, it is unlikely that the pregnancy can be saved. This can happen during the first or second trimester. A missed miscarriage (also called a delayed or silent miscarriage) occurs when the embryo or fetus stops developing, but remains inside the uterus; this type of miscarriage is most common during the first 12 weeks of pregnancy. The developing baby dies without any clear warning signs for the mother that something has gone wrong. For a

time (sometimes days, or even weeks), the baby remains in the uterus, and the mother may continue to think that her pregnancy is progressing. Or typical early pregnancy symptoms may suddenly disappear, which may alert the mother to something being wrong. If at any time you have an instinctive sense that something is wrong, call your GP.

A miscarriage is often a process rather than a single event. Sometimes bleeding may resolve itself (threatened miscarriage, see p.306) or bleeding may come and go and you may feel confused about what is happening. Alert your midwife to bleeding at any stage of pregnancy.

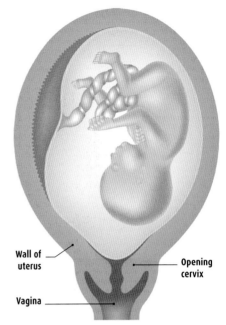

Wall of uterus

Opening cervix

Vagina

Opening cervix The most common type of miscarriage happens when the cervix opens spontaneously to stop a pregnancy that hasn't developed properly.

INEVITABLE AND MISSED MISCARRIAGES

Having an understanding of what happens in different situations can help you to process events and understand your treatment options.

TYPE	WHAT HAPPENS	SYMPTOMS
Inevitable (complete or incomplete)	The cervix starts to open up before the baby is viable, and the uterus responds by contracting and starting to push out the developing fetus or embryo. This may be complete, when all of the pregnancy tissue (the embryo, sac, and placenta) is expelled, or incomplete, when some of the pregnancy tissue remains inside the uterus.	An inevitable miscarriage may be accompanied by severe period-like pain, and is often accompanied by bleeding and clots.
Missed (also called a delayed or silent miscarriage)	The embryo or fetus stops developing, but remains inside the uterus. Eventually, the fetus dies, but with no clear warning signs, and the mother may continue to think that her pregnancy is progressing.	There may be no symptoms, or there may be a brown discharge, and pregnancy symptoms such as nausea, breast pain, and fatigue may suddenly disappear.

Q What are the causes of a miscarriage, and are there factors that increase my risk?

Around 80 per cent of miscarriages that take place in the first 12 weeks of pregnancy, known as early miscarriage, occur because there is a chromosomal irregularity with the developing fetus. The baby may have too many or too few chromosomes, which means that there is incomplete chromosomal information, and as a result the baby is unable to develop properly.

A miscarriage in the second trimester, known as a late miscarriage, is more likely to have had another trigger, and is often the result of an underlying health problem or condition in the mother. There are several possible reasons for a late miscarriage, including:

» If you develop an infection.
» If you have a pre-existing condition, such as thyroid disease, polycystic ovary syndrome, or diabetes, that increases the risk of miscarriage.
» If you have a weakened cervix.
» If you have a problem with your uterus,

such as a structural abnormality.
» If you have an immunological or endocrine disorder.

There are also several other factors that increase your risk of miscarriage. These include maternal age – you are at a greater risk of miscarriage over the age of 35 – and lifestyle choices. For example, being obese increases your risk of miscarriage, as does smoking during pregnancy, taking recreational drugs, or drinking alcohol. Drinking caffeine is also thought to be a risk factor in whether you might have a miscarriage.

Q Is bleeding in pregnancy always a concern?

Not always. There are lots of unexplained incidences of bleeding early in pregnancies that lead to perfectly healthy, full-term babies. However, bleeding in pregnancy, at any stage, should never go unchecked.

In some cases, women experience bleeding, but the cervix remains closed, the symptoms pass, and the pregnancy continues. This is known as a "threatened miscarriage". Doctors used to prescribe bed rest for this, but there's insufficient evidence that this affects the outcome. If the cervix does go on to dilate, there is really nothing you can do to stop this and a miscarriage is inevitable. Bleeding in early pregnancy can also indicate an ectopic pregnancy (see p.308). If you have any bleeding, consult your doctor as soon as possible.

12-week old fetus

Blood from the uterus

Blood travelling through cervical canal

Threatened miscarriage In this situation, miscarriage symptoms such as bleeding can occur, but the cervix stays tightly closed, and a healthy pregnancy continues to term.

Q How is an early miscarriage in the first trimester treated?

If you have symptoms such as bleeding, you will be given an early scan. If this reveals that your pregnancy isn't developing, you have a choice of letting the miscarriage happen naturally, without medical intervention, which is known as "expectant management", or of having the miscarriage medically managed, either by speeding up the process with drugs, or by surgically removing the pregnancy tissues.

Doctors often advise letting nature take its course for an early miscarriage, and the National Institute for Clinical Excellence guidelines also recommend that for a miscarriage in the first trimester so, unless you are at risk of a haemorrhage, you have a natural, or expectant, management. This gives your body a natural hormonal response to the loss, which is thought to help you adjust physically and emotionally.

It can be hard to predict the exact course of a miscarriage, but at some point you will have bleeding, and, often, painful cramps. You may be asked to take a pregnancy test two to three weeks later to see if hormone levels indicate that the pregnancy has ended. Your midwife will support you and your partner throughout, and you will be offered counselling. If symptoms persist after this time, you will

need to see your doctor again. He or she may recommend that you take a pessary or tablet to dilate your cervix to encourage the expulsion of the pregnancy tissues. You will usually begin to bleed within 24 hours of taking the medication, but if you don't start to bleed, or if a pregnancy test three weeks later indicates that you are still pregnant, you may be referred for surgery.

Surgical removal of pregnancy tissues happens either under a general or (most likely) local anaesthetic. In both cases, an instrument called a curette is inserted into your vagina. The curette has a plastic end that gently scrapes away pregnancy tissues, and a hollow tube provides suction to remove the tissues.

Q Is a miscarriage in the second trimester treated differently?

Yes, a late-stage miscarriage usually means that you will need to give birth to your baby. Although this may sound harrowing, studies show that going through birth can help women cope better long-term both physically and psychologically. You may go into spontaneous labour, but if this doesn't happen, you will be offered a pessary to trigger labour. Your midwife may ask you if you would like to hold your baby. Don't worry if you don't want to

straightaway – or even at all – you must do what feels right for you and your partner. If you would like a photograph of your baby, one of the maternity staff will take one for you.

Q Will I be able to find out what caused my miscarriage?

Sometimes, but not always. It's often hard to be certain about what caused a miscarriage, and many aren't investigated. After an early miscarriage, you're most likely to have a healthy pregnancy next time. For this reason, it's only when you have had three early miscarriages in a row, known as "recurrent miscarriage", that your doctor will consider tests to try to find out the cause. You may have investigations after one or two late miscarriages. Recurrent miscarriage may be caused by irregularities in the uterus or cervix, recurring genetic issues, or problems with the immune system, endocrine system, the clotting system in the blood, or with your partner's sperm. Or (most likely of all), there may be no identifiable reason.

During investigations, you and your partner may be asked for blood samples to test for genetic causes, doctors will check the placenta if there is one, and for a late miscarriage, you'll be asked if you would like your baby to have a post-mortem. Sometimes the examination of the placenta tells doctors all they need to know. However, it's important to prepare yourself for the fact that even after investigation, you may never know for certain what went wrong.

Q How long should we wait before trying for another pregnancy?

You should wait until bleeding has stopped before you try to get pregnant again to avoid the risk of infection. It's also advisable to have at least one period before trying again, as this makes it easier to date a pregnancy – after the uncertainty of miscarriage, it can be best to avoid confusion in a future pregnancy. Otherwise, it's up to you both. You may need more time to recover from your loss, or factors such as your age or how long you had been trying to get pregnant may mean you want to try again as soon as possible. Taking folic acid, reducing stress, eating healthily, and monitoring alcohol intake can help maximize your fertility.

Q How can we cope with my pregnancy loss and look to the future again?

After the devastating loss of your pregnancy, giving yourselves time to grieve can help you to process what has happened and to start to look to the future. You may feel a range of emotions during this time. Finding coping strategies and seeking support can help the healing process.

There are many emotions associated with grieving, and you may feel some, or all, of these at different times. It's common to feel numb at first, and this is your body's way of coping with the shock of the loss of your pregnancy. In time, feeling numb will pass and you may feel angry, cheated, or resentful. When those feelings also pass, you may feel deeply sad, withdrawn, or even depressed – not wanting to see friends or family, crying uncontrollably, or retreating into yourself. All these responses are perfectly normal and are symptoms of your intensely personal response to your loss. Eventually, though, you will emerge adjusted for life without your baby. Although "getting over it" isn't the right term – you will always remember your loss – you will be able to accept what has happened, and to start to move forwards. There are a range of things you can do, and steps you can take, to help you to cope with your loss, and throughout your grief, the most important thing you can do is to express how you're feeling – through words and actions.

» Try writing a letter to your baby Tell her how loved she was, and what you had hoped for her. Fold the letter and put it in an envelope and keep it somewhere safe.

» Keep a daily journal of your feelings Putting your thoughts down on paper can help to formalize and organize them, which can help you to feel more in control of them, if this is what you need.

» Talk it through with your partner You may not feel like doing this at first, but when you're both ready, don't shut each other out. Remember that just as you intend to parent together, you have both experienced the loss together. Try to give each other room to express your grief in your own ways, and support and comfort each other, too.

» Have a ceremony to remember your baby You might like to plant a tree in your garden or dedicate a bench in your local park so that you have somewhere to go to remember and reflect on the baby you lost.

» Join a miscarriage support group This way you can meet other couples who have experienced what you're going through. Sharing how you feel with those who truly understand provides a unique network of comfort and understanding that can reassure you that you're not alone.

While everyone deals with loss in their own way, how you respond to your miscarriage can often depend on your individual circumstances, and may be influenced by the course your miscarriage took. For example, if you had a lot of pain and bleeding, it may take longer for you to feel physically recovered. If the miscarriage played out over a relatively long period of time, you may feel particularly exhausted, though you may also feel a sense of relief that the miscarriage is behind you. Allowing yourself time to recover and to process your emotions is likely to

help you move on more completely. If, though, after a period of time you are finding it hard to shift your emotions, or you still feel below par physically, chat to your doctor, who can review your recovery and may have suggestions to help you to cope. Getting the right help and support can help you to avoid feeling isolated with your loss and give you the strength and resilience you need to look to the future once more.

Support each other Facing the loss of your pregnancy together can help you both to cope with the difficult emotions that miscarriage throws up.

Q What is an ectopic pregnancy?

This is a pregnancy in which a fertilized egg implants outside the uterus. In about 95 per cent of cases, ectopic pregnancy occurs in a Fallopian tube, but it can also happen, for example, in the cervix, on an ovary, or in the abdominal wall.

Ectopic pregnancy is a serious condition that not only means that the embryo cannot survive, but can also be life-threatening for the mother if a Fallopian tube ruptures. However, it is also very rare – occurring in just over 1 per cent of UK pregnancies.

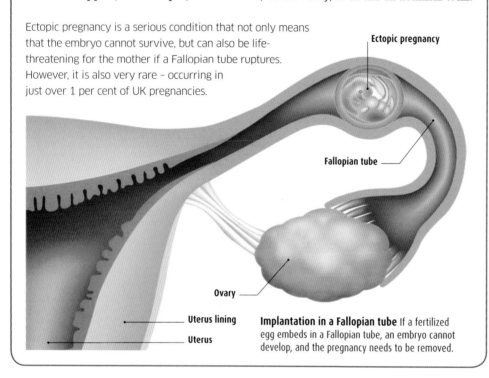

Ectopic pregnancy

Fallopian tube

Ovary

Uterus lining

Uterus

Implantation in a Fallopian tube If a fertilized egg embeds in a Fallopian tube, an embryo cannot develop, and the pregnancy needs to be removed.

Q How will I know if I have an ectopic pregnancy?

There is no one set of symptoms for an ectopic pregnancy. Some women may have no signs or symptoms at first, or the body may respond to the implantation of the egg as a normal pregnancy and respond accordingly. In this case, it can take up to 10 weeks for the symptoms of ectopic pregnancy to appear. Only when the ectopic pregnancy is discovered at a routine scan, or the blastocyst gets so big as to cause swelling or rupture at the site of implantation will you receive warning signs that something is wrong. Early symptoms can include:

» Severe cramping, similar to bad period pain.
» Pain and tenderness on one side of the abdomen.
» Vaginal bleeding.
» Stomach-upset, such as diarrhoea and nausea.
» Pain on defaecation.
» Shoulder-tip pain.

Q Are there circumstances that increase my risk of an ectopic pregnancy?

You are at increased risk of ectopic pregnancy if you have had previous problems with your Fallopian tubes, such as damage caused by an infection such as chlamydia, or a previous ectopic pregnancy; IVF treatment; patches of endometriosis that have spread to the Fallopian tubes; pelvic inflammatory disease; or an appendectomy or other abdominal surgery that left scars. Some types of contraception, the IUD and progesterone-only Pill, also increase the risk of ectopic pregnancy as they work by preventing implantation in the uterus, but they do not always prevent fertilization.

Q How will my ectopic pregnancy be dealt with?

An ectopic pregnancy is a medical emergency and you will need to go to hospital. Once there, you will be given an internal ultrasound, during which a long, thin ultrasound scanner is inserted into your vagina, to check whether there are any signs of pregnancy within your uterus. A blood sample will be taken to measure your levels of the pregnancy hormone human chorionic gonadotrophin (hCG). Depending on the level of the hormone and your symptoms, one of the following will be recommended:

» **Expectant management** means that your ectopic pregnancy will be expected to resolve itself naturally without intervention. You will be closely monitored in hospital.

» **Medical management** will be suggested if your pregnancy is in its very early stages. You will be given an injection to prevent the fertilized egg from growing any further. It will die and then be reabsorbed into your body's tissue.

» **Surgical management** will be given if there is a high chance that you will suffer a rupture in your Fallopian tube. Surgery will be performed under general anaesthetic to remove the fertilized egg and possibly to remove the affected tube. Although sometimes the tube can be saved, losing one tube doesn't affect your chances of becoming pregnant again. Unless your tube has already ruptured and you are too unwell to offer your consent, you will always be asked before you go into surgery if you agree to the affected tube being removed if necessary.

Q Will I be able to have a normal pregnancy after an ectopic one?

Yes. Although there's a slightly increased chance of suffering another ectopic pregnancy, statistically you are far more likely to go on to have a safe and healthy pregnancy next time.

65% of women have a **successful pregnancy** within **18 months** of an ectopic pregnancy. It's thought that this figure rises to **85 per cent after two years.**

Q How is stillbirth dealt with?

Stillbirth occurs when a baby dies inside the uterus after 24 weeks of pregnancy. It is the term used when the baby would have been "viable", or developed enough to have potentially survived (albeit with assistance) if he had been born living. Stillbirth may occur before labour, while the baby is in the uterus, or a baby may die during labour. In the UK, about 10 babies each day are stillborn.

Only around one stillbirth in 10 occurs as the result of a serious congenital abnormality, that is, a birth defect that has put the baby's life at risk. In most other cases where a cause can be found, stillbirth occurs as a result of a pregnancy complication rather than from the baby's genetic make-up.

They are often picked up at routine antenatal appointments, when your midwife can't detect a heartbeat. If you are in late pregnancy, you may have alerted her to the fact that you haven't felt your baby's usual pattern of movement. If your midwife is concerned, she'll immediately send you for a scan. Two sonographers will be there to confirm your diagnosis. You'll be encouraged to have someone with you for support and to listen to what the doctors tell you, as it can be hard to take in at such a sad time.

If you have a known medical condition, such as pre-eclampsia, you'll be encouraged to have your labour induced straightaway. If you are in no immediate danger, you may be able to return home for a few days to give yourself a little time to come to terms with what's happened before going through labour. After the delivery, you will be given quiet time to hold your baby if you wish to do so. You will be given a drug to stop your milk from coming in. You'll be asked if you wish for a postmortem to be done; this will be carried out only with your consent. Attending all antenatal appointments and reporting any changes in your baby's pattern or strength of movement reduces the risk of stillbirth.

POSSIBLE CAUSES OF STILLBIRTH

The chart below gives some of the possible causes of stillbirth, though in some cases a definite reason for the stillbirth is never established.

WHAT HAS GONE WRONG	WHAT DOES IT MEAN?
Pre-existing conditions	Conditions such as kidney failure, high blood pressure, diabetes (prior to becoming pregnant), and other chronic illness can cause pregnancy complications, so you will be monitored closely during your pregnancy.
Maternal age	Mothers aged over 40 years old are more likely to have a stillbirth than women who are in their 20s. This is because becoming pregnant when you're older increases your likelihood of having other risk factors for stillbirth – including congenital or chromosomal abnormalities in the developing baby, gestational diabetes, and high blood pressure.
Lifestyle factors	Heavy drinking, smoking, and recreational drug use are all risk factors for stillbirth, because they restrict the baby's access to oxygen and nutrients. Obesity can also increase the risk.
Multiples births	Possible complications with multiples may result in stillbirths, but your babies will be monitored throughout your pregnancy to ensure their wellbeing.
Pre-eclampsia	This condition causes high blood pressure in the mother, which in turn reduces blood flow to the baby, starving him of oxygen.
Problems with the placenta (including abruption)	Your placenta is your baby's life-support system in the uterus. Your midwife will check the growth of your baby at your antenatal appointments. If your baby is smaller than expected it may be due to the poor function of the placenta. If it stops working for any reason, your baby is starved of the oxygen and essential nutrients he needs for life. Placental abruption (when the placenta comes away from the uterine lining) can be why the placenta might stop working. Over 50 per cent of unexplained stillbirths are thought to be because of placental problems, but all the causes are not yet fully understood.
Haemorrhaging (including abruption)	Losing blood during pregnancy has the automatic consequence that your baby receives a restricted blood supply, increasing the risks of stillbirth.
Obstetric cholestasis	This is a rare liver condition that's been linked with stillbirth, although it's unclear why the two are related. Your midwife may suggest delivering your baby at 37 weeks if you suffer from obstetric cholestasis.
Maternal infection	Although the placenta and amniotic sac provide a barrier against many infections, in some cases bacteria and viruses can make their way into your baby's system. The most common culprits are infections that travel from the vagina into the uterus such as Group B streptoccocus, E.coli, and enterococcus, but this rarely happens before your waters break – contact your midwife at this point and she will monitor you. Many sexually transmitted infections, such as chlamydia and mycoplasma can also increase the risk of stillbirth.
Problems with the umbilical cord	If your baby becomes entangled in his umbilical cord during labour, or lies on it in such a way that the vein and arteries within it become compressed, he can restrict his oxygen supply. A prolapsed cord, which protrudes into the birth canal, is another possible cause of stillbirth.

Your newborn may need **extra care** or medical attention before he can go home if he was born prematurely, or needs to be **monitored or treated** because of occurences during his development, or the birth itself. This section looks at some **situations and conditions** that require special care, and the type of care your baby will receive.

Special-care babies

After the birth

If you had complications during pregnancy, or a problem with your baby was identified during antenatal screening, you may have been prepared for your baby to be cared for by the medical team straight after the birth. The doctors and midwives will have explained what they need to do before the birth, so you will know what to expect. You may also have had a chance to visit the special-care ward in the hospital and will be familiar with the facilities. If a problem wasn't anticipated, it can be a shock and extremely worrying if your baby needs medical attention at birth. The maternity staff may not have time to explain fully what is happening, as their priority will be your baby's health and wellbeing. As soon as possible, though, they will inform you about your baby's condition, and explain to you why your baby needs medical care.

Your role in the care of your special-care baby

Seeing your baby carried off and into the care of nurses feels totally counterintuitive for most parents – as if the important first moments of parenthood are literally taken from your hands. However, even though your baby needs extra medical help, his emotional and psychological wellbeing relies upon you. He has been listening to your voice from within your uterus, so talking to him, as well as stroking him and holding him whenever you can, ensure that his recovery is as rapid as it possibly can be.

Where special-care babies are looked after

Many hospitals have a special-care unit where babies are taken when they need help after birth. Usually this unit has three divisions, each one providing a different level of care appropriate to the seriousness of a baby's condition. Occasionally, a hospital may be unable to provide the level of specialist care your baby requires, and in this case your baby may need to be transferred to a hospital with the right facilities.

» **Neonatal intensive care units (NICU)** are for the babies that need the most help, including those who are very premature and are having difficulty breathing or regulating their heart rates.

» **High-dependency units** are for those babies who are very unwell, but who are better able to cope with life outside the uterus than those in the NICU.

» **Special-care baby units** (SCBU – often pronouced "skiboo") are for babies who just need a bit of extra help after birth. These babies might be only a few weeks premature and need some initial help with breathing, or they might have jaundice (see p.322), or just need some additional help regulating their temperature.

Q Why might my baby need medical care?

There are many reasons why a newborn might need medical care. Some relate to premature births and others may occur in full-term babies. The following is a list of the most common reasons:

>> **Respiratory disorders:** your baby may need extra oxygen or help with breathing in the short term if his respiratory system hasn't fully formed yet, or because he has an infection or meconium in his lungs.

>> **Temperature control:** even full-term babies are very bad at regulating their temperatures after birth. Your baby may need to go into an incubator until his body systems are better developed.

>> **Hypoglycaemia:** this describes a condition when your baby's glucose levels

fall too low. This can be the case in babies of mothers with diabetes, or in premature babies. Your baby's brain and body need glucose to function, so if he's unable to raise his sugar levels through feeding, he may have to go onto a nasogastric feeding drip to correct the imbalance.

>> **Jaundice (see p.322):** this is a relatively common newborn condition in which a baby's liver doesn't break down bilirubin (a by-product of red blood cells) in his blood. It occurs in around 60 per cent of full-term babies, and approximately 80 per cent of premature babies. Most cases are harmless. Your baby may need

Your reassuring presence Staying close by, talking to, and stroking your baby will help him to feel calm, and is a comfort for you, too.

treatment if he's premature, or has particularly high levels of bilirubin in his blood. Exposure to light or phototherapy might be recommended.

>> **Patent ductus arteriosus:** when your baby is born, the vessel that keeps blood-flow away from the lungs during pregnancy should close off. If this doesn't happen – your baby's lungs and heart can be put under strain (patent ductus arteriosus). See p.323.

Q When is a baby considered premature and why do some babies arrive early?

A premature (or "preterm") baby is a baby born before 37 weeks of pregnancy. In the UK, almost eight per cent of births (approximately 11 per cent in the US) are premature. It's unusual for there to be a single, clear reason why a baby arrives early; usually preterm labour is the result of a combination of factors. For up to 30 per cent of premature births, the cause never becomes clear. In a further 25 per cent of premature births, labour is medically induced before the baby is full term because a problem has been detected that means an early delivery is the safest option for the mother and/or baby. The following list sets out some of the reasons why babies are born prematurely:

>> **If you have a pregnancy condition** such as pre-eclampsia (see p.144), where your baby's growth may be restricted, or gestational diabetes (see p.145), where your baby can grow very large, you may be induced early on.

>> **Placental problems,** including placenta praevia (see p.147) and placental bleeding, can mean that labour needs to be induced early.

>> **You may have a weak cervix,** which cannot support the baby and membranes to full term.

>> **If amniotic fluid begins to leak** from the sac around the baby, known as premature prolonged rupture of membranes, your baby is at risk of infection, and labour may need to be induced.

>> **Having had a premature baby** in a previous pregnancy or having had a previous late miscarriage increases your risk of premature labour.

>> **Carrying twins or more** adds to pressure on the uterine muscles. Similarly, excess amniotic fluid can distend the uterus and trigger labour.

>> **Pre-existing maternal conditions,** such as high blood pressure, diabetes, or kidney disease, and irregularities in the shape or structure of the uterus, can mean labour is induced earlier.

>> **Being younger than 25 or older than 35** increases the risk of premature labour.

>> **Lifestyle factors,** such as smoking, drinking alcohol, taking drugs, or poor nutrition in pregnancy make premature labour more likely.

Q What will my premature baby look like?

This depends upon how close to your due date you were when you went into labour. A baby born at 36 weeks will look as you might expect a newborn to look, except smaller. A more premature baby might have very pink or reddish skin, because the fat layer under the skin hasn't formed, and he may be covered in lanugo, the soft, downy hair that protects the skin in the uterus and is shed towards the end of pregnancy. His head may seem large for his body, and, if very premature, his eyelids may be fused. The top of his skull will be soft (and his fontanelle large), as the flat bones haven't fully formed over the sides and top of his head. His limbs may seem fragile, and as his muscle tone is still quite weak, he may not be curled up as term newborns often are as he can't hold his knees to his chest. His facial features will be fully formed and he may have hair on his head.

A CLOSER LOOK
The power of touch

When a baby cries, our instinct is to pick him up and cuddle him. However, caring for a special-care baby can make soothing touch a little more complicated. When your baby goes into the special-care unit, he may be in an incubator or in a special cot and attached to machines and drips that mean you can't always pick him up when you wish to. However, simply touching your baby can be hugely beneficial for him.

Contact with your baby Studies show that stroking your baby through the holes in the sides of the special-care cot, and, once he is strong enough to be picked up, holding him whenever you can and nestling him against your bare skin as much as possible, can help with bonding and trigger the release of hormones that aid milk production.

Less stressed Being close to you and hearing your familiar voice help to reduce the amount of the stress hormone cortisol in your baby's body. Babies in special care are more tolerant of medical care, becoming less distressed during examinations, general procedures, and administration of medication, if they've felt the power of your touch.

A sense of calm When you touch or stroke your baby, you stimulate the release of oxytocin – the calming and bonding hormone – in your body and in your baby's body, promoting the bond between you and helping your baby to feel calm and secure. The release of this hormone especially helps you to feel closer to your baby if he is too tiny to be held.

Help your baby sleep Your loving touch, whether stroking him or holding him also helps to soothe your baby and promotes sound sleep. During sleep, energy is diverted away from taking in the sights, smells, and sounds of his surroundings, and from trying to keep warm, to the growth and development of his organs, limbs, and brain.

Close contact As your baby grows stronger, and with advice from your neonatal nurses, he can spend longer amounts of time being held by you outside of his incubator. Holding your baby skin-to-skin is beneficial, and even babies who are very premature can benefit from brief periods outside the incubator being held next to their mother's skin.

FASCINATING FACTS

Touch has many benefits for both special-care baby and parents, not least helping to promote a strong bond.

Boost immunity When held skin-to-skin, bacteria from the mother's skin colonize the baby, protecting him from germs.

Avoid PND Mothers of special-care babies are more likely to suffer from postnatal depression. Oxytocin, released when you touch your baby, can help you avoid PND.

Home early Premature babies held skin to skin are likely to need less time in hospital. Studies also show better neurological development scores at six and 12 months for premature babies who received kangaroo care.

Skin-to-skin contact Babies who receive kangaroo care (see below) are better able to regulate temperature, have improved oxygen levels, and breastfeed more easily.

Kangaroo care This is the practice of holding your naked baby against the skin of your chest, wrapped in a sling or cloth, snuggled upright between your breasts. The technique was first used in Colombia in the 1980s when hospitals had no incubators to keep premature babies warm. With his face turned to one side, your baby can breathe easily and, crucially, maintain a warm body temperature.

Q What can I expect in the neonatal intensive care unit?

As a parent, it's natural to feel anxious and scared when you see your baby in an incubator, perhaps with tubes attached and hooked up to lots of machines. However, all of the equipment in the unit is there to help your baby to breathe and keep him nourished to ensure he develops and grows so that in time he can cope on his own.

Support Babies who are born prematurely may spend time in an incubator. These are similar to usual hospital cots, but have a lid to keep your baby warm. Holes in the sides enable you to reach in to touch and stroke your baby.

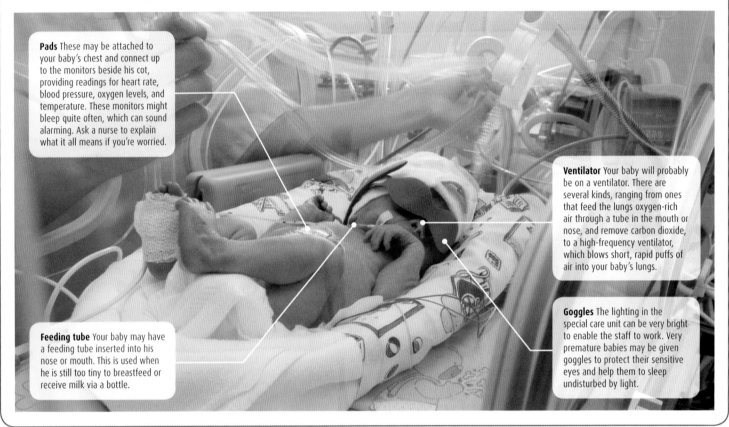

Pads These may be attached to your baby's chest and connect up to the monitors beside his cot, providing readings for heart rate, blood pressure, oxygen levels, and temperature. These monitors might bleep quite often, which can sound alarming. Ask a nurse to explain what it all means if you're worried.

Ventilator Your baby will probably be on a ventilator. There are several kinds, ranging from ones that feed the lungs oxygen-rich air through a tube in the mouth or nose, and remove carbon dioxide, to a high-frequency ventilator, which blows short, rapid puffs of air into your baby's lungs.

Goggles The lighting in the special care unit can be very bright to enable the staff to work. Very premature babies may be given goggles to protect their sensitive eyes and help them to sleep undisturbed by light.

Feeding tube Your baby may have a feeding tube inserted into his nose or mouth. This is used when he is still too tiny to breastfeed or receive milk via a bottle.

Q How will my baby be looked after in the special-care unit?

Your baby will receive round-the-clock care, specially tailored for his specific circumstances. Special-care nurses will look after your baby every minute of the day and night, with one nurse specially assigned to your baby's care. As well as the nurses, paediatricians with expertise not just in premature babies, but also in the specific issues relating to your baby, will look after him. For example, if your baby is showing signs of neurological damage, a neurologist will take care of this aspect of his care. Your baby will also be assigned to a neonatologist (a doctor specializing in the complex needs of

special-care babies) and to a social worker, who will support you through your baby's time in the unit. Other relevant specialist specialist doctors, and nurses will also all be on hand to ensure that your baby receives the best care possible.

Q Can I talk to the staff at any time about my baby's progress, and can I help with his care?

The special-care nurses are always on hand to talk to, and they will encourage you to ask questions and, when possible, to help with tasks such as washing and changing your baby. If you

have any questions that the nurses can't answer, they will ensure that the appropriate doctor or other clinician contacts you as soon as possible to talk to you. You should find that the clinicians looking after your baby are happy to have an open and supportive dialogue about his care, and you should feel involved in all the decisions that need to be made about his care. If you're worried or confused about anything and want a layperson's view, ask your social worker to put you in touch with other parents who have been through similar experiences. One of the best ways to get involved in your baby's care, and to get to know the medical staff who look after him, is to be there when the doctors visit him – the nurses can tell you at what time each day this is likely to be.

Q Will I be able to stay with my baby all the time?

You will need to check the policy in your hospital, but most hospitals allow parents to stay with their baby for as long as they want throughout the day and night. Being near to you, hearing you, and being stroked by you are all ways in which you can help your baby gain strength. Do bear in mind, though, that you and your partner need to rest, and that your body needs to recover from birth. You may have been faced with difficult decisions and have had to deal with the unexpected circumstances of your baby's arrival in the world; though you may feel guilt if you're not with your baby the whole time, some time away from the NICU, both together and separately, is important for your wellbeing.

Q Can other family members and friends visit my premature baby?

Most neonatal intensive care units will allow a few visitors at a time, and siblings in particular are encouraged to come and bond with their new brother or sister. The ward will, though, have specific visiting times for visitors, whereas parents usually can stay around the clock. Bear in mind that too many people at one time can be overwhelming, so try to keep visitor numbers small at any one time. Don't feel obliged to keep open house; you have a lot to contend with so if you prefer just immediate family to visit for the time being, this is fine. Premature babies have low immunity, so anyone who has an infection, such as a cold or bug, will be encouraged to stay away until they are completely recovered.

Q When will we be able to take our baby home?

The circumstances of every baby's special-care needs are different, and so how long your baby remains on the special-care unit entirely depends on his health at birth and his reasons for needing special care. In general, hospitals will recommend that premature babies stay in the unit at least until they have reached "full term". At this stage, your baby's organs should be well developed enough that he can cope with the demands of life outside the incubator.

In general, before your baby is ready to be cared for at home, the unit will want to ensure that he fulfils a number of criteria. First, staff need to be happy that your baby can breathe independently, which happens in stages. As he grows stronger, the nurses will take him off the ventilation equipment for short periods of time so that he can practise breathing for himself. Gradually, the amount of time your baby spends having help with his breathing will decrease, until he can breathe fully on his own.

As well as being able to breathe independently, the staff will want to see that your baby is feeding well – whether breast- or formula feeding – and gaining weight, and that he is urinating and passing stools regularly and without difficulty.

When you do leave, you may be given a follow-up appointment at the hospital in a few weeks time to check your baby's progress.

Q How can I prepare to take over the care of my baby?

Before you take your baby home, the nursing staff will ensure that you are confident about administering his medication (see box, below) and that you have support systems in place to ensure you get all the help (personal and professional) you need to care for your baby. Some hospitals will ask you to stay overnight with your baby just before you take him home so you can follow his 24-hour pattern of care with help on hand if you need it. It's natural to be nervous when your baby has been so closely monitored in the hospital, but remind yourself that the hospital are happy for him to leave as they are confident that you will be able to care for him independently now, and that home is the best place for him to grow and thrive.

Q I'm worried about administering my baby's medicines. Are there any tips or techniques I should know?

The neonatal nurses in the special care baby unit will try to make sure you're confident about administering your baby's medicines while your baby is on the unit so that you can continue once home. However, inevitably when you get home, without their watchful guidance, giving medicine can feel overwhelming. The following tips, techniques, and guidance can increase your confidence:

» **First and foremost** try to stay calm, as your baby will pick up on your stress and in turn will be less relaxed himself. Eye drops, nose drops, vitamins, minerals, and medicines all come in easy-to-administer liquid form for babies.

» **Most importantly, always wash your hands** before giving your baby any medicine. Shake any medicines before you give them, and have everything you might need, such as antibacterial wipes or cotton wool pads, within easy reach.

» **Swaddle your baby** so that his arms and legs stay still, then lie him on his back on the floor or cradle him in one arm, depending upon whether you need one or two hands to give the medicine (for eye drops, you'll need two, for example).

» **Try to avoid** any part of the medicine bottle, for example the eye drop pipette, or the tip of a bottle of nasal drops, touching your baby's skin. If you do, don't worry – just wipe the tip with an antibacterial wipe before you use it again.

» **If your baby becomes distressed**, stop what you're doing and calm him before trying again. Never miss a dose of medicine, though, unless your doctor says that it's okay to do so.

» **Make a wall chart** to remind you when to give which medicines, and check them off each day so that you don't have to rely upon your memory.

» **Bear in mind that at home** you will follow the same medication routine that your baby had during his stay in hospital, which at first can provide a helpful pattern for your day.

Q How will my premature baby be fed on the special-care unit?

This depends on how premature your baby is. The coordinated movement of sucking, breathing, and swallowing doesn't kick in until around 34 weeks' gestation, so your baby may need to be fed through a drip or tube at first.

Babies born before 34 weeks' gestation need to be fed either directly into their blood stream (a drip), or via a tube into their stomachs.

If your baby is extremely premature, she may be fed via an IV tube directly into a vein. She can be given your breast milk, donor breast milk, or specially formulated liquid food tailored to her needs, made up of carbohydrate, protein, fat, vitamins, and minerals, including electrolytes, taking into account the levels of electrolytes in her blood and her age and weight.

If your baby needs to stay on a ventilator or doesn't yet have a coordinated sucking, breathing, and swallowing movement, she will receive breast- or formula milk through a tube that passes via her nose or mouth into her stomach. The milk feeds will be small, but frequent – once every two to three hours – and you may be able to hold your baby while she feeds, and perhaps help to administer the milk. You can express your breast milk for your baby, or she can receive donor breast milk from a bottle bank, or enriched low-birthweight formula.

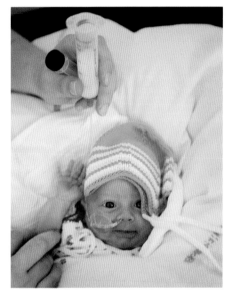

Feeding via a syringe Your baby can be fed tiny quantities of milk this way. Your expressed breast milk is nutritionally best for your baby, as your body makes it specifically for her, and it contains important antibodies that boost your baby's immature immunity.

Moving to a bottle If you wish to bottlefeed, once your baby is strong enough to suck, you can use a smaller sized teat that holds just a little milk at a time, which is easier for your tiny baby to manage.

Q When can I start expressing milk for my baby?

You can begin expressing milk as soon as you feel ready, the sooner the better. Even tiny amounts of breast milk from you contain important antibodies and nutrients specially formulated for your baby's needs. The sooner you start to express, the sooner you will establish a good milk supply, and the more likely you are to breastfeed successfully once your baby can coordinate sucking, breathing, and swallowing. While your baby is too small still to latch on to the breast, your milk can be fed to her via a tube.

Q When can I start to breastfeed my baby?

As your baby becomes stronger and gradually learns to coordinate sucking, breathing, and swallowing, you can start trying to put her to the breast. A premature baby can take time to get the hang of breastfeeding, and even once she has developed her sucking technique, they may find it hard to latch on with her tiny mouth. At first, just give your baby short periods of time to practise latching on and sucking. She may not take much milk initially, and supplements may be needed. Be guided by the neonatal nurses or midwives, who can help you ease your baby into breastfeeding. They will encourage you to hold her skin to skin so she is stimulated to breastfeed, and help her to build up her time on the breast slowly.

Q My baby brings up a lot of milk. Why is this?

It's common for babies to bring up some milk after a feed, known as reflux, and it is especially common in premature babies. This is because the muscles that control the valve at the bottom of the oesophagus, which stops food coming back out of the stomach and up to the throat again, are less likely to be well developed. Keeping your baby upright during and after a feed, spending time winding her, and, if you're bottle-feeding, switching to a slower flowing teat to avoid her guzzling down milk too quickly, can all help to minimize the problem (see p.295 for more information and advice on dealing with reflux).

Q Can my baby have normal formula milk?

If you wish to give your premature baby formula milk, she will need to have special formula that contains additional amounts of nutrients, calories, and essential fats. Your hospital will provide this for you while you are there. Once your baby has reached the due date, and is ready to go home, the hospital will probably prescribe this special high-calorie formula milk and recommend that she continues on this until she has reached a certain weight and is well enough to go on to ordinary formula. Don't switch formula without consulting your midwife first.

Latching on Be patient when you start to offer your premature baby a breastfeed, and give her plenty of time to practise latching on.

Q How can I help support my baby's development and growth once she's home?

It's reassuring to know that most premature babies will usually catch up to be at least almost as tall, strong, and heavy as their classmates by the time they are four years old. This is because premature babies have two "catch-up" growth spurts (see below) that bring them in line with their peers. For your part, making sure your baby is well nourished is essential for triggering these growth spurts.

The first months

Your medical team will discharge your baby from hospital once they are confident that she is gaining weight. If you are breastfeeding, continue to do so on demand. If you are formula-feeding, follow the advice your midwife gives you about pacing feeds. Breastfed babies (and some formula-fed ones) need vitamin and mineral supplements to ensure they receive extra dosages of all the nutrients they need for development. Your baby may need to continue taking these until she is a year old.

Catch-up growth spurts

Between the ages of one and two years, your child may have catch-up growth spurts – this will be apparent first from an increase in her head circumference recorded on her centile charts, followed by a sharp rise in her length and weight – she may rapidly start to grow out of her clothes! She may have another small catch-up growth spurt at around three years of age. After this time, she will be roughly the same height and weight as all the other children her age.

Weaning

Although advice is that babies should be weaned onto solid food at around six months of age, for premature babies this means six months from their due date rather than their actual age. So, if your baby was four weeks premature, you would wait until she is seven months old before weaning, when her digestive system will be mature enough to digest solid food. If your baby was very premature or you are in any doubt as to when to wean her, the medical team who cared for your baby can guide you.

Other ways to help

» **Encouraging good sleeping patterns – and, over time, teaching your baby to soothe herself to sleep –** will help your baby to grow and develop. Studies show that premature babies who sleep deeply in kangaroo care (see p.313) grow and develop faster than those who don't have this experience.
» **As your baby grows, periods of activity every day** will help to improve her muscle tone and skeletal strength, which in turn will help to maximize her growth.

While arriving home with your special-care baby is a joyous occasion, you may feel nervous about being in sole charge. Parents often find that it's only once they're home that the full force of what they've been through sinks in. Working through emotions and seeking support will help you to cope.

Coping emotionally

It's very normal to begin a period of grief when you arrive home with your baby after his prolonged hospital stay – for your expectations of your first days, weeks, or months of your life as a family. You may feel anxious about the responsibility of caring for your baby without constant medical support, and angry that life hasn't been as simple as it was supposed to be. Along with frustration, guilt, confusion, irritability, and helplessness, these are perfectly normal reactions to your situation. The five-step plan, below, can help you work through complex feelings.

A close bond The time your older child spends with the new arrival, talking to and touching him, will help them form an enduring bond.

Your growing family

Welcoming a new baby into the family presents challenges, and when that baby needs extra care, challenges magnify. Be careful not to shut out older children. Involve them in the baby's care if you can: perhaps they can help with topping and tailing or find a nappy bag. You are bound to feel anxious about a two-year-old "cuddling" a premature infant, so set boundaries you're happy with. Be honest, but kind, and explain that the baby is tiny and has been unwell, so only grown-ups can cuddle for now, but he loves to have his head stroked or his hand held. Sing songs to the baby together, and tell your toddler how the baby loves to hear his voice and how this helps to make him better. Older children may feel confused if you are sad or irritable, and think the baby is unwell because of something they've done. Reassure them that nothing that's happening is their fault. Say sorry if you're snappy, and explain that you're tired. Praise your children for any help they give you and try to spend dedicated time with them every day, even if this is just at bath- or bedtime.

FIVE-STEP PLAN

This simple five-step plan can help you work through the emotions you may feel about your baby needing special care. This isn't a cure-all, but one, some, or all of them may help you start to accept events and move forwards.

 1 Acknowledge your grief

 2 Express your emotions

 3 Celebrate the successes

 4 Ask for help

If you knew before the birth that your baby would need extra care, you may be grieving for the loss of an easy-going pregnancy. If your baby was premature, you may grieve for the loss of those last weeks of pregnancy. Or you may grieve for the loss of those first moments after birth when you could be alone with your baby. Acknowledging that events represent a loss of the experiences you might have wished for is the first step to coping.

The hospital can put you in touch with a counsellor or therapist who has been trained to advise and help parents of special-care babies. Talking to someone who isn't emotionally involved can help you to rationalize how you feel. You can go with your partner, on your own, or a mixture of both. Keeping a journal of your baby's progress and how you feel provides a positive reminder of how far you've come.

Successes don't have to be big things. The first time you manage a walk with your baby in the pram, to give eye drops without forgetting to keep tissues beside you, to sit down with a slice of toast in the morning, to write a thank you card or two, are all steps towards "normal" life, which makes them successes worth celebrating. They will help to remind you that every day you can achieve something.

You don't need to be strong all the time. When possible, ask for help with the practical matters of being at home, so that you can focus on your baby and yourself. Ideally, someone else can do the cleaning, shopping, and cooking. Don't be bashful about drawing upon the resources of well-meaning friends and family, and accept all offers of practical help willingly.

Time together Once home with your baby, you can enjoy a new sense of closeness.

WHERE CAN I GO FOR HELP AND SUPPORT?

There are plenty of avenues of support that you can explore to help you cope when caring for your special-care baby.

» **Your partner:** sometimes asking for help from your partner can be a trigger for him to feel more involved and positive himself.

» **Your health visitor or midwife:** once home, your health visitor or midwife will visit you within 24 hours. Ask him or her anything you need to know about your baby, or about your own health.

» **Friends and family:** ask for practical help whenever you can. Close family and good friends will want to do all they can to ease your load.

» **Other parents:** the social worker assigned to your baby in the special-care unit can put you in touch with other parents who have been through a similar situation. Many hospitals run support groups for the parents of their special-care babies.

» **A counsellor:** ask your doctor about seeing a counsellor, or, if you had a neonatal counsellor in hospital, arrange to speak to him or her. Talking things through with an impassive observer can help you to unload without fear of judgement.

» **The Internet:** look for support charities set up for parents of special-care babies. Many have online chatrooms and forums, telephone helplines, and information about local groups.

 5 Take one day at a time

Making plans or giving yourself deadlines will only add to your load. Instead, try to enjoy every moment and every day for what it is, and to relish the stage that your baby has reached. Give yourself permission to roll with the punches.

Supporting each other

Though you and your partner will react in your own ways to the pressures of caring for your baby, it's best to try to work as a team. Assign roles so you both feel valued and included, and that you're contributing your individual strengths. Your partner may also to be worried about you. Suggest practical ways for him to help, such as making you a "packed lunch" before he goes to work, or taking on responsibility for the washing. Encourage him, too, to have some skin-to-skin time with the baby to help them bond.

Mothers of babies who have spent time in intensive care have a higher risk of postnatal depression (PND), so be aware of the symptoms (see p.263). Sharing how you feel each day will help to keep you connected, and for you to feel supported.

Many midwives report that one of the most common questions when a baby is born is, understandably, **"Is everything alright?"** Here, we look at some concerns parents might face. These might be conditions that you've heard others talk about, or that you've had experience of, either in a previous pregnancy or through a family member or friend.

Issues at birth

Assessing your baby

As soon as your baby is born, her immediate wellbeing will be assessed. Then, over the following 72 hours, a paediatrician, or a midwife or GP will make a series of checks on your baby for complications or problems. Many of the conditions in this section, including ones such as cleft lip, tongue tie, and hernia, will be picked up during these checks (see p.246) – or may even have been picked up during pregnancy – and, if necessary, treatment can begin straightaway. Home visits for a further six to eight weeks – at first from a midwife, and then from a health visitor – provide a means of ensuring that all continues to be well, that your baby is growing, and that you are recovering well, too. Your care will then move solely into the hands of the health visitor, who may visit you at home, or who may invite you to "weigh-in" clinics where you can check your baby's growth and development and ask any questions you might have. While some problems are picked up on quickly, others may become apparent only after a period of time, which is why your baby's development is followed closely in these early months.

Trust your instincts

You are the person most closely attuned to your baby's wellbeing, so if you think something might be wrong, even if you're worried you might be imagining things, raise it with the midwife, health visitor, or the doctor. Concerns about newborns are always taken seriously, and no one will think you are over-anxious or overly cautious.

When a problem is found

Finding out that your baby has a problem is naturally upsetting. If a concern was identified during pregnancy, you will have had some time to adjust and find out about possible treatment. If a problem is discovered after the birth, you will have questions and concerns. Many minor concerns are easily remedied. Some do require longer-term treatment and sometimes your baby may need an operation, but most problems can be either eliminated or improved. Finding out about a condition early on means that treatment is prompt and outcomes improve.

This section looks at a range of conditions that can affect newborns, some of which may be identified or suspected during pregnancy through scans or because of concerns about a baby's growth, and many of which are detected in the days and weeks following the birth. The conditions range from those that are relatively common, such as jaundice and umbilical hernias, to those that are quite rare. In each case the implications for your baby are explained as well as the treatment and help available.

What problems or conditions might my newborn encounter?

When you consider the myriad cell divisions and biological processes that are involved in making a baby, it is little wonder that sometimes things go wrong and babies are born with conditions that need treatment in their first months of life, or that require ongoing care. The earlier a problem is identified, the sooner treatment or attention can be given, and often this lessens any long-term repercussions for your baby.

Respiratory Distress Syndrome (RDS)

» What is this?

In order to inflate properly, a newborn baby's lungs need sufficient amounts of surfactant – a fluid that keeps the lungs inflated and prevents the air sacs within them from collapsing when your baby starts to breathe on her own at birth. The air sacs begin to produce surfactant at around 27 weeks of pregnancy. Babies born before 31 weeks don't have sufficient surfactant to enable the lungs to draw in air properly, which leads to RDS. Your baby will show signs of breathing difficulties at birth, which will vary in severity depending upon how prematurely she was born, and symptoms worsen in the following days if left untreated. Some babies will need to go on to a ventilator immediately to begin breathing, while others may show signs of rasping or grunting as they try to fill their lungs.

» What can be done?

If there's time, you may be given steroids as soon as you go into premature labour to speed up the development of your baby's lungs. Once your baby is born, she may need to go into an incubator, where she can be given surfactant through a tube that goes into her mouth and directly into her tiny lungs. When she is stable, she will be put on a ventilator, which mechanically fills her lungs with air, breathing for her; or a continuous positive airways pressure machine, which allows her to breathe on her own, but prevents her lungs from collapsing between breaths.

» What does this mean for my baby?

The potential effects of RDS depend upon your baby's gestational age at birth. With swift treatment, and gentle but steady progress, your baby is likely to make a full recovery. Some babies will need help with breathing for just a few days, but if your baby was very premature, she may need assistance for weeks; sometimes it can take many months for a premature baby's lungs to work properly. Many very premature babies have RDS that develops into chronic lung disease.

Congenital infections

Viral or bacterial infections present at birth are called congenital infections, passed to the baby from the mother via the placenta in pregnancy, or during birth. The table here shows some common infections. Others include toxoplasmosis, hepatitis, HIV, and CMV.

INFECTION	WHAT IS IT?	WHAT CAN BE DONE?
Group B streptococcus (GBS infection)	A baby may contract group B streptococcus infection during birth from a mother carrying the bacteria. The baby develops blood poisoning, which can cause serious complications. Premature infants are at greater risk.	Fast treatment with antibiotics leads to no long-term effects. If the mother is a known carrier, the baby will receive antibiotics as soon as she is born to prevent the spread of infection. Where the infection isn't known about, the baby may have signs such as unresponsiveness, breathing difficulties, convulsions, poor temperature control, and pale skin.
Herpes	The herpes simplex virus comes in two forms – HSV1, which causes cold sores; and HSV2, which causes genital herpes. HSV2 is most common in newborns, who catch the virus during birth. It is a potentially serious infection that can cause severe conditions, or even neonatal death.	If you know or suspect you have genital herpes, your doctor may advise a Caesarean section to prevent the spread of the virus to your baby. If not, and your baby contracts the infection, she may have no symptoms at first, and may go on to be perfectly healthy. If the virus activates, babies may be unresponsive, have difficulty feeding, and have a fever. Your baby will need intravenous antiviral medication for up to three weeks to control the infection.
Rubella	Also known as German measles, this is a viral infection that can cause serious complications for premature infants (see p.139). Congenital rubella occurs when the baby contracts the virus in the uterus in the first trimester. It can cause developmental problems, which can affect the heart, and the nervous and musculoskeletal systems.	There is no way to treat the rubella infection itself, so treatment involves minimizing its effects. Some babies will be able to have heart surgery to correct defects. Sadly, any damage to brain tissues is permanent.

Jaundice

» What causes jaundice in babies?

Jaundice in newborns, known as neonatal jaundice, is a usually harmless condition caused by high levels in the blood of the substance bilirubin. Bilirubin is a yellow pigment that is produced when old red blood cells are broken down and metabolized by the liver, then excreted in the urine and faeces. In the uterus, your baby needed extra red blood cells to carry oxygen to her own body and the placenta. However, for life outside the uterus she needs fewer red blood cells, and has to break down the excess. At birth, the extra red blood cells mean an extra load on your baby's immature liver; the liver can't keep up and therefore bilirubin is reabsorbed back into your baby's blood stream, causing yellowing in the skin and the whites of the eyes. The condition is very common in newborn babies, affecting 6 out of 10 babies born at term, and 8 out of 10 born prematurely. Premature babies are slightly more likely to be jaundiced as their immature liver and gut are even less well equipped to deal with an overload of red blood cells. Jaundice usually arises in the first two to three days of life, and in most babies resolves itself without treatment within a week or so. In a few babies, jaundice becomes severe, and the babies require treatment to avoid serious, but rare, complications affecting the brain.

» How will I know if my baby has jaundice?

If you notice a yellow tinge to your baby's skin, press the middle of her forehead with your finger (the skin yellowing progresses from top to toe): if your baby has jaundice, the colour of the depressed skin will be yellow when you remove your finger. You may also notice a yellowing on the palms of the hands or soles of her feet. Stools may be pale (rather than brown), and urine very yellow (rather than pale). The whites of your baby's eyes may appear yellow, too.

» Can jaundice be missed?

You may not notice mild jaundice, but your midwife will check your baby regularly for jaundice if you are in hospital, and when she visits you at home over the first few days, so it's unlikely that it would go unnoticed. Your midwife will also take into account risk factors for jaundice, such as whether or not your baby is premature, if you have other children who had neonatal jaundice, whether your baby is feeding well, whether you're breast- or bottle feeding (jaundice is more common in breastfed babies), and whether your baby seems alert and responsive. Poor feeding and a disinterested baby can build up a picture of likely jaundice. Call your midwife straightaway if yellowing skin is accompanied by extreme lethargy, irritability, unwillingness to feed, or a fever.

» Will my baby have to have any tests to confirm suspected jaundice?

If the hospital is concerned about the level of your baby's jaundice, they will use a special light that shines through the skin to show up bilirubin. Your midwife may also take a small blood sample to test for bilirubin levels in your baby's blood, and he or she may take a urine sample to check for an underlying condition. If jaundice is confirmed, doctors will do further tests on your baby's blood to try to establish the cause and severity.

» Will my baby need to be treated?

If jaundice is mild, your baby will usually be left alone to allow the liver to mature and resolve the jaundice naturally – usually the liver is able to metabolize excess bilirubin by two weeks after birth. If your baby is premature, or she has very high levels of bilirubin, she will be treated with a form of light therapy called phototherapy. Treatment is usually completely successful within a few days and, assuming all else is well, your baby will be able to go home. If bilirubin levels remain high, a blood transfusion may be given in a neonatal intensive care unit. Small amounts of your baby's blood are replaced with matching donor blood until the levels of bilirubin are low enough that the jaundice dissipates.

» Is there anything I can do to prevent my newborn getting jaundice?

Ensure that your baby feeds well so that she doesn't become dehydrated. If you're breastfeeding, encourage her to feed every two hours. If you're bottle-feeding, aim for a 30 to 60ml feed every three hours. If you're breastfeeding, but your baby isn't drawing off enough milk and begins to show early signs of jaundice, your midwife may suggest you use a breast pump to express your milk for a day or so (which will also encourage your milk-flow), feeding it to your baby in a bottle.

The phototherapy lamp emits a blue-green light.

A filter removes harmful ultraviolet rays.

A special eye patch protects your baby's retinas from the light.

Your baby is undressed to her nappy, so that a wide area of the skin is treated by the light. Sometimes, babies are placed on a light mat, too, to treat the back of the body.

Phototherapy treatment Your baby is placed under a special lamp that changes the chemical make-up of bilirubin to make it easier to break down.

Cleft lip and palate

» What is this?
Parts of your baby's face develop independently in the uterus and then grow together. However, if they don't join up successfully, a cleft lip and/or palate is the result – these are gaps in the top lip and in the roof of the mouth. A baby may have a cleft lip or a cleft palate, or both. The conditions are often inherited and can hamper your baby's ability to feed successfully, and eventually to talk. This affects around one in 700 babies in the UK.

» What can be done?
Your baby will need surgery to bring the two sides of the mouth together, both for the upper lip and the palate. This is usually done by your baby's first birthday; the correction of a cleft lip may be done as early as three months and is followed by a procedure to correct the palate. A few babies may go on to have slight difficulties forming some words or to have a nasal tone to their voice; most recover to have perfectly normal speech. Further operations may be needed.

Umbilical hernia

» What is this?
This occurs when the baby's intestine pushes out through the hole in her abdominal wall where the umbilical cord was attached, and when this hole fails to close up spontaneously after birth. It is painless, and you may notice the protrusion only when your baby cries or strains. Umbilical hernia is a common conditions in newborns, affecting around 3–5 per cent of healthy term babies. Premature babies are at slightly increased risk.

» What can be done?
Unless your baby's hernia is large or has become infected, it will probably be left to clear up on its own. Eventually the hole closes over and the protruding portion of the intestine goes back into position. Large or infected hernias may need treating, possibly with surgery. As long as any infection is treated before it affects the intestine wall, there are no long-term implications.

Inguinal hernia

» What is this?
In around one in six premature babies, part of the small intestine protrudes through a hole in the abdominal wall near the groin, in the space called the inguinal canal. You may notice this hernia only when you see a swelling under the skin near the groin when she cries or strains.

» What can be done?
Your baby will need surgery to push the hernia back into position and close over the hole into the inguinal canal in order to prevent a reoccurrence. This will usually be done as soon as possible after the hernia has been diagnosed.

Congenital heart problems

» What kinds of defects can occur?
Up to nine in every 1000 (almost 1 per cent) of babies born in the UK have a congenital heart defect, so heart problems in newborns are rare. Among the most common is one relating to a special blood vessel – the ductus arteriosus – that enables blood to bypass the baby's lungs while in the uterus. This vessel should close within 24 hours of the birth, but occasionally this doesn't happen, overloading the lungs and heart with blood (see p.311). Other congenital heart problems include:

Atrial septal defect (ASD) and ventricular septal defect (VSD). Commonly referred to as "a hole in the heart", this is when the two sides of a baby's heart fail to become distinct from one another, causing oxygenated and deoxygenated blood to mix. This is often easily resolved with surgery, and small holes may close up on their own.

Coarctation of the aorta occurs when the aorta (the heart's main artery) is narrowed, limiting blood flow. It can become a serious condition, but is treatable with the insertion of a stent (a small tube that opens the artery), or with surgery to remove the affected part of the aorta.

Stenosis of the valves occurs when the arterial or ventricular valves are narrowed, hampering blood flow between the chambers of the heart and causing a heart murmur. The condition usually requires surgery to correct.

Some babies may have more serious problems such as failure of one side of the heart to develop fully, or the arteries and veins of the heart "transposing" – developing the wrong way round.

» When will heart problems be spotted?
Some heart defects are picked up by the sonographer at your antenatal scans, others develop at birth. If a problem is spotted, a cardiac specialist will explain the implications of the condition and what treatment, if any, your baby will need when she is born. Ask as many questions as you need to. Your midwife will be able to give you details of support groups, and other parents who have been in a similar situation.

KEY

→ Oxygen-rich blood
→ Oxygen-poor blood
→ Mixed blood

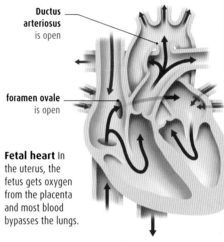

Ductus arteriosus is open

foramen ovale is open

Fetal heart In the uterus, the fetus gets oxygen from the placenta and most blood bypasses the lungs.

Ductus arteriosus has closed

foramen ovale has closed

Healthy newborn heart At birth, a hole (foramen ovale) between the chambers and another at the ductus arteriosus closes – normal circulation begins.

Ductus arteriosus has closed

foramen ovale has remained open

Open foramen ovale If the hole between the chambers remains open at birth, oxygenated blood returns to the lungs, making circulation less efficient.

Ductus arteriosus remains open

foramen ovale has closed

Open blood vessel If the ductus arteriosus fails to shut at birth, oxygenated blood meant for the body is diverted back to the lungs again.

Hip dysplasia

» What is this?

The long bone of the thigh (the femur) connects to the pelvis in a ball-and-socket joint at the hip, which gives us full range of circular movement in our legs. In around 2 per cent of births, babies are born with femur joints (one or both) that completely or partially malform outside the socket. Your baby's hips will be tested for this condition within three days of birth – a doctor or midwife will manipulate her upper thighs in the hip sockets to check for freedom of movement. The condition tends to run in families and is more common in baby girls than in boys.

» What can be done?

Sometimes it's just a matter of ligaments tightening up around the joint to hold the femur bone in place, which can happen naturally. If your baby has hip dysplasia caused by malformation in the bone, however, she may need to wear a special harness to hold her legs in position so that as the bones of the pelvis harden, the socket forms properly around the top of the femur bone. If hip dysplasia isn't picked up until after your baby is six months old, or if treatment with the harness

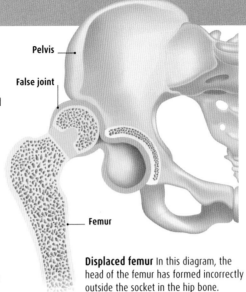

Pelvis

False joint

Femur

Displaced femur In this diagram, the head of the femur has formed incorrectly outside the socket in the hip bone.

hasn't worked, your baby will need surgery to position the femur correctly within the socket. After surgery, your baby will need to wear a cast until the bones have reformed around the corrected femur, a process that usually takes about three months.

Undescended testes

» What is this?

During the third trimester of pregnancy, a baby boy's testes should descend into the scrotal sac. However, in up to 4 per cent of baby boys, the testes fail to descend and the baby is born with an empty scrotum. This doesn't cause any pain.

» What can be done?

Most of the time, the testes will descend without any intervention before the baby is six months old. If they don't, your baby will need to have an operation to move them into the correct position. The operation usually takes place before he reaches the age of five.

Talipes

» What is this?

More commonly known as club foot, this occurs when the tendons on the inside of a baby's lower leg are tighter and shorter than those on the outside. The result is that the foot (or feet – about half of all cases of talipes show up in both feet) turns inwards. Usually, the bones of the ankle are also poorly formed. It's more common in boys, and occurs in around one in 1000 babies. The condition runs in families. There are several types of club foot, ranging from isolated

conditions that can be easily corrected to types that are an indication of other, chromosomal abnormalities.

» What can be done?

Soon after birth, your baby will begin a weekly programme of manipulation and casting to coax the foot into the correct position as the bones grow. Once this process is over, he may need a simple operation to release the tension in his Achilles tendon. To prevent re-tightening in the tendon, he will probably have to wear special harnesses on his feet continually, and then only nightly, until he is four or five years old. After this, children usually recover fully.

Syndactyly

» What is this?

Your baby's hands and feet form in the early weeks of pregnancy. At around five weeks, they look like paddles, with fingers or toes joined together. They begin to separate around two to three weeks later. Syndactyly occurs when two or more of the digits of the hands or feet fail to separate properly, leading to a webbed appearance. The effect may be superficial, in just the skin, or the bones may have fused. It affects around one in 2000–3000 babies, and can run in families.

» What can be done?

Your baby will need surgery to separate the bones and/or

skin of the fingers or toes that are joined together. If she has more than two conjoined digits, she will need more than one operation, because only one side of each digit can be operated on at a time in order to preserve the blood flow to the whole hand or foot.

Tongue-tie

» What is this?

Tongue-tie occurs when the frenulum, the small piece of tissue that lies beneath the tongue, connecting it to the bottom of the mouth, is too far forward, so the tongue can't move forward or from side to side effectively. This can make breastfeeding especially difficult and can sometimes cause sore and ulcerated nipples for the mother if the baby is unable to achieve a good latch. If your baby is feeding well, you may never notice that she is tongue-tied. However, if you are having problems feeding, perhaps finding that your baby doesn't latch on to your nipple properly, tongue-tie could be the cause. Tongue-tie affects 4–10 per cent of newborn babies and is more common in boys than girls.

» What can be done?

If your baby is having problems with feeding and it's thought that tongue-tie is the problem, doctors may perform a tongue-tie division, a procedure that involves a painless snip in the tightened frenulum to enable the free movement of the baby's mouth and tongue.

Retinopathy of prematurity (ROP)

» What is this?

Images are formed on the back of the eye, at the retina. Babies born before 31 weeks are at risk of developing abnormal blood vessels leading to the retina, impairing its ability to receive information and so distorting vision. It occurs in around 20 per cent of premature births. There are no outward signs of the condition and diagnosis relies upon assessment by an ophthalmologist at birth.

» What can be done?

After birth, a specialist eye doctor will shine a torch into your baby's eyes to assess the health of her retinas. Your baby may have drops put into her eyes to give the doctors a better picture of what's going on. Laser surgery may prevent the advancement of the condition and save sight.

» What does it mean for my baby?

Mild forms of ROP, which are the most common, will correct themselves in time, as the blood capillaries feeding the retinas settle down. More severe forms may lead to the retina detaching from the layers beneath it; laser surgery may correct this but it isn't always successful, and often babies will have at least some form of visual impairment, particularly in their peripheral vision.

Hypospadias

❯❯ What is this?
This condition occurs in around one in 300 baby boys when the urethra exits the penis along the shaft, rather than at the tip of the penis. Depending upon where the hypospadias occurs, the penis may not be able to straighten properly, and the foreskin may not develop normally on the underside.

❯❯ What can be done?
If the urethra appears close to the tip of the penis, the condition is considered mild and often it is left as it is. However, more severe forms of the condition, which can cause pain on urination and later difficulties with erectile function, are usually treated with surgery before the baby reaches 18 months old.

Pyloric stenosis

❯❯ What is this?
Around one in 500 babies are born with this condition. The pylorus is a muscular tube that connects the stomach to the bowel. Sometimes a baby may be born with a section of overdeveloped pylorus muscle and this means that milk can't pass beyond the stomach. This causes the baby to vomit back up her feeds (sometimes violently) and in turn she becomes dehydrated and undernourished. It can sometimes be a hereditary condition, and tends to affect more boys than girls. It usually develops at around six weeks after birth.

❯❯ What can be done?
Your baby will need to have an operation (often keyhole surgery) under general anaesthetic to cut through the muscle and create a passage for milk to pass into the bowel from the stomach. There tend to be no long-term side effects, and babies make a full recovery, going on to feed perfectly normally throughout life.

Imperforate anus

❯❯ What is this?
This is a rare condition affecting around just one in every 5000 babies. In the uterus, the whole of your baby's digestive system begins, essentially, as one long tube, separated by thin membranes that gradually break down as necessary as the different sections of the gastrointestinal tract form. Sometimes, the sections that form the large intestine, anus, and rectum don't form properly, making it impossible for your baby to pass a stool. This is an imperforate anus.

❯❯ What can be done?
Imperforate anus is corrected using surgery, usually as soon as the problem is discovered (or at birth – as often it shows up on an ultrasound scan). Your baby will need to wear a colostomy bag until the bowel has healed. Most children go on to have a perfectly healthy and well-functioning bowel, but occasionally a child may need to go on to a special diet to relieve constipation.

Fetal alcohol syndrome

❯❯ What is this?
Fetal alcohol syndrome (FAS) occurs when the levels of alcohol a mother drinks during pregnancy affect the development of the baby. A newborn with FAS often has a small head with distinctive facial features, including droopy eyelids with skin folds in the upper inner corners, and small eyes. Ears may be set low down and the mouth may have an underdeveloped jaw, a thin upper lip, and only a shallow or indistinct groove above the lip (called the philtrum). The bridge of the baby's nose will seem low when compared with the position of the eyes, and the nose itself may seem short and upturned. In addition, FAS can cause heart problems and learning difficulties. It is estimated that around one in 1000 children are affected by FAS.

❯❯ What can be done?
There is no treatment for FAS itself, although any heart abnormalities may be operable, and the baby will need support throughout childhood for any learning or behavioural difficulties.

Cerebral palsy

❯❯ What is this?
Cerebral palsy is the result of lack of oxygen to the brain, which can occur before a baby is born (causing damage directly to the neurons in the brain as the brain forms), during birth (as a result of haemorrhage), or as a consequence of an illness such as meningitis after birth. It affects areas of the brain that control muscle movement (including those for speech and swallowing), hearing, vision, and learning.

❯❯ What can be done?
There is no cure for the condition, but it is not progressive – that is, it doesn't get worse over time. This means that management can be uniquely tailored to each individual child. Once your child has been diagnosed with cerebral palsy, you will have a team of health professionals involved in her care. You will also have one key worker, who may be your point of contact and will help to coordinate the management of your child's condition. There is a wide range of therapies for cerebral palsy that help deal with different aspects of the condition, with the aim of relieving symptoms and maximizing your child's independence. Physiotherapy is one of the main treatments, which is important to prevent muscles weakening further and movement becoming more restricted. Occupational therapy may be given to help your child manage everyday activities and

Massage therapy Complementary therapies such as massage gently manipulate soft body tissues, helping to relax and relieve muscle stiffness.

tasks. Speech therapy provides exercises to help your child communicate more clearly if needed. Speech and language therapists can also help children to reduce drooling. If the muscles are very stiff, your child may need medication to relax them. Occasionally surgery is needed to treat bone and joint problems.

Cerebral palsy occurs in around **1 in 400** births in the UK, and it is more common in **boys** than girls. More than half the cases each year occur as a result of **premature births**.

Occasionally, a baby is born with or develops a condition that requires **lifelong support**. It may be caused by a faulty **chromosome or gene**, or may have no known cause. You may have found out in pregnancy that your baby had a problem, or it may become evident only **after the birth**, or in the first months of your baby's life.

Special needs

What is meant by "special needs"?

Special needs refers to any condition that means a child, or an adult, needs extra support to reach their potential. If your baby has special needs, she may need help to maximize her opportunities to develop not just physically, but emotionally, socially, and mentally, too. Some conditions present physical or neurological challenges, others require a special diet, or a particular medication to control the condition. Essentially, special needs is an umbrella term for myriad conditions, from those that affect a baby physically, such as chronic illness or malformations in limbs or organs, to those that affect psychological or mental wellbeing, such as memory disorders or learning difficulties. Chromosomal conditions such as Down's syndrome fall under this umbrella term, too, as do some inherited illnesses, such as cystic fibrosis. This section looks at some of the most common special-needs situations, as well as some rarer conditions that are tested for with the heel prick blood test in your baby's first week of life (see p.250).

Readjusting your outlook

In many cases, babies born with special needs aren't "suffering from" anything, but are living with and often overcoming the challenges of conditions that carve their and your lives into a different kind of normality. Understanding your baby's condition, and knowing about its causes, features, symptoms, and prognosis, can help you to come to terms with it so that you can nurture your baby in the most positive and fulfilling ways possible.

Your role

If your baby has a condition that requires ongoing care, it can be easy to feel marginalized against the whirling backdrop of medical care, especially in the early years. However, you lie at the heart of your baby's life, and your understanding of her needs is instructive. While doctors can discuss and treat her physical condition, you know best how to ensure her emotional and social wellbeing. This means that doctors and midwives will look to you to take charge of your baby's care, following their advice so that it works for your family. Never underestimate the importance of your opinion, or be afraid to share it, and never be afraid to ask as many questions as you need to.

As your baby grows and gains an understanding of her situation, talk to her about her treatment or the challenges that she faces in age-appropriate terms. Involve siblings and other family members, too, ensuring that no subject, appropriately discussed, is off-limits, and having open discussions, which will draw you together.

Q How can we build up an effective support network?

Having a baby with a life-limiting or special-needs condition can be overwhelming for a parent. It's important that throughout your baby's diagnosis and treatment, you accept all offers of help and support available to you.

Caring for your special-needs baby presents many new challenges, and the early years are likely to be a steep learning curve. Not only are you adjusting to being a new parent, with the lifestyle changes this throws up, but you are also finding out about and coping with the additional special needs of your baby. The right help and support can be crucial.

HELP AND SUPPORT

Accessing all the help and support that is available to you and your baby can provide you with essential practical and emotional back up, making it easier to cope with your baby's particular needs and enabling you to provide the best possible care for her.

» Communicate with your partner. Although at times you may respond to challenges differently, no one knows what's going on as intimately as your partner. Don't judge each other and listen to each other's point of view. Set aside some time for just the two of you, and know when to give each other space.

» Call on your family frequently – they have a vested interest in you and your baby, and ensuring a grandparent, aunt, or uncle is fully involved in the details of your baby's special upbringing will give you a babysitter you can completely trust, so that you can have a break when you need it.

» Having friends to talk to can provide welcome relief and a sense of normality. If a friend offers to grab the shopping, bring round a meal, or pick up your dry cleaning, take up the offer willingly and gratefully.

» Support groups can provide a new perspective from someone with experience of the situation you're in and provide solutions to challenges that seem hard to fathom when you're trying to cope. Even if there are no solutions, talking to someone who has been through similar events and knowing you're not alone is often enough to keep you positive.

» Counsellors are trained at helping you to explore and rationalize your emotions. Caring for a sick or special-needs baby comes with a whole range of emotions, and talking to a counsellor can help you channel these for positive effect. Talk to your healthcare professional about finding a counsellor with an approach that will suit you.

» Your GP is there to support you and your baby. He or she can offer advice, give you a referral to a specialist if you feel you need one, and will also know about schemes in your area that offer respite care to give you a break every now and then. He or she can also advise on your entitlement to financial allowances and grants from the Government.

» Try to have someone with you who can act as an extra pair of ears when you go to hospital appointments and meetings with therapists. This might be your partner, or a close family member or friend. Making notes will help, too, giving you something to refer back to that will help you to formulate questions for next time, or even for a follow-up call.

Q What causes Down's syndrome?

Down's syndrome, also known as Trisomy 21, is a chromosomal abnormality. Healthy babies are born with 23 pairs of chromosomes, with one chromosome in each pair received from each parent. Down's syndrome occurs when a baby has an extra version of chromosome 21, creating a group of three chromosomes. In the UK, Down's syndrome occurs in approximately one in every 650 to 1000 births, and the chances of having a baby with Down's syndrome rise with increasing maternal age (see p.97).

Q What are the signs of Down's syndrome?

A person with Down's syndrome has distinctive facial and anatomical characteristics, and will have some degree of learning difficulties. Some babies may be born with heart problems and a closed section in the small bowel (known as a duodenal atresia), as well as problems with hearing and vision. Characteristics include:

» Rounded face with a broad brow.
» Folds at the inner corners of the upper eyelids.
» Slanted appearance in the openings for the eyes.
» Low-set ears.
» Weakened muscles in the legs and arms.
» Flattened bridge of the nose, set low down compared with the position of the eyes.
» Single crease across the palms of the hands.
» Short little finger that may curve inwards.
» Protruding tongue and overly arched palate.
» Gap between the big toe and the toe next to it.
» Short neck with loose skin.

Recognizing Down's Each baby with Down's has an individual appearance, though there are a number of physical characteristics that are common to the condition. These are not always immediately evident at birth.

Q Will my Down's baby need to stay in hospital for longer?

Most likely, yes. Even if you were given a strong indication during pregnancy that your baby was likely to have the condition, Down's syndrome won't be officially diagnosed until after the birth, when tests and checks will be done in hospital to confirm it. Firstly, a paediatrician will examine your baby to look for anatomical features that suggest Down's syndrome is present. Then, he or she will take a blood test to see if your baby has an extra chomosome 21. Only once you have this chromosomal analysis – which may take up to 48 hours to come back, although timings vary from hospital to hospital – is the diagnosis given. Furthermore, babies with Down's syndrome may have trouble feeding as a lack of muscle tone in the tongue can make sucking difficult. Like any mother of a newborn baby, you will be encouraged to stay in hospital until you and the midwives are confident that your baby is feeding well.

Once you have the final diagnosis, your baby will need further tests to try to establish the degree to which she is affected by the condition. Effects can range from mild to severe – in the former case you may be allowed to go home soon after diagnosis, in the latter, your hospital stay may be longer.

Q What are the likely long-term challenges for babies with Down's syndrome?

Although life expectancy for people with Down's syndrome was once limited to middle age, men and women are now expected to live well into their 50s, and sometimes 60s. Increasingly, individuals with Down's syndrome can live full lives, even leaving home once an adult to live independently. Nonetheless, the condition does pose certain challenges.

» Weakened immunity: your baby may be more susceptible to everyday infections, such as coughs, colds, and respiratory illnesses, although no one is really sure why this should be the case. Your baby is also more susceptible to serious conditions, such as leukaemia.

» Thyroid problems: your baby is more likely than children without the condition to have to take medication for hypothyroidism (an underactive thyroid). Even though this is relatively straightforward to control, this will be something that your baby will have to have monitored throughout her life.

» Learning difficulties: all babies with Down's syndrome grow up to have some level of learning difficulties. Obviously, the more severe your baby's learning difficulties, the greater social and behavioural challenges she will then face. Problems such as impaired hearing and vision can exacerbate issues with cognitive function, as these can further delay several developmental stages, such as learning to talk, read, and write. Difficulty sleeping is also a trait of the condition, and this too can further impede learning.

» Dementia: studies indicate that people with Down's syndrome are more likely to suffer from dementia after the age of 40, which can lead to the need for long-term residential care.

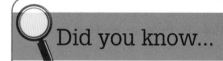

Did you know...

Down's syndrome is named after the 19th-century English doctor John Haydon Down, who first registered the condition in 1862.

Q What can I do to help my baby in the future?

Like any parent, your job is to help your baby reach her potential, not just in terms of learning, but also by helping her develop confidence in herself and to become as independent as possible.

Try to avoid comparisons with other babies without Down's syndrome born at the same time, and instead celebrate your baby's successes as they happen. Tailor your parenting methods to her own unique learning styles – if she is creative, get creative with her; if she finds it hard to form words, teach her sign language; if she loves music, take her to music groups and as she gets older even learn an instrument together. Show her that she has unique talents, just like any other child, and in this way watch her grow in confidence and independence. Give her lots of opportunity to meet and play with other children, both with and without Down's syndrome. Teach her social skills, such as manners and sharing, and offer her plenty of opportunities to socialize.

Finally, it's essential that throughout your parenting you work in partnership with the medical staff who are looking after your baby – not just for her physical wellbeing, but also because this can help you to allay her fears or anxieties about any tests or procedures she may need to have.

Loving support With your constant support and love, your baby will grow in confidence and flouish, ready to take on challenges, knowing that you are there for her.

Q Will I know straight away if my baby has cystic fibrosis (CF)?

About one in 10 babies with CF have a condition called meconium ileus at, or shortly after, birth, which causes a bowel blockage and requires surgery. Other symptoms of CF usually emerge in the first year of life, so it may not be obvious immediately that your baby has CF. However, most cases of CF are now diagnosed shortly after birth as CF is one of the conditions screened for with the heel prick test (see p.250), carried out at around five days old. Signs of CF include difficulty breathing, a raspy, hacking cough that doesn't go away, and coughing up a lot of phlegm. If the condition affects your baby's pancreas, she'll be unable to produce the right level of enzymes to break down her food sufficiently, and her digestive juices will be too thick to draw out nutrients properly. As a result, she may show signs of malnutrition, such as having pale skin, a thin and small frame, and a distended tummy, and may pass fatty-looking stools. Her skin may taste salty, as your baby's sweat has a high concentration of salt.

Q Can cystic fibrosis (CF) be treated?

There is no cure for CF. However, although it is a life-limiting condition, advances in medicine over recent decades mean that life expectancy has dramatically improved, and now more than 80 per cent of babies born with CF will live into their 50s. Treatment involves relieving symptoms, and is tailored to the individual's needs. Physiotherapy, oxygen therapy, and inhalers can be used to ease breathing, while vitamin and mineral supplements, replacement digestive enzymes, and a high-calorie diet can help to improve nutrition and growth. Your baby will be more vulnerable to infections, so may also be prescribed prophylactic (preventative) antibiotics. In more serious cases, a heart and lung transplant may be needed.

There are certain characteristic effects of CF on the sufferer's body, including, most significantly, impairment of the function of the lungs and pancreas.

» Damage to the pancreas can not only cause problems with digestion, but also lead to diabetes as the pancreas is responsible for making insulin, which controls sugar levels.

Q What is cystic fibrosis, and how does it affect babies?

Cystic fibrosis (CF) is a condition caused by a faulty gene, called CFTR. The gene needs to be inherited from both parents for someone to suffer with CF. The faulty gene causes a build-up of mucus that in turn affects breathing and feeding.

The condition primarily affects the lungs and digestive system, causing a build up of mucus in these organs. The faulty gene affects the way in which salt and water move in and out of cells in the body; an excess of salt enters the cells of certain organs, causing an imbalance of salt and water. Eventually too little water remains in the fluid surrounding the affected organ's cells, resulting in a build-up of thick mucus that impairs the organ's function. The condition affects one in 2500 babies born in the UK every year, although one in 25 babies will carry the faulty gene.

Mucus build-up Here, mucus (in green) can be seen clearly in a CF sufferer's lung, blocking airways and causing difficulty breathing.

HEALTHY AIR SAC   INFECTED AIR SAC

Air sacs This artwork shows how the build-up of mucus seen in the lungs of a cystic fibrosis sufferer clogs up the multitude of air sacs (alveoli). This affects the flow of oxygen in the lungs and causes difficulty with breathing.

» The intestine can't absorb nutrients properly from food.

» Increased likelihood of infertility, particularly for men.

» Poor nutrition can lead to osteoporosis later on, especially in women.

» Sinus infections are common, as well as polyps (small growths) inside the nose.

» The lungs fill with mucus, which leads to breathing difficulties, repeated chest infections, and increased coughing.

» Risk of liver damage.

Q Will cystic fibrosis affect my baby's growth?

This partly depends upon how severely she has the condition. Mutations in the gene that causes cystic fibrosis mean that it varies in its effects. Mild forms of the disease may affect only the lungs, and her pancreas may remain relatively stable. This will mean that she won't suffer the nutritional deficiencies associated with more severe forms of the disease and is more likely to grow normally. Even in more severe cases, most sufferers are able to take supplementary pancreatic enzymes that help to do the job that the pancreas is failing to do. This can help with the breakdown of food and has been shown to greatly improve growth in those with CF.

Q What can I do to help ease the symptoms of cystic fibrosis?

First and foremost make sure you get all the information and support that's available to you. Then, follow the guidelines from your specialist doctor with care. These will be tailored to your child's individual requirements and can help you to manage her condition. Importantly, give your baby all her medicines, including any that help her to digest her food properly, as this is essential for growth and development. In consultation with your doctor, make sure that she gets all her immunizations at the correct times, as she is especially susceptible to illness.

You will also have a physiotherapist involved in your baby's care. He or she will teach you age-appropriate techniques that help to clear the lungs, so that you can give your child essential care at home. Ask plenty of questions while you learn the techniques until you're fully confident about using the methods on your own. Try not to panic when your baby experiences breathing difficulties as she is more likely to be anxious if she senses that you are panicking, which can worsen her symptoms. Be reassuring and matter of fact while you carefully administer the procedures you've been taught. However, if at any point you are very concerned about your baby's breathing, call the hospital – or an ambulance.

It's a good idea to extend your trusted network of friends or relatives who can use CF techniques so that you have support to call upon when you need it.

Q I've been told my baby has phenylketonuria. What is this?

This rare genetic condition, referred to as PKU, occurs when the body lacks or is unable to make an enzyme called phenylalanine hydroxylase (PAH).

The enzyme PAH is needed to convert the amino acid (the building blocks of protein) phenylalanine into another amino acid, tyrosine. Tyrosine helps regulate moods, aid concentration and memory, and maintain energy levels. A build-up of phenylalanine can lead to severe neurological damage. Although potentially serious, once detected, PKU is completely treatable with a special diet (including special infant milk), which needs to be maintained throughout life. The heel prick blood test (see p.250) carried out in the first week of life screens for PKU, and if your baby is found to have it, early treatment is given. The condition affects only one baby in every 10,000 born in the UK each year.

Inherited genes For a baby to have PKU, she must inherit the affected gene from both parents. Inheriting the gene from only one parent will make her a carrier of PKU, but she won't show the effects herself, as shown in this diagram.

FATHER (CARRIER)

MOTHER (CARRIER)

Both genes A child who inherits both

NORMAL CHILD

CARRIER CHILD

CARRIER CHILD

AFFECTED CHILD

Q I've been told CF may affect my baby's growth. How can I help her growth?

As well as giving your baby supplements to assist her digestion (see p.329) to ensure she absorbs essential nutrients, you'll probably need to wean her on to solid foods slightly earlier than is usually recommended – perhaps as early as three months old – to make sure she gets the calories she needs to grow properly. As she gets older, keep plenty of high-calorie snacks in the cupboards and encourage her to eat them regularly, as well as her usual meals. Also encourage your older child to take part in sports and other physical activities to help strengthen her lungs. It can seem counterintuitive, but exercise is an important part of her therapy. Not only that, but running, playing, and competing at sports with friends is essential for giving her as normal a life as possible.

Q How does phenylketonuria (PKU) affect babies?

A baby who inherits PKU may begin to show symptoms in the first few months of life if the condition goes undetected. Symptoms include convulsions, a musty odour on her skin or in her urine, a pale complexion and eye colour, slow growth rate, a small head, and eczema. In time, if PKU goes untreated, children may develop severe learning and behavioural problems, and hyperactivity.

Q Will my baby develop healthily, even though she has PKU?

As long as you adhere to her dietary regime (and she continues to follow it when she's older), evidence suggests that PKU has no obvious effects on growth, emotional and social development, or mental agility. A PKU diet is low in protein and includes some carbohydrates, as well as supplements of the amino acid tyrosine that supports certain brain functions (see box, left). Your baby will have regular blood tests during childhood to monitor the levels of phenylalanine in her blood to ensure they are within safe limits.

Q What are the characteristics of Turner's syndrome, and can it be treated?

This rare chromosomal condition affects only girls and occurs when there is one X chromosome missing from the pair that determines her gender. It affects around one in 2000 baby girls born in the UK every year and is named after the American doctor Henry Turner, who first described it in 1938. One of the main characteristics of the condition is short stature, and most girls with Turner's syndrome are also infertile. The condition results in several other distinctive physical features, including a broad neck, ears that are set low on the sides of the head, nipples that appear far apart, a low hairline, and swelling in the hands and feet. Other problems may include hearing problems, short fingers, thyroid problems, and diabetes.

Although there is no specific treatment for Turner's syndrome, growth-hormone supplements and supplements of oestrogen can help to stimulate growth and bring on puberty, though most girls still remain infertile. The side-effects of the condition are treated on a case-by-case basis.

Q What causes the condition congenital hypothyroidism?

Congenital hypothyroidism (CH) is a rare condition, occurring in only one in every 3,500 births in the UK each year, and is slightly more common in girls than in boys. It is thought to be caused by malformations in the thyroid gland during development in the uterus (usually because the gland doesn't move into a forward position in the throat), or perhaps the absence of the thyroid gland altogether. Occasionally, an inherited gene mutation may be the cause. The condition means that babies are born without the ability to make thyroxine, an important growth hormone, and if left untreated, hypothyroidism can lead to long-term growth problems and neurological damage.

Your baby will be tested for levels of thyroxine as part of the standard heel-prick test taken at five days old. If your baby has CH, she will be given thyroxine supplements that she will need to continue throughout life. As long as the dosage remains accurate, the condition has no long-term consequences for your baby.

Q What is neurofibromatosis?

This rare genetic condition affects the nervous system, causing non-cancerous tumours to grow on and along the nerves. The condition has a range of symptoms, (and is also associated with learning difficulties).

Babies may have clusters of freckles around the groin and armpits, and flat, light-brown pigmented patches of skin elsewhere on the body. Sometimes freckles appear on the whites of the eyes, and benign tumours may occur on the optic nerve. All over the skin, along nerve pathways, small lumps – as a result of the neurofibromas growing on the nerves – may appear, which can be significantly disfiguring. Children with the condition may have an unusually large head, and may develop convulsions, learning or behavioural problems, and hearing and sight may be affected. There is no treatment for this progressive disorder, although doctors may use chemotherapy or surgery to remove tumours that become cancerous, as well as surgery to remove benign tumours if these start to affect bodily function. Sufferers are offered counselling to try to come to terms with their appearance, especially if the neurofibromas are too numerous to consider removing for cosmetic reasons.

Neurofibromatosis This "dominant" gene disorder means a baby needs to inherit the gene from one parent only to develop the condition, as shown below.

Dominant genes A child who inherits an infected gene

PARENT (NON-CARRIER)   PARENT (CARRIER)

UNAFFECTED CHILD   UNAFFECTED CHILD   AFFECTED CHILD   AFFECTED CHILD

Q Is sickle cell disease the same as sickle cell anaemia?

Sickle cell disease is the umbrella term for a group of conditions that includes sickle cell anaemia. It is an inherited blood disorder in which red blood cells are shaped like a crescent moon – or a sickle. Healthy red blood cells are disc-shaped and bendy, enabling them to pass freely through the body's network of veins and arteries. Conversely, sickle cells are rigid and sticky, which means they become trapped in the junctions between blood vessels. This causes blockages in the circulation, starving bones, muscles, and organs of the oxygen and nutrients they need to grow and develop. In turn, organ damage, low growth rate, and pain in the joints and muscles occurs. A person with sickle cell disease will go on to develop sickle cell anaemia, because sickle cells have a short life-span and they die off faster than bone marrow can manufacture new cells to replace them. The result is anaemia, which is characterized by a pale complexion and causes extreme tiredness and fatigue.

Your baby is screened for sickle cell anaemia as part of the heel-prick test at five days old. There is no certain cure for sickle cell disease, though occasionally bone marrow and stem cell transplants can work. Nonetheless, there have been major advances in the understanding of how to treat the symptoms and to minimize its effects, including prolonging life expectancy.

Building a relationship Even the sickest babies benefit from their parents' love and attention – the touch, smell, and sound of you will all comfort your baby. She recognizes the sound of your heartbeat and your voice from her time in the womb, and they soothe and relax her.

Glossary

Abruption Premature separation of the placenta from the wall of the uterus.

Active positions An approach to childbirth that involves upright positions and movements during labour.

Active labour The point during labour in which the cervix begins to dilate more rapidly and contractions are stronger, last longer, and are closer together.

Alveoli Milk glands in the breasts, which produce a flow of milk when they are stimulated by prolactin and the baby's sucking.

Amniocentesis The surgical extraction of a small amount of amniotic fluid through the pregnant woman's abdomen. This procedure is usually carried out as a test for fetal abnormalities.

Amnion The thin inner membrane surrounding the fetus and the amniotic fluid. It's also known as the amniotic sac.

Amniotic fluid The fluid that surrounds the fetus in the uterus. Ultrasound scans may be carried out in late pregnancy to ensure that enough fluid is present.

Amniotomy The surgical rupture of the amniotic sac, often done to speed up labour. This is referred to as ARM (artificial rupture of the membranes).

Anaemia A condition in which there is an abnormally low percentage of haemoglobin in the red blood cells. It is treated by taking iron supplements.

Anaesthetic Medication that produces partial or complete insensibility to pain.

Anaesthetic, general Anaesthetic that affects the whole body, with temporary loss of consciousness.

Antenatal Before birth.

Antibiotics Substances capable of destroying or limiting the growth of micro-organisms, especially bacteria.

Antibodies Protein produced naturally by the body to combat any foreign bodies, germs, or bacteria.

Anti-D An injection of antibodies given to women who have a rhesus negative blood group if they may have been exposed to rhesus positive fetal blood cells.

Apgar score A general test of the baby's wellbeing carried out at 1, 5, and 10 minutes after the birth to assess the baby's heart rate and tone, respiration, blood circulation, and nerve responses.

Areola The pigmented circle of skin surrounding the nipple.

Bilirubin Broken-down haemoglobin, normally converted to nontoxic substances by the liver. Some newborn babies have levels of bilirubin too high for their livers to cope with (neonatal jaundice).

Blastocyst An early stage of the developing egg after fertilization, when it has divided and subdivided into a group of cells.

Braxton Hicks contractions Practise contractions of the uterus that occur throughout pregnancy, but which may not be noticed until towards the end of pregnancy.

Breast pump A device for drawing milk from the breasts.

Breech presentation When the position of the baby in the uterus is bottom down rather than head down.

Caesarean section (C-section) The delivery of the baby through an incision in the abdominal and uterine walls.

Cardiotocograph (CTG) An electronic monitor that is used to measure the progress of the mother's contractions and the baby's heartbeat during labour.

Carpal tunnel syndrome Numbness and tingling of the hands arising from pressure on the nerves of the wrist. In pregnancy, it is caused by the body's accumulation of fluids.

Cephalic presentation The position of a baby who is head down in the uterus. The most common presentation.

Cephalopelvic disproportion A state in which the head of the fetus is larger than the cavity of the mother's pelvis. Delivery of the baby must therefore be by C-section.

Cervical dilation See *Dilation*.

Cervical insufficiency A disorder of the cervix, usually arising after a previous mid-pregnancy termination or damage to the cervix during a previous labour, in which the cervix opened up too soon, resulting in repeated mid-pregnancy miscarriages. It is sometimes treated by stitching to hold the cervix closed during pregnancy.

Cervix The lower entrance to the uterus, or neck of the uterus.

Chorion The outer membrane tissue that envelops the fetus and placenta.

Chloasma Pigmentation of the skin that causes darker patches, often on the face. Also known as melasma.

Chorionic gonadotrophin See *Human chorionic gonadotrophin (hCG)*.

Chorionic villus sampling A method of screening for genetic disease by analysing tissue from the small protrusions on the outer membrane enveloping the embryo (chorion), which later forms the placenta.

Chromosomes Rod-like structures containing genes. They occur in pairs within the nucleus of every cell. Human cells each contain 23 pairs.

Cleft palate A congenital abnormality of the roof of the mouth and upper lip. It is often treated with reconstruction surgery.

Colostrum A kind of milk, rich in proteins, formed and secreted by the breasts in late pregnancy and gradually changing to mature milk some days after the birth.

Conception The fertilization of the ripened egg by the sperm and its implantation in the uterine wall.

Contractions The regular tightening of the uterine muscles in labour as they work to dilate the cervix and press the baby down the birth canal.

Cordocentesis Fetal blood sampling or umbilical vein sampling. A diagnostic test to detect fetal abnormalities.

Crowning The moment when the baby's head appears at the entrance of the vagina during labour and does not slip back again.

Cystitis Infection of the bladder.

Diabetes Failure of the body to metabolize glucose, indicated by excess sugar in the blood and urine.

Dilation The progressive opening of the cervix caused by uterine contractions during labour.

Dizygotic See *Twins*.

Domino scheme A scheme operated by some hospitals, in which community midwives provide antenatal care and are present at hospital for the delivery.

Doppler A method of using ultrasound vibrations to listen to the fetal heart.

Doula A paid helper who provides support before, during, and after childbirth.

Drip See *Intravenous drip*.

Ectopic pregnancy A pregnancy that develops outside the uterus.

EDD The estimated date of delivery.

Electroencephalogram (EEG) A test where electrodes are placed on the scalp to record the electrical activity of the brain.

Embryo The earliest form of the baby in the uterus, from 4 weeks of pregnancy until around 10 weeks of pregnancy, after which it is termed a fetus.

Endometrium The lining of the uterus.

Engaged When the baby descends into the pelvis and three-fifths of his head have moved below pelvic bone. Usually a sign that labour is imminent.

Engorgement The over-congestion of the breasts with milk. If long periods are left between feeds, or the baby is not latched on well, painful engorgement can occur. This can be relieved by putting the baby to the breast or expressing the excess milk.

Entonox A mixture of 50 per cent oxygen and 50 per cent nitrous oxide, breathed in through a mask during labour, that gives pain relief as contractions peak. Also known as gas and air.

Epidural anaesthesia A method of numbing the nerves of the lower spinal cord to ensure pain-free labour.

Episiotomy A surgical cut in the perineum to enlarge the entrance to the vagina.

External cephalic version (ECV) The manipulation of the fetus by gentle pressure into the cephalic (head down) position. This may be done by an obstetrician or midwife at the end of pregnancy if the baby is in a breech or transverse position.

Fallopian tubes Two tubular structures (one on each side of the uterus) leading from the ovaries to the uterus.

Fertilization The meeting of the sperm with the egg to form a new life. See also *Conception*.

Fetus The developing baby in the uterus, known by this name around 10 weeks of pregnancy until birth.

Fibroids A benign (non-cancerous) growth of muscle in the uterus, usually spherically shaped.

Flavonoids A group of compounds with antioxidant properties (also known as bioflavonoids).

Fontanelle The soft spot on top of a baby's head, which closes after about one and a half year's of age.

Forceps A tong-like instrument that fits on either side of the baby's head and is used to help deliver the baby.

Fundal height The distance from the pubis to the top of the uterus. It's measured regularly throughout pregnancy and is used as a marker of fetal growth.

Fundus The top of the uterus.

Gas and air See *Entonox*.

Hepatitis Viruses (named A, B, C, E, and others) that infect the liver, causing jaundice and generalized illness.

Hormone A chemical messenger in the blood that stimulates various organs to carry out specific actions.

Human chorionic gonadotrophin (hCG) A hormone released into the woman's bloodstream by the developing blastocyst after implantation. Its presence in the urine means that she is pregnant.

Hypnobirthing A type of self-hypnosis using visualization and breathing techniques to achieve a deep state of relaxation during labour.

Hyperemesis gravidarum Persistent, excessive nausea and vomiting that prevents the woman eating and drinking adequately.

Hypertension High blood pressure. During pregnancy this can reduce the fetal blood supply.

Hypotension Low blood pressure.

Implantation The embedding of the fertilized egg within the wall of the uterus.

Induction The process of artificially starting off labour and keeping it going.

Intravenous drip The infusion of fluids directly into the bloodstream by means of a fine catheter introduced into a vein.

In vitro fertilization (IVF) A type of assisted conception where fertilization occurs outside the body and embryos are transferred back into the uterus.

Jaundice, neonatal The yellow colour noticed in the eyes and skin due to an increased level of bilirubin (a substance produced when the liver breaks down red blood cells).

Kangaroo care A technique, adopted especially with premature babies, where baby and parent have prolonged skin-to-skin contact. This is thought to provide warmth, stimulation, and to encourage the baby to breastfeed.

Lanugo The fine soft hair that grows on the body of the fetus.

Let-down reflex The flow of breast milk into the nipple.

Lie The position in which the baby is lying within the uterus.

Linea nigra A line of dark pigmentation that appears on the skin of the abdomen in some women during pregnancy. It runs down the centre of the abdomen over the rectus muscle.

Lochia Postnatal vaginal discharge.

Longitudinal lie The position of the fetus in the uterus in which the spines of the fetus and the mother are parallel.

Low-birthweight baby A baby who weighs below 2.5kg (5lb) at birth.

Meconium The first contents of the bowel, present in the fetus before birth and passed during the first few days after birth. The presence of meconium in the amniotic fluid before delivery is usually taken as a sign of fetal distress.

Melasma Dark, uneven patches of skin on the cheeks, forehead, nose, and chin during pregnancy. Sunbathing makes it worse. See also *Chloasma*.

Membranes Two layers of protective sacs enclosing the fetus, called the amnion and the chorion.

Meningitis A serious infection of the meninges, layers of tissue covering the brain.

Miscarriage The spontaneous loss of a baby before 24 weeks of pregnancy.

Monozygotic See *Twins*.

Morula A stage in the development of the fertilized egg, 3–4 days after fertilization, when it has grown into around 16 cells.

Multigravida A woman in her second or subsequent pregnancy.

Neonatal A baby less than 28 days old.

Nuchal scan A special ultrasound scan that can check for risk of Down's syndrome.

Nucleus The central part or core of a cell, containing genetic information.

Occipital anterior The position of the baby in the uterus when the back of its head (the crown or occiput) is towards the mother's front (anterior).

Occipital posterior The position of the baby in the uterus when the back of its head (the crown or occiput) is towards the mother's back (posterior).

Oedema Swelling caused by water retention and blood pooling in the lower body. In rare cases this can be a sign of pre-eclampsia.

Oestrogen Hormone, levels of which rise rapidly in the first weeks of pregnancy, thickening the lining of the uterus, swelling breasts, and keeping hair and nails in a growth phase.

Opioids (Narcotics) Painkilling drugs that induce drowsiness and stupor.

Ovary One of the two female glands, set at the entrance of the Fallopian tubes, which regularly produce eggs until the menopause.

Ovulation The release of a ripe egg by the ovary.

Oxytocin Hormone that triggers the uterus to start contracting in the first stage of labour. If you are very overdue, you may be given an extra dose of synthetic oxytocin via a drip.

Palpation Feeling the parts of the fetus through the mother's abdominal wall.

Pelvic floor The springy muscular structure set within the pelvis that supports the bladder and the uterus, and through which the baby descends during labour.

Perinatal The period from the 24th week of gestation to one week following delivery.

Perineum The area of soft tissues surrounding the vagina and between the vagina and the rectum.

Placenta A flat, thick disc-shaped organ that supplies the fetus with oxygen and nutrients.

Placenta praevia A placenta situated over, or near to, the entrance to the cervix. This makes a vaginal delivery unlikely.

Postnatal After the birth.

Postpartum After delivery.

Postpartum haemorrhage (PPH) Excessive bleeding following delivery.

Pre-eclampsia A condition that features high blood pressure and excess proteins in the urine. May be mild or serious.

Premature A baby born before the 37th week of pregnancy.

Presentation The positon of the baby according to the part of the fetus that is nearest to the cervix before and during labour.

Preterm See *Premature*.

Primigravida A woman in her first pregnancy.

Progesterone A hormone produced in the ovaries and then by the placenta.

Prolactin Hormone that stimulates milk production.

Prostaglandins Natural substances that stimulate the onset of labour contractions. Prostaglandin gel may be used to soften the cervix and induce labour.

Quickening The first sensations of your baby moving. Generally felt for the first time at around 20 weeks.

Rhesus (Rh) factor A distinguishing characteristic of the red blood corpuscles. All human beings have either rhesus positive or rhesus negative blood. If the mother is rhesus negative and the fetus is rhesus positive, rhesus disease (the destruction of the red corpuscles by antibodies) may occur; usually in a subsequent pregnancy unless prevented by an injection of anti-D gamma globulin.

Rooting The baby's instinctive searching for the breast in order to feed.

Rubella (German measles) A mild virus that may cause congenital abnormalities in the fetus if it is contracted by a woman during the first 12 weeks of pregnancy.

Show A vaginal discharge of bloodstained mucus occurring before labour, resulting from the onset of cervical dilatation. A sign that labour is starting.

Sonographer Medical professional who operates ultrasonic imaging devices.

Spider naevi Tiny new veins noticeable on your cheeks, breasts, and legs, required to help your body disperse the extra heat generated in pregnancy.

Spinal anaesthesia An injection of anaesthetic into the spine for pain relief.

Startle reflex Also known as the Moro reflex. Newborns are tested for this reflex to check the nervous system is working.

Stillbirth The delivery of a deceased baby after the 24th week of pregnancy.

Stretch marks Shiny lines that sometimes appear on the skin after it has been stretched during pregnancy.

Surfactant A creamy fluid that reduces the surface tension of the lungs so that they do not stick together when deflated. Premature babies may have breathing difficulties if surfactant has not developed sufficiently.

Suture The stitching together of a tear or a surgical incision.

Thrombosis A blood clot, commonly occurring in the calf; most dangerous if in the lungs (pulmonary embolus).

Thrush A yeast infection that can form in the mucus membranes of the mouth, genitals, or nipples.

Toxoplasmosis A parasite infection that can be caught from cats or other pets. It's also found in soil and it can be present on fruit and vegetables. If it crosses the placenta during pregnancy, it can cause eye or central nervous system damage in the baby.

Transcutaneous electronic nerve stimulation (TENS) A method of pain relief that uses electrical impulses to block pain messages to the brain.

Transducer An instrument that translates echoes of high-frequency sound waves, bounced off the developing fetus in the uterus, to build up an ultrasound image on a monitor. See also *Ultrasound scan*.

Transition A phase between the first and second stages of labour when the cervix is dilating to between 7 and 10cm (2¾–4 in).

Transverse lie A sideways position of the fetus in the uterus.

Trial of labour A situation in which, although a Caesarean section may be necessary, the mother labours in order to see if a vaginal delivery is possible.

Twins The simultaneous development of two babies in the uterus. If two eggs are fertilized independently by two sperm, dizygotic or fraternal twins result; more rarely, one fertilized egg divides to produce monozygotic or identical twins.

Ultrasound scan A way of building up a picture of an object by bouncing high-frequency soundwaves off it. Ultrasound scans are used during pregnancy to show the development of the fetus in the uterus. See also *Transducer*.

Umbilical cord The cord connecting the fetus to the placenta.

Urinary tract infection (UTI) Infection affecting the kidneys and/or bladder.

Uterus (or womb) The hollow muscular organ in which the fertilized egg becomes embedded. Once implanted the egg develops into an embryo and then a fetus.

Vagina The channel between the uterus and the external genitals. It receives the penis during intercourse and is the passage through which the baby is delivered (also called the birth canal).

Varicose veins Swollen veins in the legs that occur late in pregnancy.

VBAC Vaginal birth after Caesarean section.

Ventouse An instrument, used as an alternative to forceps, which adheres to the baby's scalp by suction and helps guide the baby out of the vagina.

Vernix A thick, greasy substance that covers and protects the fetus's skin in the uterus.

Vertex presentation When the top of the fetus's head is the part nearest the cervix.

Vulva The external part of the female reproductive organs.

Water birth Birth of a baby under water.

Yolk sac The first source of nutrients for an embryo until the placenta takes over at around 12 weeks.

Zygote The single cell, formed by the merging of the egg and sperm.

Useful resources

WEBSITES AND HELPLINES

Here are contact details for charities and organizations that offer support, advice, and guidance for conception, pregnancy, and life as a new parent.

Fertility

Foresight (The Association for the Promotion of Preconceptual Care)
http://www.foresight-preconception.org.uk

Getting Pregnant
www.gettingpregnant.co.uk

Human Fertilization and Embryology Authority
www.hfea.gov.uk

Infertility Network UK
www.infertilitynetworkuk.com

IVF treatment
www.ivf-infertility.com and
www.ivf.net

Pregnancy

ARC (Antenatal Results and Choices)
www.arc-uk.org

Association of Radical Midwives
http://www.midwifery.org.uk/

Babycentre
www.babycentre.co.uk

British Pregnancy Advisory Service
www.bpas.org

Family Planning Association
www.fpa.org.uk

Maternity Action
http://www.maternityaction.org.uk

Midwives Online
http://www.midwivesonline.com

Royal College of Midwives
www.rcm.org.uk

Labour and birth

Active Birth Centre
www.activebirthcentre.com

AIMS Association for Improvements in Maternity Services
www.aims.org.uk

Birth Trauma Association
www.birthtraumaassociation.org.uk

Caesarean Section Organization
www.caesarean.org.uk

Doulas www.doula.org.uk

Homebirth www.homebirth.org.uk

Hypnobirthing
www.hypnobirthing.co.uk

Independent Midwives' Association
http://www.imuk.org.uk/

Midwives online
http://www.midwivesonline.com

National Childbirth Trust
http://www.nct.org.uk/

Royal College of Midwives
www.rcm.org.uk

Breastfeeding

Association of Breastfeeding Mothers
www.abm.me.uk
Helpline 0300 330 5453

Baby Cafe
http://www.thebabycafe.org/

Baby Friendly Initiative
www.babyfriendly.org.uk

Breastfeeding Network
http://www.breastfeedingnetwork.org.uk/

La Leche League (Great Britain)
www.laleche.org.uk

Midwives online
http://www.midwivesonline.com

National Childbirth Trust
http://www.nct.org.uk/

Support groups

APEC (Action on Pre-eclampsia)
www.apec.org.uk

ASBAH (Association for Spina Bifida and Hydrocephalus)
www.mencap.org.uk

Asthma
www.asthma.org.uk

Association for Postnatal Illness
www.apni.org

BLISS (Baby Life Support System)
www.bliss.org.uk

Child Bereavement UK
http://www.childbereavementuk.org/

CLAPA (Cleft Lip and Palate Association)
www.clapa.com

Contact a Family
www.cafamily.org.uk

The Continence Foundation
www.continence-foundation.org.uk

The Compassionate Friends
www.tcf.org.uk

Cruse
http://www.crusescotland.org.uk/

Cry-sis
www.cry-sis.org.uk

Cystic Fibrosis Trust
www.cftrust.org.uk

Diabetes UK
www.diabetes.org.uk

Down's Syndrome Association
www.downs-syndrome.org.uk

Eczema
www.eczema.org
Helpline 0800 089 1122

FSID (The Foundation for the Study of Infant Deaths)
www.sids.org.uk/fsid

MENCAP (Understanding Learning Disability)
www.mencap.org.uk

MIND
(National Association for Mental Health)
www.mind.org.uk

The Miscarriage Association
www.miscarriageassociation.org.uk

Postnatal depression
www.pni.org.uk
www.pandasfoundation.org.uk

SANDS
(Stillbirth and Neonatal Death Society)
www.uk-sands.org

SENSE (National Deaf-Blind and Rubella Association)
www.sense.org.uk

Parent groups

4Children
http://www.4children.org.uk/

Fatherhood Institute
http://www.fatherhoodinstitute.org/

Gingerbread (groups for single parents)
http://www.gingerbread.org.uk/

MAMA (Meet-A-Mum Association)
www.mama.org.uk

Mumfidential
www.mumfidential.com

Netmums http://www.netmums.com/

TAMBA
(Twins and Multiple Births Association)
www.tamba.org.uk

Tommy's (The Baby Charity)
www.tommys.org

Twins UK http://www.twinsuk.co.uk/

Rights and benefits

Maternity action
www.maternityaction.org.uk

Working Families
www.workingfamilies.org.uk

General

ASH (Action on Smoking and Health)
www.ash.org.uk

British Acupuncture Council
www.acupuncture.org

British Chiropractic Association
www.chiropractic-uk.co.uk

British Homeopathic Association
www.trusthomeopathy.org
http://www.britishhomeopathic.org/

British Osteopathic Association
www.osteopathy.org

Department of Health (Advice for travellers)
www.dh.gov.uk

FRANK (drugs helpline)
www.talktofrank.com

NHS
http://www.nhs.uk/

Nutritional wellbeing
www.nutrition.org.uk

QUIT smoking
www.quit.org.uk

Vegetarian diets
www.vegsoc.org

APPS

There are a multitude of apps available to download that can help with your pregnancy, labour, and caring for your newborn. However, remember that while apps are fun and useful, never rely on them for medical advice and always consult your healthcare professional first.

Pregnancy Plenty of apps are on offer to assist you throughout your pregnancy journey. Certain ones contain personal diaries with space to upload photos of your growing bump and images from your ultrasound scans. Others have integrated communities with forums where you can connect with fellow mums-to-be.

There are apps that send you alerts for antenatal appointments, give you daily and weekly digests, monitor your baby's movements, track your weight gain, chart your pregnancy milestones, and prompt you with daily reminders for doing your pelvic floor exercises.

Labour and birth There are a variety of apps that prepare you and your partner for the big day. They encourage you to think about what will happen from start to finish. Most labour apps have a contraction timer and a place to write out your birth plan. Some apps include suggestions on how to have a natural birth, birthing positions to try out, and videos showing various labouring techniques. These apps often list the pros and cons of different birthing methods, helping you to consider all the available options. Many apps help prepare you mentally for delivering your baby – they demonstrate how to utilize meditation, relaxation, and visualisation.

There are also lots of handy apps with checklists of what to pack in your hospital bag that you can tick off as you pack the items in your bag. There are several apps with a birth announcement tool to help you share your happy news and upload photos of your new arrival.

Life with your baby Once you have your baby, there are apps with a range of tools to assist you with life as a new parent. Some give daily guidance during the first 6 months. You can communicate with other new mums and dads in your area through certain apps that include forums. If you're feeling tired and forgetful, there are apps to help track your baby's feeds, nappy changes, and sleeping patterns.

There are specific apps devoted to calming and soothing your baby through white noise, lullabies, or nursery rhymes. There are a few apps that find your nearest nappy changing facility when you're out and about. Users can rate their experiences of cleanliness, accessibility, and location.

As your baby grows, there are apps for baby weaning available to download with tips, trackers, and recipes. There are even some that demonstrate baby signing, so you can teach your baby the basic signs for milk, sleep, eat, play, and teddy bear.

Index

Acknowledgments

Publisher's acknowledgments

Creative Publishing Manager Anna Davidson
Proofreaders Jemima Dunne, Claire Cross, and Jamie Ambrose
Indexer Hilary Bird
Art Direction for Photography Isabel de Cordova, Peggy Sadler
Models Adam Dicuru, Raquel Dicuru, Abby Dorrian, Indiana Dorrian, Myles Dorrian, Justyna Duggan, and Adele Roche
Location Agency www.1st-Option.com

Picture credits

Most of the scans and photographs of the developing baby in this book are of the embryo and fetus live in utero, pictures using endoscopic and ultrasound technology. When this has not been possible, images have been taken by reputable medical professionals as part of research or to promote educational awareness.

The publisher would like to thank the following for their kind permission to reproduce their photographs:

(Key: a-above; b-below/bottom; c-centre; f-far; l-left; r-right; t-top)

4 Photolibrary: Digital Vision. **12 Maxine Pedliham:** (tr). **Science Photo Library:** P. Saada / Eurelios (br). **37 Corbis:** MedicalRF.com (tr). **49 Science Photo Library:** Anatomical Travelogue (ca). **82 Dreamstime.com:** Monkey Business Images / Monkeybusinessimages (bl). **93 iStockphoto.com:** M_a_y_a. **94 Dreamstime.com:** Ngo Thye Aun / Ngothyeaun. **95 Dreamstime.com:** Monkey Business Images / Monkeybusinessimages (bl). **Getty Images:** RJ Sangosti / The Denver Post (cl). **96 Science Photo Library:** Dr. G. Moscoso (tr); Sovereign, ISM (bl, br). **99 Wellcome Images.** **100-101 LOGIQlibrary. 100 Science Photo Library:** Living Art Enterprises, LLC (bc, br). **101 Getty Images:** LM Photo / The Image Bank (tl). **102 Dreamstime.com:** Natasnow. **103 Science Photo Library:** Dr. Najeeb Layyous (cra, bl, bc, br). **107 Corbis:** Tomas Rodriguez. **110 Alamy Images:** View Stock. **111 Alamy Images:** Jose Luis Pelaez Inc / Blend Images. **113 Alamy Images:** Jose Luis Pelaez Inc / Blend Images. **121 Corbis:** B2M Productions / Ocean (bl). **127 Alamy Images:** OJO Images Ltd (l). **130 Dreamstime.com:** Ana Blazic Pavlovic (c). **134 Corbis:** Tomas Rodriguez (tl). **136 iStockphoto.com:** momcilog (b). **140 Corbis:** JGI / Tom Grill / Blend Images (crb). **141 Getty Images:** Westend61 (br). **142 Getty Images:** Caroline Purser (cl). **143 Science Photo Library:** (br). **145 Corbis:** B. Boissonnet / BSIP (tr). **146 Science Photo Library:** Gustoimages (cb). **158-159 Science Photo Library:** Edelmann. **163 Science Photo Library:** Neil Bromhall (t). **164-165 Science Photo Library:** Neil Bromhall. **167 Corbis:** Bernd Vogel (cr). **Getty Images:** Marc Romanelli (ca). **iStockphoto.com:** PonyWang (cra). **193 Dreamstime.com:** Indigolotos (br). **209 Mother & Baby Picture Library:** Ian Hooton (l). **218-219 Alamy Images:** Lionel Wotton. **220 Corbis:** Juergen Effner / dpa (cr). **221 Corbis:** Rune Hellestad (br). **223 Alamy Images:** Chloe Johnson (br). **225 Science Photo Library:** David Parker (r). **228 Science Photo Library:** Ian Hooton (l). **229 Science Photo Library:** Ian Hooton (cb). **230 Alamy Images:** Phanie (cra). **234 Alamy Images:** Martin Valigursky (b). **237 Alamy Images:** philipus (tr). **243 Alamy Images:** Purestock (crb). **245 Getty Images:** Layland Masuda (cl). **246 Alamy Images:** Phanie (bl). **247 Getty Images:** Siri Stafford (cra). **248-249 Dreamstime.com:** Aynur Shauerman (b). **249 Alamy Images:** Family (tl). **Science Photo Library:** Dr. P. Marazzi (cra, cra/strawberry, cr, cr/skin spot); (crb, crb/mole). **253 Getty Images:** Comstock (cr). **255 Alamy Images:** Phanie (tr). **258-259 Getty Images:** Alistair Berg. **264-265 Getty Images:** LWA. **272 Dorling Kindersley:** Antonia Deutsch (br, cr, tr). **273 Getty Images:** Jamie Grill (tr). **276 Getty Images:** Mecky (br). **290 Getty Images:** Science Photo Library (bl). **291 Getty Images:** Tetra Images (br). **293 Getty Images:** Frederic Cirou (bl). **295 Science Photo Library:** Gustoimages (br). **299 Getty Images:** ONOKY - Eric Audras (cl). **300-301 Getty Images:** Marina Raith. **311 Corbis:** ERproductions Ltd / Blend Images (tr). **312-313 Getty Images:** Science Photo Library. **313 Getty Images:** Guillermo Legaria / AFP. **314 Corbis:** Glowimages (tr). **Getty Images:** BSIP / UIG (c). **315 Corbis:** JGI / Tom Grill / Blend Images. **316 Getty Images:** Todd Bates / E+ (bl); Cultura Science / Marc Fluri (ca). **317 Science Photo Library:** Antonia Reeve. **319 Getty Images:** Focus_on_Nature / E+. **322 Getty Images:** Fertnig / Vetta. **327 Getty Images:** Leanne Temme / Stockbyte. **328 Corbis:** JGI / Tom Grill / Blend Images. **329 Science Photo Library:** Photostock-Israel. **332-333 iStockphoto.com:** IvanJekic.

All other images © Dorling Kindersley
For further information see: **www.dkimages.com**